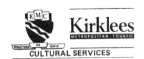
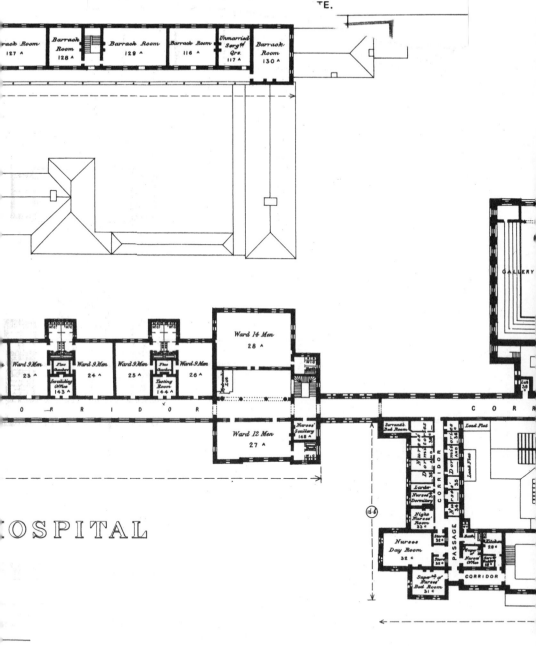

SPIKE ISLAND

Also by Philip Hoare

Serious Pleasures: The Life of Stephen Tennant

Noël Coward: A Biography

Wilde's Last Stand:
Decadence, Conspiracy and the First World War

Icons of Pop

(ed.) The Sayings of Noël Coward

SPIKE ISLAND

The Memory of a Military Hospital

PHILIP HOARE

FOURTH ESTATE • *London*

First published in Great Britain in 2001 by
Fourth Estate
A Division of HarperCollins*Publishers*
77–85 Fulham Palace Road
London W6 8JB
www.4thestate.co.uk

10 9 8 7 6 5 4 3 2 1

A catalogue record for this book is available from
the British Library

ISBN 1-84115-293-5

Typeset by Rowland Phototypesetting Ltd,
Bury St Edmunds, Suffolk
Printed in Great Britain by
Clays Ltd, St Ives plc

For Leonard, Andrew and Peter

CONTENTS

PROLOGUE   1

PART I

      Spike Island   15
      In a Lonely Place   34
      Southern Gothick   52

PART II

      Pray Stop All Work   89
      In the Very Best Style   112
      A Remarkable Improvement   135
      Enter His Gates with Thanksgiving   175
      Remembrance Day   196
      D Block   216
      Towards a Better Britain   263

PART III

      His Dark Estate   299
      The World is Infinitely Forgiving   329

EPILOGUE   352

Acknowledgements   365
Illustration Credits   368
Source Notes   369
Index   399

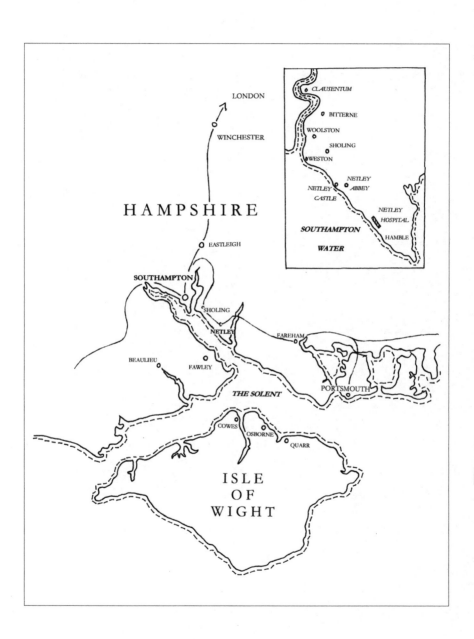

Prologue

To the unsuspecting visitor approaching from the seaward side, it looked like any other large country estate. Next to the great iron gate topped with glass lanterns was a low porter's lodge, but on the other side of the drive stood a sentry box, occupied by a uniformed soldier.

To that newcomer, the first intimation of the extraordinary building that lay ahead was the glimpse of Italianate towers over the parkland's newly-planted firs. As he walked up the lane, the vastness of Netley's Royal Victoria Military Hospital would suddenly be revealed. Rising over Southampton Water was a classical skyline, dominated by a central dome. From this sublime eye-catcher the visitor's gaze ranged in disbelief, scanning an edifice so wide that he had to move his head to see it – no one glance could take it all in.

Flanking the grandiose verdigris dome in either direction were great arms of Welsh granite, Portland stone and Hampshire brick – indeed, the clay to make the bricks had been excavated from the site itself – each crowned with their own spires and turrets. At their ends, these elongated wings bent back on themselves – as if too long for their own site – to form galleried barracks at the rear; as one architectural historian was to note, 'each would make reasonable major buildings in themselves'. In their deceptive embrace, the hospital was actually twice as big as it first appeared: it was as if it stretched into infinity.

Everything about the place was monumental. Its architecture aspired to eighteenth-century rationality, yet it spoke of nineteenth-century imperialism. Somehow the sense of proportion had been subtly overbalanced, as though designed by a team of architects whom no one had told to stop, its creators having suffered a fit of megalomania. If there had been a soundtrack to that revealing first sight of the hospital, it might have been provided by Richard Wagner, then composing his equally grandiose Ring Cycle.

But the building was also the product of bureaucracy, dwarfing the mere human like some enormous town hall conceived by committee. From a dark interior of the War Office, orders had been issued to E. O. Mennie, Surveyor of the Royal Engineer Department, and his army of assistants in Pall Mall, an architectural sweatshop producing sheet after sheet of plans, measurements and specifications. This was a building under royal patronage, created by the richest and most powerful nation on earth, and nothing was to be spared in realising its imperial vision.

The exhaustive plans demanded 'the best hard, sound, well-burnt and square stock bricks', 'the piers and arches to be of the best Portland stone', 'the whole of the ornaments, carvings and enrichments to be done in the very best style, with spirit, boldness and without blemish'. Nor was the interior neglected. In true Victorian tradition, every item was specified in a manifesto published for the contractors, E. Smith of Woolwich. Each fixture and fitting was defined: from 'blue pointing mortar' to 'fresh air tubes', from 'Rufford and Finch's baths' to 'Anglo-American stoves', from 'wine bins' to early washing machines; every article of equipment, ironmongery and furnishing was listed *ad infinitum*. In an age of mass production, this was architecture by multiplication, as though the hospital had been built by a great Victorian machine. Its façade reached one quarter of a mile in length, pierced by row upon row of arched windows, more than two hundred of them, regimented along three cliff-like storeys. The detail was overwhelming, almost hypnotic in its rhythm.

The new hospital was a statement of imperial intent, an advertisement in brick and stone of the country's international standing; it would make Netley a household name. A later report would note that 'Passengers by Cape and American line steamers, and those who journey up and down Southampton Water, are familiar with the immense façade of the hospital, built in red brick and Portland stone, with pillared porticoes of granite, and towers and windows which in some way suggest stately Venetian palaces.' Half-imaginary engravings of the building created before its completion depicted it as a kind of waterside Versailles, complete with parterres and decorative sheep cropping its neat turf, and gravel drives along which carriages could take the air, as if on some elegant gentleman's estate.

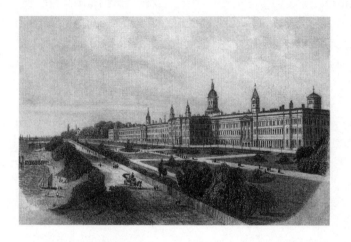

Framed by its greensward and, set back from the sea, looking out magisterially over the empire it was built to serve, the hospital straddled its 200 acres with immutable solidity. A remarkable aerial photograph taken soon after its completion reveals the scale of a building that had to be measured in yards and furlongs rather than feet. The balloon-borne camera rose smoothly into space above Southampton Water, the only way to capture the extent of the hospital as it stretched along the shore, set on some vast pedestal for display to the passing yachts and oyster boats, troopships and liners. Like the *Great Eastern*, which moored alongside it in 1861, reflecting the new building in Brunel's enormous million-pound creation – five times bigger than any other ship afloat, part-yacht, part-factory, part-hotel, with its stovepipe

3

chimneys like his stovepipe hat – Netley's hospital was a grand, if not arrogant display of technological progress.

For the *Great Eastern*'s passengers, as for the soldiers on troopships en route for foreign postings, Netley was a reminder of Britain's greatness, a symbol of power and potential succour as they sailed down the water to extend or defend the Empire. But for those inside the building, the hospital held different

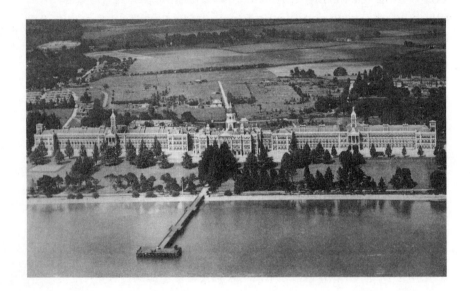

prospects. For all its glittering window eyes, it remained faceless, impenetrable, keeping its own secrets. Yet viewed in perspective from the literal height of nineteenth-century technology, the entire undertaking appeared almost shimmering in its new brick and stone; a magnificent delusion, a Victorian vision for a miraculous age.

Having paused to take in the enormity of the view that confronted him, the awed visitor would walk along the hospital's façade, counting the rows of arched windows as he went. Reaching the central portico, he would pass through the great double doors and into the building itself. Here, in a high-ceilinged and panelled hallway reminiscent of a railway hotel,

4

he would be greeted, not by scurrying nurses and doctors in white coats, but by the bleached white bones of a full-size elephant.

This was the hospital's Museum of Natural History, a room-sized cabinet of curiosities guarded by its ghostly and eyeless pachydermic porter. Ranged above the stone staircase was a cluster of spiky antelope horns and deer antlers – the kind of display you'd find gathering dust in any country house of the time, trophies of exotic shooting parties in the bush or the veldt. But crocodiles also crawled the walls, and a school of stuffed fish swam under the stairs, frozen mid-stream in the plaster. Other animal remains had been cemented in their death rictus, and on the shelves of one long vitrine, the length of a wall, stood tens of glass specimen jars, each containing the spiralled pickled corpse of a snake. It was hardly the kind of exhibition to calm the fears of a nervous hospital patient.

Yet this gloomy dissection of the natural world had an even more gothic counterpart in the hospital's other collections. One was devoted to military surgery, and had been started in Dublin in 1846 by a retired army surgeon, Professor Tufnell, as 'a museum of appliances for the transport and treatment of the wounded'. Brought to Netley to grace the new hospital, it displayed 'native' weapons next to surgical instruments, described in lugubrious nineteenth-century tones as 'the implements by which man ingeniously shortens his neighbour's life and the appliances by which he seeks to preserve his own' – in other words, a visual lesson in the survival of the fittest. One item on show was a broken lance which had passed through the body of a lancer after his horse threw him. 'The lance had to be sawn in two before it could be withdrawn', it was noted, 'but marvellous to relate, the man survived and was perfectly cured.'

In one corner stood an antler-like hatstand festooned with headgear from the battlefields of the Crimea, resplendent with red plumes and glossy cockades like stuffed birds of paradise. Meanwhile in another nearby case, neatly stacked on shelves like bowling balls waiting for a game, was a collection of decapitated

5

and mummified heads. These represented indigenous peoples from around the imperial world: the inhabitants of Java, New Zealand, Malay and Africa, arranged for anthropological identification and scientifically labelled – 'Kaffir: Tambuki tribe'; 'Kaffir: Amulosali tribe'; Hottentot and Maori. Like the animals in the entrance hall, they too were endangered species: Tasmanians killed off by the colonial process or the South Africa San 'bushmen' who would even a hundred years later still be regarded as suitable subjects to be hunted.

This index of Victorian anthropology had come from the catacombs of Fort Pitt, Kent, where the director, Sir James McGrigor, had assembled no less than 458 skulls, 29 casts, 7 dried heads and 2 mummies. Expanded by an appeal, made in 1833, for new specimens of 'Monstrosities', 'the bodies of foetuses at different ages', 'crania of various races of mankind', and 'snakes and lizards from the Colonies, preserved in spirits', the collection had acquired a national reputation, visited by 'distinguished surgeons and naturalists'. It had been transferred to Netley when the hospital opened, 'rather a gruesome sight', admitted a contemporary account, 'but to the student of anthropology the facial characteristics of the different peoples are full of interest'. The 'ghastly array' was, 'for those not accustomed to such display . . . not very agreeable', agreed another Victorian guide, 'but people come from far and wide to see it; from Germany, France, America, for it is one of the best collections of Asiatic and African skulls in the world'. Whatever its scientific merits, the ironies of this gothic ossuary in the entrance hall of their hospital were not lost on the inmates. They nicknamed it 'Skull Alley'.

In a burgeoning scientific age, the new theories of evolution and natural history had spread even to the officers' quarters at Netley. A gracious villa-like building with twin Italianate towers (a deliberate echo of Queen Victoria's holiday home, Osborne, just across the Solent on the Isle of Wight), its well-appointed rooms fit for gentlemen were separated from the hospital by fir trees.

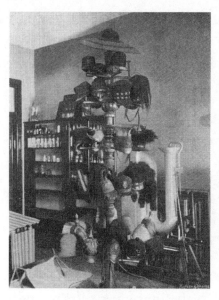
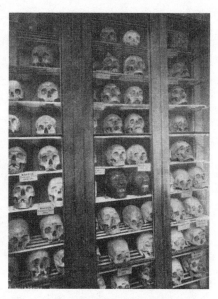

Battle Relics   *'Skull Alley'*

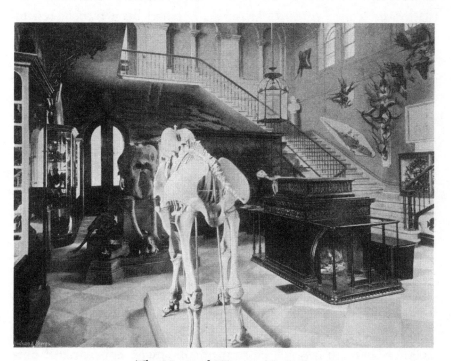

The Natural History Museum

These had been planted not only for decoration, but for their medicinal qualities: the healthy scent of pine oil provided a barrier between their quarters and the miasmas of the great building across the lawn.

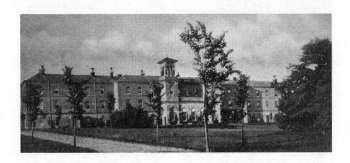

In this refined white contrast to the hospital's red-brick rigours, surgeons and doctors dined to a theatrical backdrop of aspidistras, palms and a huge decorative screen embellished, not with nineteenth-century 'scraps' of ladies in décolletage and blowsy roses, but with florid recreations of Victorian dinosaurs. Besporting themselves in an antediluvian jungle, these monsters were the cousins of those at Crystal Palace, where Benjamin Waterhouse Hawkins's saucer-eyed ichthyosaurs and arched-neck plesiosaurs reared out of the primordial swamp in a London park. Hawkins had begun his dinosaur theme park in 1853, shortly before work started at Netley, and had invited Richard Owen – the inventor of the name and concept of the dinosaur – to dine with him in the cement carcass of an iguanadon under construction; Netley's officer doctors would have to make do with eating in the shadow of prehistoric monsters.

As they sat at their mahogany dining table, these men of science doubtless discussed Mr Darwin's theories, published in 1859 and exemplified by the living dinosaurs of the Galapagos, the lumbering swimming lizards which he called 'imps of darkness', just as he called himself the 'Devil's chaplain'. Only later would Netley bear witness to the more problematic offspring of evolutionary science: social Darwinism.

8

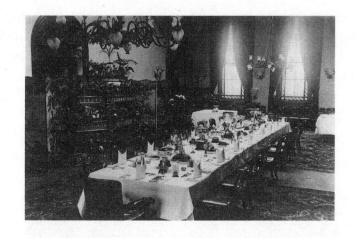

Victorian man was busy digging into his past to explain his present, the reason for his supremacy. If 'Skull Alley' and the expanding Empire provided living proof of one aspect of the theory, then dinosaurs were the prehistoric exemplars of another. Indeed, the two sensibilities combined in Alfred Waterhouse's secular gothic cathedral of the Natural History Museum, built ten years after the hospital in 1873, complete with demonic terracotta pterodactyl gargoyles hanging by their leathery wings from a façade which, like Netley's, appeared to emulate geological strata in its layers of brick and stone, yet which, like the Gothic Revival, also referred back to a medieval past.

That had been an age of unwavering faith. Now the search for an explanation of Man's origins became a metaphor for the loss of faith, in an age in which science and religion battled for the hearts and souls of Victorian man. In that battle the hospital would become a resonant symbol. For a hundred years it would bear testimony to the rise and fall of the Empire; to reason and rationality subjected to forces of superstition and fear; to issues of class and sex; to experimentation and scientific advance – sometimes at the expense of human beings. This vast building would stand for a century of British history, but it too was a dinosaur, excavated from Hampshire clay; the monster on Netley's shore.

*　　*　　*

When I was twelve years old, my family went on holiday to Scotland. It rained most of the time, and we took shelter in a series of guest houses and caravans. At Inverness we spent the night in a bed and breakfast seemingly constructed from a series of extensions joined together by skewed corridors and acrylic carpet. We younger children – myself and my two younger sisters, my brothers now too old for family holidays – were bedded down in a creaky room covered in white-painted woodchip wallpaper. I was excited: the next day we would be arriving at Loch Ness. We were already at the head of the huge body of water which, as I was at pains to tell my parents, was twice as deep as any of the water around Britain. I seemed to feel its nearness and its depth; and in that depth, the presence of its alien denizen, the reason for my excitement.

Ever since I could remember seeing pictures in the newspapers or hearing jokey items at the end of the news, I'd felt affronted by the cynics who rejected its existence, the so-called experts from the Natural History Museum who were trundled out every time there was a new sighting. Implacable in my belief, I knew what it was; a childhood spent with my head in dinosaur books told me as much. Their vivid reconstructions of prehistory were photographically real to me, and as scary as the pictures of deep-sea fish in my encyclopaedias which I could not touch – I had to turn the page with my fingertips, as if the lithographic image could, by a process of osmosis, drag me to unfathomable depths and into the nightmare jaws of the angler fish. My faith in the loch's monster was a gesture of defiance against the sceptical adult world. At home in Southampton, living within the sound of the sea yet encircled by suburbia, I was always fascinated by monsters and ghosts; by the bottomless ocean and the endless forest; by derelict buildings and damaged beauty; by loss and memory – by the memory of things and places I'd never seen. Myths and legends seemed more real to me than the reality around me. I sought to glamorise my everyday life; to find something strange and perhaps even mystical beyond it – to populate those ruinous buildings with ghosts, and to fill the sea with monsters.

That night, as I slept in my Inverness bunk, I looked down, not into unknown depths, but on the shallow end of the loch, where the waters petered out into reedy marsh. The scene was sunlit, the reeds yellow-russet, the sky blue, the water clear and still. It was picture-postcard bright, not gloomy and grey like other images I'd seen of the place. And as I watched from my elevated position, looking down, as it were, as though filming the scene from a camera on a crane, a slow-moving greenish-brown form slipped up and out of the water beneath me; obscenely snakelike and sinewy, its massive, muscular bulk was not out of place in the natural landscape, but somehow part of it, or lord of it. It undulated through the shallows, its full serpentine length visible through the clear water, its indiscernible lower reaches stirring the silt below. It moved powerfully and swiftly on, its broad slow-worm head held high as it swam towards the open loch.

Then it was gone, and I woke up.

PART

I

Spike Island

What greatness had not floated on the ebb of that river
into the mystery of an unknown earth! ... The dreams
of men, the seed of commonwealths, the germs of empires.

JOSEPH CONRAD

O n a foggy autumn morning in Southampton's eastern
suburbs, you can hear ships' horns cutting mournfully
through the thick air like sonorous sheep lost in the mist. By
night the clank-clank of the dredger takes over, as it gouges out
a passageway from the sea bed. In the still air sound bounces off
suburban walls, and behind curtain-darkened windows families
gather round flickering TV sets, just like families all round the
country, in other suburbs of other provincial towns.

This is Sholing, where I grew up. There was little to distinguish
it from other suburbs, still less as an adjunct to a port; a transient
place which people passed through rather than visited for itself,
Sholing had little claim on the national consciousness. A jumble
of Victorian villas, 1920s semis and post-war estates, its name –
Anglo-Saxon, meaning 'the hill by the shore' – may have dated
back to the Domesday Book, but the place no longer had any
discernible centre, its borders only vaguely marked by vestigial
streams and river valleys once wide enough to earn the area its
ancient title. Once the sea came closer to these hills; more

15

recently, this was still open countryside, Hampshire heathland rolling gently eastwards from Southampton, yielding soft fruit from its fields, shingle from gravel pits, bricks out of clay seams, water from its springs. For centuries its common land was used as a military camp, as archery grounds and shooting ranges, a place for soldiers, travellers and horse traders.

Then, gradually, its population began to grow, shifted here by the industrialisation of the eighteenth and nineteenth centuries. For the incomers this indefinable area needed an identity, something to give it meaning; the one it acquired came from a past which its more genteel residents would have preferred to forget: Spike Island.

Ask any local of a certain age or disposition and they'll come up with various explanations for the nickname. Some cite the heathland's characteristic gorse, *Ulex europeaus*, which still sprouts up wherever it can, spiky and resilient, once collected by furze-cutters for fuel or cattle fodder. Its toughness has its own romance as 'one of the great signature plants of commonland and rough open space, places where lovers can meet, walk freely and lose themselves, if need be, in its dense thickets'. Others attribute the name to the spike shape of the area itself, a memory of the time when the sea did indeed come closer to its hills, yet an island now only within the extended boundaries of the rivers Itchen and Hamble which separate this peninsula from the rival city ports of Southampton and Portsmouth.

Of little agricultural benefit, until 1796 the heath was marked on maps as 'Nomans Land', and held just forty-three permanent inhabitants. Only in the last years of the eighteenth century, as the common land began to be privatised by the Enclosures Act, did houses appear in any number: low brick cottages built by travellers attracted by the troops stationed on the common with whom they could trade.

Marked out by the caravans in which many of them still lived, they were looked down upon by the inhabitants of the older villages of Weston, Woolston and Netley nearby. Perhaps it is no coincidence that 'spike' was also argot for the workhouse, or that the gypsies called themselves 'pikeys', another potential

16

source for the nickname. Long established in Hampshire and its New Forest, they were living outside the confines of normal life on this furzy heathland, its spiny gorse somehow expressive of their own resilience, and perhaps this sense of being outside, of being beyond the law and civilisation, informed the most romantic of the explanations for Sholing's nickname. It was claimed that convicts being transported to Australia were held on its common, chained by their feet to a great spike.

Transportees convicted at Winchester's courts were certainly marched to the ports of Southampton and Portsmouth, and could have been stabled for the night there, just as their fellow inmates from Dorchester gaol were held overnight in a prison-like barn with slit windows and oak studded doors, 'all chained to a central post'. The place became known as 'Botany Bay Farm', just as the first part of Sholing to be settled in the 1790s was nicknamed 'Botany Bay' after the new penal colony of New South Wales.

From 1831 to 1840, more than 50,000 men and women were transported from England. The gypsies were particular victims of these purges, subject to persecution in the Southampton area in the tumultuous first few decades of the nineteenth century. With a population driven by the enclosures from the country to the city, crime rates and a general instability necessitated the invention of a new sort of English colony, an 'official Siberia'. These penal settlements came to occupy some impossibly remote part of the public imagination, places of horror and damnation where men made pacts to kill themselves in order to escape the appalling conditions.

If Sholing's Spike Island had witnessed the export of unwanted Englishmen and women to become colonial forced labour, then perhaps it was a mirror image of the slave trade that had been carried out from other British ports, at Bristol and Liverpool, where other Spike Islands would be found. But if Botany Bay was the slavery of Britons by any other name, then the most likely explanation for Sholing's nickname seemed both to reflect this sense of a prison colony on the other side of the world, and to relate it closer to home.

Across the Irish Sea, a small island off Cobh in Cork Harbour had been settled by monks in the seventh century. Its name was Inis Pich – Spike Island – depicted on early maps as a spike-shaped piece of land. Used since Cromwellian times for holding Irish rebels, by 1847 Spike had become a dedicated penal colony, a nineteenth-century Robben Island for deportees, 'From th'emerald island/Ne'er to see dry land/Until they spy land/In sweet Botany Bay.' Up to 4,000 convicts at one time were held here, clad in grey jackets, moving great mountains of earth and rock to construct the island's fortifications, building their own prison walls. Many would be buried in the bleak 'convicts' grave-yard' in one corner of the island, marked only by numbered headstones. In 1916 Spike would be used to confine the insurrec-tionists of the Easter Rising and the seeds of modern troubles. The island was handed back to the Irish in 1938, but its inmates could still be identified by particular tattoos indelibly marking its provenance on their hands, as indelibly as the island was marked with its past.

There was, I now realise, an almost genetic reason for my mythologising of my suburban surroundings, for my fascination with these tenuous traces of local history: their arcane details seemed to reference a greater story; a personal thread which linked the legends of Sholing-as-Spike Island. My maternal fore-fathers had been involved in the slave trade in Liverpool, while my father's ancestors had fled Ireland during the potato famine. Such dark romantic notions counterpointed the ordinariness of present-day suburbia, and seemed to ally me to Sholing's shad-owy epithet. They gave my rootlessness an identity.

By a strange process of insult and immigration, the infamy of Ireland's Spike Island, wreathed in crime, insurrection and its terrifying consequences, had been transposed to an odd little suburb hundreds of miles away in southern England. In the mid-nineteenth century, Irish workers were attracted by the ship-building industries of Southampton and Woolston's dock-yards, and by the shipping lines which had begun to ply between Southampton and New York. Just as the gypsies had acquired the slur of 'Botany Bay', so the incoming Irish brought with them the reputation of Spike Island – used either in half-ironic humour by themselves for their southern exile, or by their suspicious neighbours as a slur on their supposedly criminal characters. They would come to glory in the nickname, perhaps as a rebellious gesture against the moneyed class which also began to move into the neighbourhood.

Courtesy of the railway and Southampton's growing port, land here had begun to command a premium, and in the 1850s came more houses, constructed from the products of the local brickworks and gravel pits; slowly at first, then moving more swiftly along the new railway line from Southampton to Portsmouth, over a horizon as yet undarkened by brick and slate. Then grander houses appeared, wide double-fronted houses in yellow brick, as if their colour marked them out from the commoner product of Spike Island's clay and its brickworks. Invested with authority and capital, their inhabitants aspired to gentility, with their mock turrets, conservatories and brick walls. Sholing acquired the veneer of respectability; the institutions of church, freemasonry and local politics. Its pines and cedars and holly hedges set out the social status of its merchants, vicars, doctors, shop-keepers, all firm in their expectations of the future.

Then the unthinkable happened, and Armageddon intervened on this complacent scene. After the First World War the serried ranks of 'homes for heroes' marched over the land, their strip-like plots providing every Englishman with his own piece of land. The larger, older houses shrank into flats or nursing homes, or disappeared into rubble and rhododendron; gypsy cottages became bungalows or crumbled back into the dirt from which they came. After the Second World War, developers finished what the bombs had started. Spike Island was swallowed up by modern suburbia and the discrete identity of Sholing was blurred – a process almost complete by the time our family moved there in the early 1960s.

On my way to school, I used to walk past a cottage around the corner from our road, one of the low little homes that dotted the neighbourhood. In its garden stood a round summerhouse, ingeniously constructed to turn heliotropically, like a flower following the sun. Its windows were empty, the green paint peeling from the wooden slats. I'd imagine some frail elderly lady sitting inside, dressed in lace like tea-stained curtains, the pale sun falling on her papery skin. Then one day the summerhouse disappeared, and in its place grew a bed of blinding French marigolds.

Along these avenues and cul-de-sacs, the comforting icons of stained-glass sunbursts and galleons on wavy seas would soon give way to the bland stare of plastic windows, and the porches which welcomed the milkman or postman would be boarded up against the world. But for now the corner shop still sold Fruit Salad and Blackjack chews, the grocer sliced cooked meat with scything machines ready to take off an inattentive finger, and the chemist had huge bottles of blue and red water in the window and cream and chrome scales on the counter for weighing babies like quarter-pounds of sweets.

On the other side of the road from the cottage and its summerhouse ran a ribbon of woody valley where a meandering, rusty stream sought the freedom of the sea. Around it lay the vestiges of Sholing Common, the traces of its ancient provenance marked only on old Ordnance Survey maps in the gothic script of tumuli and Roman roads. The valley was crossed by Church Path, a narrow lane which descended steeply to the stream, then rose up towards a stone and slate church with a modest steeple, described in *Pevsner's Buildings of England* as 'prettily set in a pine-backed churchyard in a strange Victorian rural backwater of suburban Southampton'.

Those pines were less covered by sinuous ivy than they have since become, but even then Church Path was a shadowy place. My mother would point out tiny gravestones in its churchyard, memorials to Romany children from Botany Bay, where the dark-faced inhabitants, looking like ancient Britons, spat at us while we waited in the family car as our parents went to buy some plants from their father. Their caravans stood next to their bungalows, and sometimes we'd hear the sound of horse hooves clattering down our road, and run out to see the young blades riding past on a pony and trap.

Invested with the strangeness of the people who lived beyond Church Path, this wilderness at the bottom of our road both fascinated and terrified me. It was where, in my imagination, chained convicts awaited their criminal exile, languishing on the scrubby grass, indolently desperate figures out of Gustave Doré's *Dante*. During the war, barrage balloons had been set up on the common, leaving behind rusty iron rings which in my mind became tethers for the manacled prisoners. Now they secured two lonely gypsy ponies, slow-moving, semi-wild beasts with shaggy manes, big round bellies and a sad look in their big black eyes, as if to plead for their release.

Sometimes, on the bus from school, I'd go on a stop and walk back through Church Path. It was a self-consciously daring act. The way home led through a green tunnel overhung by yew, ivy and laurel, dipping steeply into the damp valley before the distant light at the end; the pathway was dark and scary even on a sunny day. I once found a dead mole there, its black velvet unbloodied, tiny pink fin-like paws sticking out stiffly at right-angles to its lifeless and blind body, like an abandoned soft toy dropped from a passing pushchair. On the other side of the path from the churchyard – where a girl from up the road once told me I'd be haunted that night because I'd walked across a grave – was a derelict house. Its garden contained a large rectangular pit roughcast in concrete, apparently a pre-war swimming pool. It may have been the same girl who told me that the house had been owned by a Dr White, and that he had invented something called the tampon. In fact, the owner was a plain Mr White, undistinguished by the invention of anything at all.

Below the churchyard, where dead wreaths and old prams were chucked over the iron railings into the valley's dip, was another low cottage with a tiled roof and green wooden door; smoke could sometimes be seen coming from its chimney. It looked like a farmhouse left over from a previous century, still standing firm in the last vestiges of wild land as the modern

21

world closed in; or like the old railway carriage in which we used to take our holidays at Gunard on the Isle of Wight, around which the bats flew at night.

Chickens pecked about in the small patch of cultivated land in front of the house, and there was a tethered goat with curly horns and bulging eyes with demonic slits for pupils. Another Church Path legend claimed someone had been murdered in this valley, blasted at short range with a shotgun; I saw the act replayed in slow motion, the blue smoke of the weapon's discharge, the recoil of the body, the red of the victim's blood. Although I had no reason to suspect the inhabitants of this cottage – which, like the rotating summerhouse, disappeared sometime later in my childhood – I was scared of the seldom-seen old man who lived there. Sometimes he would stand by his cottage door, white-haired, bent double and propped up with a stick. Perhaps his wife joined him, in a white pinafore, her hair done up in a silver bun. Or perhaps I invented the scene, like the psychic timeslip in *The Man Who Fell to Earth*, when the orange-and-yellow-haired alien, Thomas Jerome Newton, is driven through countryside and glimpses a family of nineteenth-century hillbillies outside their shack, its chimney smoking, a burst of inter-bred banjo on the soundtrack.

Like the privet cutway that ran up the back of our house where my brothers used to catch bucketfuls of slow worms, these wild places produced tales of innocence and loss, of murder and abandoned babes in the wood. From Church Path, the stream flowed through the old clumps of bamboo planted by the inhabitants of the cottage, past Mr White's concrete pool and widening out into Miller's Pond, a still, deep pool overshadowed by the tall brick arches of a railway viaduct. There were tadpoles and sticklebacks in the water, and it froze solid in winter, its glaucous ice spiked with dead bullrushes. On our way to the park we would walk past the pond, and I'd lean over the low wall and look down into its brackish water, imbued as it was with another local legend.

One Sunday in February 1909, Alfred Maurice Mintram, the

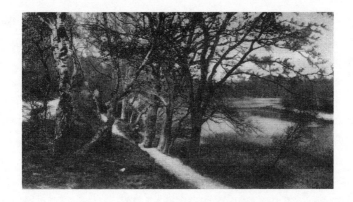

fourteen-year-old son of Charles Mintram, a coal porter who lived at Fir Grove Road – the road which crossed ours – was spending the afternoon sliding on the iced-up pond. A witness to the subsequent enquiry was walking round the pond 'when someone shouted that there was a boy drowning'.

> He ran round the bank, and saw a constable taking his tunic off, and together they went to the lad's assistance. They got to within four yards of him, and witness called out that they would soon get to him. Deceased replied, 'Hurry up, I can't hold on much longer.' The next minute, the ice gave way, and they were all struggling in the water. There was ice between them and the boy, and it was impossible to reach him. There were no ladders or ropes or anything they could have used. The boy threw up his hands and went down . . .

Reported to the coroner, in the still, formal air of the court-room, the boy's last words – plaintive, panicking, banal – seemed to presage a forthcoming tragedy which would strike the inhabitants of these streets and households. The melodramatic fatalism of the scene is compounded by postcards depicting the boy's funeral, his classmates clumped together on a cold day in February, dressed in their Sunday best, bearing wreaths. Another card shows Alfred's humped grave in Sholing churchyard, surrounded with laurel leaves and a row of five bouquets laid along its top, each protected by an odd wire frame like an upturned hanging basket. Three years later, the same families would lose brothers, fathers and lovers who foundered, like Alfred Mintram, in icy water, uttering similarly plaintive cries as *Titanic* sank.

I have only a vague memory of the house in which I was born, in Portswood, on the other side of the Itchen which divides Southampton as clearly as the Thames divides London. 'Akaba' had been the home of an army officer, and had been empty for some time when my newly-married parents discovered it in 1941, and managed to lease it, for one pound a week, from the major's widow.

The house was a large, semi-detached, red-brick villa; the names engraved on its lintel and those of its neighbours – 'Rahwali', 'Gwalia' – were as redolent of the last century as the street itself, named Osborne Road after the late Queen's Isle of Wight retreat. The monkey puzzle tree that stood along the road was a further mark of Victorian gentility, its spiky exoticness somehow reminiscent of a colonial past. Superstitiously, we'd hold our breath as we passed it, for fear something awful might befall us.

Set on the corner of the road and raised above pavement level with a walled garden, Akaba had a turret which loomed proprietorially over the junction on which it stood. It also had bellpulls to summon servants from its kitchen and scullery, and a wide mahogany staircase which turned at right-angles past a stained-glass landing window. Not that I remember much of this. My only memory – indeed, my very first memory – of Akaba is of waking in my cot; I must have been less than two years old. Gripping the wooden bars, I hauled myself out of prison and, reaching up to the bedroom doorknob, carefully descended, with a toddler's halting step, the big, wide, dark stairs illuminated by pale coloured light, looking for my mother. It must have been summer – it was still daylight – and as I made my surprise entrance in the sitting room downstairs, I saw the upturned and startled faces of my parents and three brothers. Amused at my audacious jailbreak, my mother scooped me up in her arms and carried me back, with certain praises for my adventurousness, to bed. It is a virgin memory, of a life light and uncluttered and untainted by anything other than love. The dark red brick of the house in which I lived did not register on my consciousness.

In 1962, our house – which my parents had by now bought – was compulsorily purchased to make way for a bypass which would remain unbuilt for twenty years. When it was finally constructed, the planners had no need of the land freed by Akaba's demolition, which was promptly acquired by a neighbouring garage and yet became a victim of the combustion engine as a forecourt dedicated to the display of used cars. In the meantime, saddled with an empty property, the council had tried to rent out Akaba, but found it difficult to lease. Tenants complained that it was haunted and called the police; later an exorcism was performed. Perhaps we'd left our spirits behind, although as my mother pointed out, the ghosts may have been due to the fact that we had left an unwanted upright piano buried in the garden which still tinkled as you walked over it.

So we left Osborne Road and its monkey puzzle tree, holding our breath, driving in a family convoy – mother, father, my three brothers and their vehicles, my baby sister and our dog – for the sunny suburb of Sholing, away from the urban traffic which was already swallowing up Portswood. For my mother, it was a homecoming. Born that side of the Itchen, schooled in Sholing, she knew its valleys and lanes and funny little corner shops, its peculiar character, its strange mixture. It was a place where she felt at home.

My second-ever memory is of the house in which I would grow up. Ruddy cheeked, round headed, blond haired and four years old, I ran excitedly through the front door and up the uncarpeted stairs accompanied by Bimbo, a blackish mongrel of erratic temper who later grew so wild and savage that when he eventually ran off, his absence went unregretted, at least by my parents. Having reached the top, we both promptly fell all the way back to the bottom, landing, unharmed, at the foot of the stairs. Soon after I had another accident, in the corrugated iron Anderson shelter which still stood in the garden. Trying to reach a large metal and wood model locomotive about half my size on an upper shelf, the train fell on my head, and – in my remembrance, at least – momentarily knocked me unconscious.

The incident left me with an abiding image – as though knocked into my head – of the metal and wood of the toy and the metal and wood of the shed and its dark interior where a family had sheltered from falling bombs. But life in Sholing was quiet now, following the pre-ordained, uneventful rites of suburbia. I went to a Catholic primary school a mile away in Woolston. St Patrick's had been founded in 1879 by Fr Henry Patrick Kelly, the chaplain to the military hospital at Netley; its school hall was the old Edwardian 'tin church' of green-painted corrugated iron, and the rest of the school buildings consisted of the remains of what had once been the local police station. The boys' toilets were roofless and open to the air, but dark and smelly inside, and in the grounds stood a bunker-like concrete air raid shelter, overgrown with brambles like barbed wire. A pair of classrooms were housed in corrugated iron huts like extended versions of our Anderson shelter, while in the far corner of the playground stood another shed, a smaller cousin of the tin church, also painted dark green. 'Miss Enright's hut' had also come from Netley, where it had been the matron's quarters in the First World War.

It was in this little hut, with its tilting floor, that on my first day of school I answered the register by calling out 'Yes, Mummy', and shortly afterwards wet myself; the water trickled slowly down the slope to the back of the classroom. I was not easily reconciled to leaving home: no sooner had my mother put me on the bus in the morning than I got off at the next stop and promptly walked back again. An ex-police station, a military hut and open air toilets did little to allay the fears of a knock-kneed boy in a home-knitted green jumper and grey shorts; still less an elderly teacher with an iron calliper on her leg.

In our tin classroom we would dutifully copy out Miss

Clements' copperplate writing from the blackboard, dipping our nibs in china inkwells filled by the ink monitor from a giant bottle of Quink, inevitably staining our fingers and our shirts dark blue. We recited our times tables, and on Wednesday mornings we'd file next door for Mass in the big 'new' church, built in 1939 (and promptly gutted by incendiary bombs in 1940). Now refurbished, with its green stained-glass windows, a stone statue of St Patrick over the entrance and, inside, another huge portrait of the saint driving the serpents out of Ireland, it was as invested with Irishness as were our green school uniforms and the bunches of shamrock which would mysteriously arrive from Ireland on St Patrick's Day. They were symbols of a state-hood I did not share, except by the association of faith, and, somewhere in my green eyes, the faint traces of a genetic Irishness.

Class by class we'd troop across a parquet floor dented by a decade of Sixties stilettos, file into our seats and pull down the kneelers. Crouching, I'd look through my fingers to the wounded, contorted figure of Christ above the altar, and the glass mosaics on either side, art deco versions of Byzantine icons. On one side, Jesus pointed to the exposed and radiant heart, red and glowing in His chest; on the other, in front of me, was the Blessed Virgin, her oval face surrounded by a gold tesseral halo. Like her grown-up son, her body lay full length against the wall, floating in space and impossibly attenuated; but in the folds of her transcendent blue gown she clasped an unwounded and perfectly formed Christ Child holding up His baby hand in blessing. Sometimes, as I stared, I felt I too could float into the air, to be suspended above the congregation, to the amazement of my fellow pupils. At the end of term we would return for Benediction and its Latin litany intoned in clouds of intoxicating incense, and on May Day we would process through the church gardens behind a statue of Our Lady carried on a wooden stretcher, her beautiful neat head crowned with a garland of flowers as we sang, 'Ave, ave, ave Maria'.

One dinnertime I ran down to the school gate to see my father arrive in the big old family car with my beaming little sister, her brown hair in bunches, not yet old enough for school, jumping excitedly up and down on the passenger seat. We drove home to see our new baby sister, pink and bawling in crocheted wool and carry cot by my mother's bedroom window. She was as blonde as my elder sister was dark; they were a perfect pair, and I loved them and they loved me. The world seemed as safe and secure as our new baby swaddled in her cot, her tiny fingers clasping the wool like soft pink bird's talons. I read the *Beano* on my father's knee on dark winter evenings and he cut my finger- and toenails.

The house was yellow and warm, but one day I came home from school to find my mother airing clothes on a wooden clothes horse in front of the coal fire, upset by the news she had just heard on our old valve radio (with its illuminated dial and place names as strange as the lunchtime shipping forecast). Many children had died after a mountain of coal had fallen on their school in Wales. Later, on TV, there would be grainy black and white images of a destroyed building in a mining village, and men in coats picking over what looked like a bomb site. In my mind's eye I saw the black soot engulfing the high ceilings of my classroom, pouring in through the big wide window, silently crashing and crushing.*

But mostly life and death carried on over my pudding-basin-haircut head. I went to school as the sun rose at one end of the street, and went to bed as it set at the other. I saw my first streak

---

* In 1998 the artist Linder Sterling filled a derelict Catholic school in Widnes – close to the Mersey's Spike Island (site of the Stone Roses' 1990 concert) – with forty-two tonnes of industrial salt. The effect of a half-glazed classroom filled to its windows with the luminous, snow-like mineral was beautiful, but disturbing. Sterling's 'Salt Shrine' was about the abusive nature of institutions (somehow reinforced by the statue of St Bernadette in a nearby corridor which the pupils believed came to life at night); but for me it resonated with the memory of Aberfan.

of lightning make an electrified crack in the sky, and ran home for cover. I played soldiers and feared hospitals, and once visited the dentist's in an Edwardian house opposite our school to have a tooth pulled out. In grey shorts, another green home-knitted jumper, and a permanent scab on my knees, I saw the brass plate at the entrance, the venetian blinds at the windows, the unadorned front garden: all too neat, too clean, too white to be a home. I panicked as the black rubber mask descended, halo'd by the yellowy examination light that shone on the steel instruments laid out in a tray at my shoulder. The nauseous smell of the rubber was pressed down on my memory with the hiss of the gas as it was clamped over my small face, the dentist's white coat and stubble and glasses above. The next thing I remember was staggering out of the porch, spitting gobs of gelatinous blood like leeches, reeling on to the front lawn and lying there, the world turning above me as I experienced my first intoxication, mixed with medically-induced pain from a suburban house of torture.

If these were the worst things in my life, the rest of it must have been pretty good. But then everything changed.

It was a Saturday morning. I remember coming downstairs and looking over the banisters – another aerial view, as if I were removed from these proceedings in my life, these out-of-body experiences – and watching my parents moving about in the front room. They were not doing the housework; they were not moving in the way parents should move.

My brother had been injured in a car crash. He was twenty-three years old. After a week in a coma, my mother and his young wife staying at the hospital to be at his bedside, Andrew died.

The news permeated the house like an invisible gas. I remember being told about it while standing by the kitchen door; I knew it had happened, but I must have appeared as if I didn't. Crouching down to my eleven-year-old level, my brother explained in slow, clear tones that Andrew was dead. 'I know',

I said, and ran out, down to the bottom of the garden, where the snakes hid in the privet hedge.

Everything seemed thrown in the air, as though the atmosphere itself had buckled and warped. Nothing was right; everything was wrong. It was almost exhilarating, as though you were moving backwards at speed, removed from the events that were taking place, that you knew you were witnessing and yet could not feel.

Later, I tried to access the emotion I should have felt. I tried to remember Andrew, with his thick, dark spiky hair and round head, shaped like mine, and which my parents said was as hard as a bullet. I thought of his kind face, his stocky body, his sports shirt, the tinned steak and kidney puddings he sold from the back of his van, even though he was a vegetarian. But all I could remember was the day he took my sister up to the corner shop and filled her dolls' pram full of sweets for her birthday. For that act alone he was a hero. He became the lost connection that would have made the rest of my life happy.

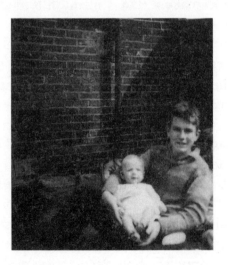

In the back garden of Akaba, sitting against a brick wall, my dead brother cradles me proudly in his strong arms, my plump little baby's fingers in his. He grins at Dad's camera, his arms full of me: pale and pudgy, I look straight ahead, eyes unfocused, nonplussed, still vaguely embryonic, as though I'd only just emerged into the world. Over in our new suburban home, with its smaller rooms and without my brother's wide arms, I would grow like a goldfish grows to the size of its bowl; knees bent as I crouched by the gas fire in grey wool dressing gown tied with a twirly cord, chilblains on my feet in winter, burning ginger biscuits in front of the ash-white ceramic that glowed luminous red with internal heat as the wind whistled up the chimney.

The shadow of loss lay over us, but I can only remember the funeral, which I insisted on attending, dressing myself and running round to Andrew's house to join the cortège. Shortly afterwards, my eldest brother – still only in his twenties – separated from his wife and came with his two young daughters to live with us. It became crowded in our three-bedroom semi. My mother had to cook for two families: big aluminium saucepans held pounds of peeled potatoes, sitting in their starchy water ready to be boiled like blind white fish. Life was as normal as my parents could make it, but I was a different boy.

From Lance's Hill in Bitterne, Sholing's neighbouring suburb, you can look across the dual carriageway to an opposing rise in the land and the tree-surrounded site of St Mary's College. Its white stucco mansion, with bay windows like the bows of a man-o'-war, is the last great house of the estates which once studded the banks of Southampton Water. Like many of its counterparts, the house reacted to the social changes of the twentieth century by becoming an institution, a seminary for Catholic monks expelled from France; they added a slate mansard roof, giving the building the air of a Normandy chateau. In 1922, a new order, the De la Mennais brothers, took over, adding a utilitarian four-storey brick block to accommodate their school, with a chapel between marking the religious transition from the house in which they lived to the secular block in which they worked.

I'd won a scholarship to St Mary's in my last year at primary school. All three of my brothers had been there, and in the wake of Andrew's loss, a sense of tradition, if not duty, settled on me. After a summer of freedom came the day in September when my brother, who wore gold crushed velvet flares and had met his girlfriend at the Isle of Wight festival, drove me in his pre-war Austin, complete with running boards, to my new school.

At the end of a long gravel drive shouldered by rhododendron was the playground, a desert of grey tarmac surrounded by high chain-link fencing. Inside this giant cage was a teeming horde in a strange new uniform of brown and gold. With his hand on my shoulder, assuming his appointed role just as I must assume mine, my brother introduced me to the deputy headmaster. Dressed in a cassock edged and elbowed in black leather, the monk regarded me through his steel-rimmed spectacles: he had the raw, overshaved face of the early-rising religious, Brylcreemed hair and a wide toothy grin that belied his school nickname – 'Crippen'. I was left in the playground, waiting for the whistle, abandoned to my fate. It was a recurring nightmare, of being lost in some unknown place, not knowing how to get home; it was the same sense of abandonment I felt when, lying in my top bunk in the bedroom I now shared with my two grown-up brothers, I heard in my head 'The Green, Green Grass of Home', and realised for the first time, with a sudden and sharp pain, the reality of loss.

Marshalled into lines and into the building that was to be home for half my waking life, we filed into long glazed corridors of creaking floorboards smelling of polish and chalk and ink and leather. At the end was the hallway to the chapel, and as we trooped down to Mass we would catch sight of the dark interior of the old house beyond. To cross this point was forbidden. Occasionally, a monk would pass through the connecting door, allowing a glimpse of a stark domesticity. I imagined the monks' bedrooms to be bare, with iron bedsteads, crucifixes and bedside tracts – whereas the prosaic truth was probably the deputy head-master with his feet up, reading *Sporting Life* over a glass of whisky.

Crippen was said to have tailor-made leather straps hanging on the wall of his office, each whimsically named after his 'girl-friends' and ready to punish any transgression. He was the most worldly in an eccentric staffroom of characters easily baited by the ingenious cruelty of schoolboys: the shell-shocked language teacher whom we'd tease by imitating exploding bombs; another well-meaning brother who taught maths and whose fury was kept under control only by his undoubted devotion; and a physics master who, it was claimed, had helped invent the aerosol. He may have been a genius, but we could hardly care less. It was our duty, like prisoners of war, to taunt a chalky-cassocked and leather-patched cast who would not have been out of place in *Nicholas Nickleby*. The sense of them and us, of prisoners and wardens, was emphasised by our uniforms and their cassocks. The wooded grounds provided cover for our transgressions, a place to smoke illicit cigarettes and conduct other experiments, not all of them the kind that even the deputy's girlfriends could dissuade.

In front of the school buildings, once gracious but now shaggy lawns sloped down to a series of turf banks dividing the school from its playing fields below. We were barred from the manicured grass in front of the White House itself, under which it was rumoured tunnels ran. One came out under the library; others we could only speculate about in our prisoner-of-war fantasies. As my best friend, Peter, and I trespassed in the cellars, he told me – and I had no reason to doubt him – that one tunnel led far out under the playing fields, down and down until it reached the distant shore of Netley.

In a Lonely Place

... The shores fringed with oak to the very margin, and
studded with the fairest vestiges of magnificence and
modern comfort, seem to connect the past with the present, like the wild yet bewitching imagery of a poet's
dream.

MARY RUSSELL MITFORD
visiting Southampton Water, 1812

From its shore, the slow-moving estuary seems like the Loch
Ness of my dream. The gently rippling surface belies its
length and width, a foreshortened trick of the eye as deceptive
as the calm surface of the fathomless Scottish lake. It is a liminal
space, a place of possibilities, evocative of the deep oceans that
lie beyond.

But Southampton Water is an unlikely place to find a sea
monster, although occasionally the sinister, half-submerged
black bulk of a submarine slips silently out of its military port.
Neither sea nor river, this sinuous inlet reaches deep into England's underbelly like a gynaecologist's finger. Stoppered at one
end by the Isle of Wight, the island is believed to bounce the
moon-dragged sea back up the estuary, creating the watery *déjà
vu* of Southampton's unique double high tides (in fact it is the
result of the port's midway point on the Channel, combined

with the Atlantic Pulse and the relative positions of the sun and moon).

Fed by the Atlantic Pulse, it is a fortuitous piece of geography. 'A seaport without the sea's terrors, an ocean approach within the threshold of the land,' extolled one nineteenth-century promoter of its virtues. Here the great Hampshire rivers of the Itchen and the Test conjoin, their chalk-filtered fresh waters mingling in the salt of the seaway. Like the Pool of London at the beginning of Marlow's journey in *Heart of Darkness*, in which 'the sea-reach of the Thames stretched before us like the beginning of an interminable waterway', Southampton Water has always promised adventure and commerce, a country's past and future. To incomers it was the Gateway to England; to the inhabitants, it became the 'Gateway to the Empire'. From here too England reaches out into the dark heart of other lands.

Centuries have passed through this inseminal conduit. From Roman barges to ocean liners; from plague ships to Pilgrim Fathers; from French marauders to Hollywood film stars; from Francis Drake's *Golden Hind*, laden with Spanish gold for the Virgin Queen, to Goering's bombers, heavy with a deadlier cargo. Enemies or tourists, missionaries or immigrants, they all entered or left the land here, and in some other age their phantoms are still processing along Southampton Water: the stately red and black hulk of *Titanic*, crewed by the men of Spike Island; the speed boat piloted by T. E. Lawrence, the doomed hero of Arabia; the flying boat in whose leather seats was strapped the aesthete, the Honourable Stephen Tennant, on course for the tamarisk-lined shores and pink sunsets of the Riviera. Here they pass for ever, these pale, mortal, glamorous ghosts, unobserved by the cars that speed along Weston Shore.

When Weston's housing estate was built in the 1950s, the council tried to turn the shore into a resort. Like the strand made in the shadow of the Tower of London for Cockneys to swim off, a beach was created and an esplanade was constructed, studded at intervals with shelters built like waiting rooms for a railway which would never come. Old photographs show holiday makers in their Sunday best, strolling the prom, children paddling at the water's edge.

Nowadays Weston Shore, at the bottom of the hill from Sholing, seems a grey parody of a place. The shelters' windows were long ago shattered and the beach reclaimed by banks of shingle and scrubby grass. Here the land lies low, and often floods, as if to mark its transition from the city's edge to the woods ahead, where the road inclines to leave the shore through a tunnel of trees, and from where it rises then falls again, gently and without due ceremony, into the village of Netley. Even now, those few hundred yards act like a timeslip, a fault in the chronology; as though, having passed through this interzone, you have left one world for another. The concrete tower blocks at your back and the ancient woodland ahead only serve to make Netley's past all the more extraordinary.

Netley extends the tongue of land that begins at Sholing, bounded by the Itchen and Southampton Water on one side and the Hamble river on the other, the borders of Spike Island. Half ceded from the coastline, this peninsula is occupied by villages which long ago lost their discrete identities to new housing and the out-of-town developments spreading along the motorway corridor – the visible symptom of what Nikolaus Pevsner called 'subtopia'. Subsumed by light industry, yachting marinas and modern estates, it is a place of retreat and recreation; a faithless culture that seems to have no other aim than the nearest shopping opportunity. It is as though England lost its way in this cul-de-sac; as if it gave up keeping the barbarian at bay.

Nothing happens here now. But once it did.

In 1826, during one of his 'rural rides', William Cobbett called on the Chamberlaynes at Weston Grove, their marine villa on the shores of Southampton Water. The estate is now only discernible by stately cedars among the council houses and the traces of a carriage drive in neighbouring Mayfield Park, but in its brief century of existence it epitomised the area's Georgian gentility, a time when the eastern banks of the water were studded with such mansions.

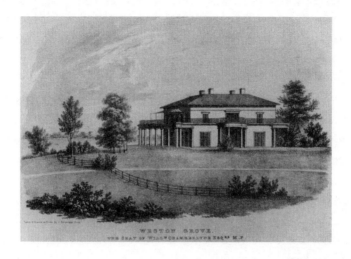

William Chamberlayne had built the house, where he lived with his sister, in 1802, on land inherited from his close friend and neighbour, Thomas Lee Dummer of Woolston House. Already a major landowner in the area, Chamberlayne had used his friend's bequest to extend his domain down to the shore and inland through Sholing's valleys, where the houses around Church Path were 'Chamberlayne's cottages', humble dwellings for his subjects (as we, living on roads named after our masters, still seemed to be). He had also demolished several houses to 'improve' the landscape, in the current parlance. Cobbett, a Tory-turned-radical and famed for his polemics against industrialisation and its consequences for rural England, considered that Chamberlayne 'and his equally benevolent sister' had set 'a *striking and a most valuable practical example*' for their fellow land-owners. 'Here is a whole neighbourhood of labourers living as they ought to live; enjoying that happiness which is the just reward of their toil.' In such a setting England's green and pleasant land could be reinvented, the broken connexion between land and man remade.

Yet as Cobbett may have suspected, the threat to that idyll was irrevocable; it had been for some time. In Chamberlayne's grounds, in the wooded valley which continued from Church Path through his parkland and down to the sea, was Walter Taylor's mill, a modern, industrialised version of the windmill which stood above it on the hill, its site now surmounted by a stone obelisk. Established in 1762 and powered by the water from Miller's Pond, there had been a mill here since at least the fourteenth century. Now a new machine had been installed, a circular saw invented by Taylor for cutting ships' blocks out of hard lignum vitae imported from the West Indies and South America. It was a significant marker in the Industrial Revolution and Britain's expanding empire: here, in this damp valley where kids now chuck empty Coke cans, the rigging for HMS *Victory* was made.

Chamberlayne's estate dominated the peninsula, the ruler of Spike Island in all but title, and Cobbett's description read like the literary equivalent of a nineteeth-century watercolour:

> To those who like water scenes (as nineteen-twentieths of people do) it is the prettiest spot, I believe, in all England ... The views from this place are the most beautiful that can be imagined. You see up the water and down the water, to Redbridge one way and out to Spithead the other way. Through the trees, to the right, you see the spires of South-ampton, and you have only to walk a mile, over a beautiful lawn and through a not less beautiful wood, to find, in a little dell, surrounded with lofty woods, the venerable ruins ... which make part of Mr. Chamberlayne's estate ...

Those venerable ruins represented the old England; a fantasy which would inspire a new cult – that of the gothic. Set back from the sea like a series of theatrical flats behind the green drapery of trees, the medieval remains of Netley Abbey might have been designed as a piece of stage scenery by William Kent, the gothic taste-maker who once planted a dead tree in Kensington

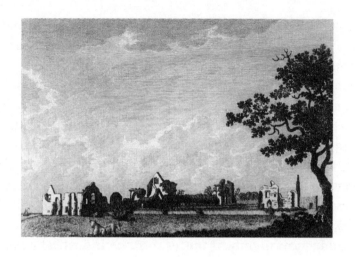

Gardens. It was a place which had ever been wreathed in a sense of its own mystery. Throughout its history, it seems, this wooded site had a gloomy, perhaps even a terrible charm.

'Netley Abbey ought, it seems, to be called *Letley Abbey*', wrote Cobbett, 'the Latin name being Laetus Locus, or Pleasant Place. *Letley* was made up of an abbreviation of the *Laetus* and of the Saxon word *ley*, which meant *place*, *field*, or *piece of ground*.' But like Spike Island, the provenance of Netley's name was disputed, its very identity surrounded in myth. Some writers considered *Laetus Locus* a play on the name of Letelie, which was already recorded in the Domesday Book; others believed that it originated from 'Natan-leaga, or Leas of Naté, a wooded district extending from the Avon to the Test and Itchen'. Yet other sources attribute another old English meaning to the name: lonely, or desolate place.

For thousands of years these river valleys had been used as routes into England's interior, through primeval forest with its wild boar, bear and wolves, and into the uplands; Bronze Age axes and tumuli have been found in Sholing's heathland. When the Romans came, they set up their military base and strategic port of Clausentum on a bend in the River Itchen, building a tall lighthouse to make plain their dominion. Half a millennium later it would crumble with the rest of their empire in the Dark Ages. When in turn the Saxons built their settlements, Hamwih and Hamtun, on the opposite bank, they would merge to become Suthhamtun, and give their name to the county, Hamtunscire.

In the Viking raids of the ninth and tenth centuries, the inhabitants would retreat behind the remaining Roman walls; those that did not were slain, enslaved, or, in the coy words of one nineteenth-century historian, used by the invaders 'to satisfy their insatiable cupidity'. Medieval Southampton learned from such lessons, building defences to the north and east, yet leaving the waterside disastrously open to attack. One Sunday morning in 1338, while most of Southampton was at Mass, a fleet of fifty galleys 'crowded with Normans, Picards, Genoese, and Spaniards' sailed up the water to launch an ungodly assault. Many died as they came out of St Michael's Church, clubbed or stabbed on the threshold of their place of worship; others were hanged in their own houses. The invaders took arrogant leisure in their destruction and stayed overnight to burn, rape, pillage and plunder – a fatal mistake, as by that time the King's men had arrived to drive them back to their ships, killing 300 in the process. Their leader, Carlo Grimaldi, however, escaped to the Mediterranean, where he used the spoils to establish his Monte Carlo principality.

Netley, meanwhile, remained on the sidelines of these events, looking on as its neighbour suffered successive invasions. Set in its woods, the place kept to itself. This uncanny sense of timelessness was marked by the Seaweed Hut which once stood on Weston Shore. A weird dome of worm-eaten wood, draped with turf and seaweed like a maritime haystack of flotsam heaped up on the beach, it was described by the *Victoria History of Hampshire* in 1903 'to be of considerable antiquity' and celebrated on Edwardian postcards as a local curiosity. Some claimed it was a fishermen's lookout, shelter and store, or perhaps an old ferry shelter, but to me it resembled nothing so much as a tribal hut.

As children we used to creep inside, the sky showing through the gaps in its roof, the interior dark and damp and smelling of salt and seaweed. I imagined it tenanted by a Father Neptune

40

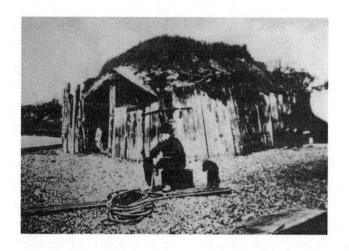

figure, holding court and garbed in kelp like a sea voyager crossing the Equator, half-hermit, half-warlock. Even to the end, the
hut retained its secrets: crumbling and weather-beaten, when it
finally fell apart in the 1960s its age was unknown. Roman coins
had been discovered in the field behind; perhaps the hut was
there to witness the imperial arrivals in their shiny helmets and
red tunics, subjugating the natives and their shamanistic rites in
the woods. Perhaps it was a Celtic temple, there when Christian
missionaries first arrived to battle with the pagan gods of the
forest. But whatever dark spirits had occupied this gravelly shore,
they were to be firmly supplanted by a new invasion.

Like the old religion, the order of the Cistercians was born in a
wood, founded in the Burgundian forest of Cîteaux as a more
austere version of the Benedictines. In the late twelfth century
the monks crossed the Channel to establish houses in England
and, encouraged by King John, founded an abbey at Beaulieu in
the New Forest in 1204. Soon after, the Bishop of Winchester
commissioned the Cistercian abbots to investigate the site at
Netley, and on 25 July 1239, an advance party arrived from
Beaulieu, sent from the beautiful place to the sad place across
the water – a journey still made by fallow deer, only to be felled
by poachers, an ill-return for these animal asylum-seekers.

Cut off as it was by dense woodland from the interior, with the sea the only practicable means of access, it was Netley's isolation which attracted the ascetic Cistercians. Their order characteristically sought sites 'of horror – a vast wilderness', 'far from the concourse of men', as they had at Fountains Abbey on the Yorkshire moors. They would go to great lengths in their search for 'lonely, wooded places': if the chosen site wasn't empty enough then, like later landowners, they made it so, evicting the resident population and levelling cottages. As Walter Map, Archdeacon of Oxford, noted, 'they make a solitude that they may be solitaries'.

Built out of stone from the Isle of Wight quarry of Quarr, by 1251 the order had run out of money, and work on their new church ground to a halt. To fund its completion, the monks applied for, and were granted, state aid. The result was a rather more sophisticated building, its importance plain from the inscription on the chapel's foundation stone – '*H: DI. GRA. REX ANGL.*', 'Henry, by the grace of God, king of England' – and the ornate tracery windows modelled on those of Westminster Abbey, which the King had recently rebuilt, in a style which the Cistercians themselves had imported to England. At a time when architecture was an expression of man's creativity by God's grace, gothic had become the predominant aesthetic of an age predicated on religion.

One hundred years before, Abbot Suger had built the first gothic structure, the Abbey of Saint-Denis outside Paris: his *opus modernum* in stained glass and stone. The Cistercians appreciated its sharp pointed arches, functional rib vaults and flying buttresses as a reaction against the ungodly excesses of rounded Romanesque arches and their writhing serpents and mythological beasts. They agreed with the reforming mystic St Bernard of Clairvaux, who declared, 'What are these fantastic monsters doing in the cloisters ... What is the *meaning* of these unclean monkeys, these savage lions, and monstrous creatures? To what purpose are here placed these creatures, half-beast, half-man, or these spotted tigers?' In decrying such 'semi-human beings', the serpents and monsters which may still have lurked in the woods and lakes, St Bernard looked to a new image of God, exorcising the creatures in which a 'crypto-pagan' people hardly out of the Dark Ages still half-believed. This was the aim of the Cistercians' misson: to convert this pagan shore. Their new order would convey the clarity of God's vision, and conquer the mythical denizens of a wild forest.

Gothic was as innovatory and as modern as anything by Mies van der Rohe. Like twentieth-century architecture, its buttresses and pillars openly displayed its technological achievements. Load-bearing ribs – a technique later used in skyscrapers – allowed the thin walls between them to be cut away to let in light. The result was a luminescent box, charged to uplift the human soul into sanctity. As God's light pierced the 'cloud of unknowing' between Heaven and Man, so His holy rays shone through the stained glass set in arches that pointed Heavenwards; rays almost as visible as those emitted by a halo'd Christ in a medieval illumination. Abbot Suger named it the 'new light', *lux nova*; a transcendent vision for those who beheld it, at a time when the sense of sight was regarded as so powerful that it could affect the object at which you looked, and vice versa. To look upon the true image of God, for instance, would, were it possible, mean instant destruction, so He was represented by a colour, 'the strange blue of twelfth-century glass which seems to filter to our souls the essence of other skies in other worlds'. Light itself was God-given. Thus mediated, Netley's abbey was also acknowledging its dedicatee, the Blessed Virgin, herself known as the 'window of Heaven', *fenestra coeli*, an image through which, like an icon, the unseeable God might be vouchsafed.

As its aspiring gothic windows pierced the walls like thorns in her son's heart, their glass stained with the sin of the world, so the chapel impressed its cruciform plan, Christ's mark, into the Hampshire soil. And by granting the monks 'free warren in their demesne lands of Netley, Hound, Sotteshall [Satchell] and Sholing', Henry III's patronage gave them full authority to impose their Christian order on the land.

It may have been suitably 'horrible' as a site, but there were also good economic reasons for the monks' choice of Netley. Here were lush pastures for their sheep and cattle, fertile land for their crops, and plentiful fish and oysters in Southampton Water, supplemented by the abbey's own freshwater stewponds. A grange farm was set up, along with a lodge to receive lepers barred from entering Southampton – an isolation ward in which the afflicted could be tended by novice monks in an already isolated site. Thus did the Cistercians reinvent the land in their own image – the image, by association and intent, of God.

The result was a self-sufficient community, maintaining its distance while continuing Christ's mission in caring for the sick. Its proximity to water was an important spiritual aspect: water held traditional healing powers for the body and the soul, and Netley's abbey would provide for both. And just as their new settlement sought to express Christ's message, so the monks emulated their Saviour's simplicity. They wore white habits and black scapulas without shirts underneath, slept on straw beds, rose at midnight to pray and remained silent for most of their day; they ate no meat unless in sickness, and transgression could result in solitary confinement or flogging. Such a regime was more like that of a prison, a medieval Spike Island, but their ordered lives and monastic traditions set the precedent for the industrialised society to come, just as their beliefs determined the order of life around them.

Bound by their vow of silence, protected by royal patronage and geographically removed from the sometimes dangerous nearby port (though trading with it in wool and other produce), the abbey's monks could remain secure in their wordless isolation, as though their own castle walls, gothic rationality and implicit faith could keep out the barbarian world. They escaped the bloody raids of the 1330s, protected by their religious status and French origins, although not immune to the prevailing sense of instability as the taxation returns for February 1341 noted, being short of '8s of their usual value as a good part of the corn land lies left fallow through dread of foreign invasion and the marauding of the king's sailors'. But then came an invasion no one could ignore.

According to the contemporary historian Henry Knighton of Leicester, the bubonic plague of 1348 entered England through Southampton, via fleas carried on the backs of rats and men up the estuary, injecting the country with its terrible bacillus. Other ports would lay claim to this dubious honour, but a later historian noted that 'the town suffered much from a destructive pestilence which, beginning in China, had swept over the face of the whole discovered globe, and, entering into this island, spent its first fury in this neighbourhood'. The plague would kill half of Southampton's population, while upriver at Winchester the townspeople were persuaded to parade around the marketplace reciting the seven penitential psalms three times a week; all to no avail as half its populace too would perish.

As *Pasteurella pestis* infected the rest of Britain with its flesh-corrupting buboes and noisome stench, culling three million – half the population – Netley's Cistercians lived on in their lonely place. Around them England was pulled down by the calamity; fields were left untended, entire villages died. The plague was the hell of medieval imagining come to life, an evil miasma that lurked in the air itself, and in turn culture became infected with mortality, disease and decay. It was the plague that gave gothic its darkness: the images of St John's Apocalypse, *memento mori*, and most vividly the Dance of Death, a skeleton leading bishops, kings, merchants and beggars alike to their graves in a *danse macabre* prompted by the shattered nervous systems of the disease's victims.

Even Netley's institutional self-sufficiency could not resist the inevitable change – not least the decline in lay-brothers, either from mortality or desertion, attracted by better working conditions to a world in which labour was at a premium. As the devils of disease punished the wicked, the halt in civilisation's progress became manifest in its buildings. Before the epidemic, gothic had begun to develop a decadent enflorescence of ornate foliage and lascivious curves. The plague curtailed such extravagance (not least by decimating the workforce). It was God's retribution for Man's decadence – a moral decay which also appeared to have afflicted Netley, succeeding where the bubonic bacillus had failed. Society became more materialistic and more sceptical, paradoxes which made the religious orders prey both to apostasy and their own sensuality. By the end of the fifteenth century, Pope Sixtus IV had relaxed the rules governing closed orders, and the populace now began to turn against its white-robed neighbours, accusing them of laxity of observance and immorality. When Henry VIII began his move towards reformation, his supporters agreed that such orders had become corrupted by their own privilege.

Yet Netley was hardly a wealthy estate. By 1535 the population of monks had fallen to just seven, with thirty-two staff, £43 worth of plate and jewels, and an annual income of just £100. Establishments of its size were easy targets for suppression – especially by those who might stand to gain from the release of their land and resources – and the 1536 act of Parliament which began the process justified itself 'forasmuch as manifest sin, vicious, carnal and abominable living is daily used and committed amongst the little and small abbeys, priories and other religious houses of monks, canons and nuns . . .'

All around England statues and stained glass were smashed and destroyed, and in 1536 the wreckers came to Netley. The abbey's lucent wonder was demolished by the sons of those who had built it, and with its dissolution, the Cistercians' lonely place became an empty ruin.

The legend of tunnels running from underneath our school to Netley was irresistible. Ignoring its improbabilities, we crept into the school cellars and in the cobwebby gloom imagined a journey to the centre of the earth, or at least to the ruined abbey, where a workman by the name of Slown was said to have died of fright when he was sent down such a tunnel, his last words being, 'Block it up! In the name of God!' Netley bred these myths: the abbot's treasure trove was said to lay buried in the grounds after the monks' flight from the Dissolution, jealously guarded by his ghost.

Peter actually lived next to the abbey. I'd met him in my first year at St Mary's, when he seemed a glamorous figure, with his sophisticated manner, anarchic humour and jet-set air (he had been to New York); he brought out the aspirational in me. Peter lived with his parents in a detached house next to the abbey ruins, and claimed it had been built on the monks' graveyard, pointing out, as proof, the bumps in the lawn. That was a scary enough story, but the unmade driveway to his house passed the abbey itself, thrilling on moonlit nights with its great broken walls and gothic arches rising out of the trees. In their fantastic ruins you could reinvent yourself as any romantic figure of the past.

For a boy from Sholing, this gothic vision was captivating; the abbey seemed able not only to conjure up the past, but to invite the creation of a new identity – just as the ruins had reinvented themselves.

In 1540 Henry VIII had granted Netley, its buildings and lands – including Sholing – as a reward to his courtier, Sir William Paulet, for good service. To the outspoken William Cobbett, however, this was less good service than political manoeuvring quite equal to the corruption of which the abbey's former owners had been accused. Paulet, later first Marquis of Winchester, was a nationally important figure: royal minister, Master of the King's Wards, Comptroller of the Household, Lord Treasurer and sheriff of Hampshire; his mansion at Basing was one of the largest private houses in England. He was also 'a man the most famous in the whole world for sycophancy, time-serving, and for all those qualities which usually distinguish the favourites of kings like the wife-killer', said Cobbett.

With the deterioration of relations with France, and Henry VIII's determination to pursue a glorious war, the King ordered the fortification of Southampton Water. In return for under-taking to build twelve castles along the Solent, Paulet was given certain manors and lands – including those of Netley Abbey. It was a shrewd piece of business. The dissolution of the monasteries freed up valuable building material, and the waterside abbeys of Quarr, Beaulieu and Netley were convenient to plunder and recycle as Henry's new castles at Yarmouth, Cowes and Hurst. Yet by 1542 – just three years before an invading French fleet of 200 ships would mass off the Isle of Wight – Netley had acquired only a small fort, built on the site of the abbey's sea gate with stones from its refectory. Evidently Paulet was conserving the rest of the abbey for a palatial dwelling. He created a new grand entrance flanked by polygonal turrets like Hampton Court, then levelled the cloisters to make an open courtyard with a fountain; the nave was turned into one enormous banqueting hall. Thus were the abbey's holy spaces expanded to make room for Paulet's ego. Ironically, however, it was this secularisation that helped preserve the holy site: Paulet's selfish scheming resulted in posterity's gain.

William Paulet would live through four Tudor reigns, dying in 1572 at the remarkable age of ninety-seven, a testament to the acquisition of riches and his own swiftly-changing political and religious allegiances. In the meantime, Netley continued in its new function as a grand house. In 1560 it passed to Edward Seymour, the Earl of Hertford, son of the Protector Somerset, who that August entertained Elizabeth I on one of her royal progresses, as Southampton's mayor proudly – or perhaps nervously – observed: 'The Queenes Maiestees grace came from the Castle of Netley to Southampton on the XIII of August.'

For the next century or so, the building remained somewhere between an abbey, a mansion and a castle, a fortified retreat secure enough for Seymour's Royalist son to be confined there during the Interregnum. The abbey retained some sacred duties – one of the Seymours was baptised in its chapel in 1665 – although when it became the property of the Earl of Huntingdon, the new owner converted the west end of the chapel into a kitchen and 'other offices'. But by the eighteenth century, this draughty architectural portmanteau had become decidedly old-fashioned, and its latest owner, the apparently disinterested Sir Berkeley Lucy, began to sell off chunks of the ruins for building materials.

Abbey stones had already found their way into local houses and churches, but these came from secular parts of the building, not its consecrated chapel. In 1703 an eminent Southampton builder, Walter Taylor, grandfather of the mill-owning industrialist, made a deal with Lucy 'for the purchase of so much of its materials as he could carry away in a certain space of time'; other chroniclers record that Sir Berkeley 'sold the whole fabrick of the chapel'. Taylor's God-fearing family urged him 'not to be instrumental in destroying an edifice which had been consecrated to the worship of the Deity', and although such imprecations did not persuade Taylor to abandon his plans, 'they dwelt so much on his mind as to occasion a dream one night, that the arch key-stone of the East window fell from its situation, and fractured his skull'. Another version has the ghost of a monk appear to the transgressing developer, threatening him 'with great mischief if he persisted in his purpose'.

Taylor duly reported his dream to his friend Isaac Watts, schoolmaster and father of the Methodist composer, who, like Taylor, was a Dissenter, and had been gaoled for his beliefs. Watts gave what the Victorian historian William Howitt frowningly described as 'somewhat Jesuitical advice', instructing Taylor 'to have no personal concern in pulling down the building'. Ignoring his friend's warning, Taylor went ahead and 'tore off the roof (which was entire, till then) and pulled down great part of the walls'. But,

in an exertion to tear down a board from the window loosed the fatal stone, which fell upon his head, and produced a fracture. The wound was not, at first, deemed to be mortal, but the instrument of the surgeon unhappily slipped, in the operation of extracting a splinter, entered the brain, and caused immediate death.

The moral of the story was plain: human greed invited God's retribution, and the abbey's ghosts would avenge the destruction begun by an ungodly king. The tale became part of the growing myth of Netley. Even a century later, William Howitt's proposal that the tragedy actually benefited the abbey seemed to infer that Taylor had been a sacrifice required for its perpetuation: 'the accident had the good effect of staying the demolition of the Abbey, which has since been uninjured except by time and tourists'. Netley had again managed to save itself by another lucky circumstance, just as Paulet's domestic conversion had stopped it falling down. Taylor's hapless fate – wrapped up in the abbey's legends – had preserved these crumbling stones.

By the mid-eighteenth century Netley's ruins had taken on an increasingly feral air, as though Nature had appointed itself as the abbey's new guardian. Ivy crept up over the walls as if to hold them together, and mature trees grew to create a leafy new canopy for the now roofless nave; descendants of the sheep originally kept by the monks wandered the ruins. Beyond, the grounds ran down to a view of the open water, decoratively framed by more trees. It was a truly picturesque sight, a natural focus for those who sought the sublime sensation of 'ruins, ivy, owls, moonlight, musing melancholy and life's passing pageant'.

The century had in turn seen Nature tamed: 'Enclosure like a Buonaparte let not a thing remain', as the poet John Clare wrote from his asylum, driven there by the predations of the enclosures which prevented him from making his living either as farm-worker or poet. And with Nature thus controlled, men could indulge their taste for the sublime and the picturesque, as though England were a panorama spread before them, framed by their own aesthetic. Tiring of 'improved' landscapes, they now looked for something more thrilling, and found it in gothic.

Eighteenth-century art historians believed that gothic architecture was inspired by the tall forests of northern Europe; they saw its sacred arches, crockets, spires and columns as stone versions of ancient woodland – the antiquarian James Hall even built a wicker 'cathedral' in his garden to demonstrate the ancient provenance of the style. For the rarefied tastes of the eighteenth-century connoisseur, it was a delicious meeting of art and life to be savoured: this gothic abbey returning to its arboreal inspiration, shaped by the deep, dark, mysterious woods themselves, still surrounded by the very pagan spirits which its Cistercian builders had sought to dispel.

When it was built, Netley's abbey must have stood out from the landscape like a piece of ostentatious modern architecture, but it had now been subsumed by the land, made decrepit by Nature and blunted by Time, and in the process had become a place of myth and legend. And within that myth, the abbey found its new identity by reaching back, through its medieval past, and into the dark ages of Europe's forested depths – perhaps even to their old gods and rituals, their supernatural mysteries. In an era of cool rationality, Netley reacted by becoming a natural artifice, a set-piece of theatrical bravura composed by Man and framed by Nature – a fantastic escape from that rational age.

Southern Gothick

In fact they are not the ruins of Netley, but of Paradise
– Oh! the purple abbots, what a spot had they chosen to
slumber in! The scene is so beautifully tranquil, yet so
lively, that they seemed only to have <u>retired into</u> the
world . . .

HORACE WALPOLE, 1755

————

In the summer of 1755, Horace Walpole, dilettante son of
Britain's first prime minister, undertook a tour of Hampshire
with his friend, John Chute. Along with their mutual friend, the
architect and artist Richard Bentley, this bachelor trio formed a
'Committee of Taste' to supervise the creation of Walpole's
house on the banks of the Thames at Strawberry Hill, where he
was reinventing gothic in stone and stained glass. With its romantic name, castellated turrets and towers and strange chapel in the
woods, Strawberry Hill was a three-dimensional expression of
the imagination which would inspire the first gothic novel, *The
Castle of Otranto*, written by Walpole in 1764.

As a maligned victim of the Renaissance, gothic was ready for
a revival. Scathingly coined by Vasari in the sixteenth century to
represent the barbarian destroyers of classical Rome and Greece,
Walpole's rehabilitation of a pejorative term was an act of genteel
subversion. 'His taste as expressed in Strawberry Hill was one of

a deliberate rebel counter-culture', wrote Walpole's biographer, Timothy Mowl. 'He was delighted by his own identity and concerned, like a public relations expert, to communicate it to us down the years . . .' Walpole was, wrote Mowl, 'one of the most successful deviant infiltrators that the English establishment has ever produced', and his Committee of Taste both used and hid behind the fantasy of gothic in the same way that later 'decadents' used it to both promote and mask their identities.

The dandyism of Walpole and his successors stood against an age of mass production. It was an individuality symbolised by the romantic figure of the Solitary or the Outsider; the roots of the modern cult of the individual, first discerned in Thomas Gray's 'Elegy Written in a Country Church-yard'.* Gray had been Walpole's Eton intimate, and the aristocrat would employ his Committee of Taste to frame Gray's work in the gothic arches of Bentley's 'exquisitely irreverent' illustrations, making the poet the personification of their cult, an early media superstar.

It was the beginning of a new gothic lineage that would merge with a self-conscious sense of decadence, from the macabre costume drama of the Revolutionary *incroyables* and *merveilleuses* of France, to Wilde's *Salomé* and its Edwardian interpreter Maud Allan posing as a graveside angel cloaked in black chiffon as she danced to Chopin's *Marche funèbre*; from the Sitwells as gothic figures on catafalques, to Diana Cooper as the statue of a gothic nun imprisoned in Oliver Messel's medieval plaster in *The Miracle*; from Rex Whistler photographed by Cecil Beaton as Thomas Gray from Bentley's portrait of the poet in the nude, to Stephen Tennant as a dead Romeo in his silver-foil-covered room, to the silver walls of Andy Warhol's Factory and its

---

* Like John Clare, Gray's elegy also 'apostrophised' the 'human fodder of transportation' driven out of the land by enclosure, a social awareness that contrasted sharply with the epicene obsessions of the Committee of Taste: 'Some village-Hampden that with dauntless breast/ The little tyrant of his fields withstood.'

Electric Chair, modern icons produced in a 1960s version of Strawberry Hill: a succession of silver walls, like Walpole's hall of mirrors, reflecting its decadent narcissists.

Deep-dyed in narcissism, gay and addicted to gossip (although also a serious man of art and letters), Walpole both represented and recorded a frivolity which pervaded English culture – a decadence which gothic, as the extreme expression of romanticism's counter culture, would embody. Yet this was essentially seen as an unEnglish disease, as the poet Charles Churchill (himself a doomed young hedonist) wrote: 'With our own island vices not content/ We rob our neighbours on the continent.' For Walpole, his unhappy Grand Tour of Europe, taken with Gray in tow and in pursuit of his *inamorata*, the bisexual Lord Lincoln, had served both to encourage his gothic tendency and to import foreign perversions to England.

That summer of 1755, Walpole and his circle embarked on a new tour which would confirm their deviant identities. To them, gothic – Suger's *opus modernum* – represented an indefinable, fantasy past; its pointed arches were a rubric for a romantic rebellion which queried the rational progress of their age. When they discovered its ruins, sleeping unawares on the shores of Southampton Water, Netley Abbey would become a locus for their subversive masquerade. The Cistercians' 'horrible' site became an historical reference for what Walpole and his friends were doing at Strawberry Hill. By the time they had finished with it, it would seem as though Netley itself had been redesigned by their Committee of Taste in a new importation of foreign vice to this English shore.

Walpole had been alerted to 'all the beauties of Netley' by Gray's visit to the abbey that July. The place had deeply inspired the poet in his taste for the antiquarian and the 'romantick'. On 6 August 1755 Gray had written, with an idiosyncratic disdain for punctuation and spelling, to another close friend, Dr Wharton. It was the first of a series of descriptions written that year which fixed Netley as a modern gothic site:

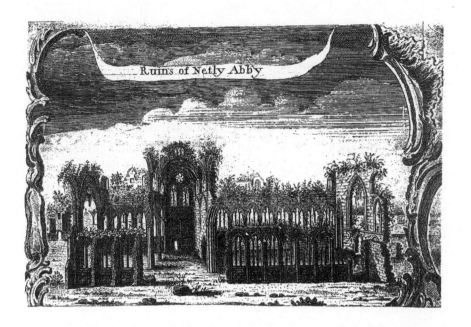

Ruins of Netly Abby

I wished for you often on the Southern Coast, where . . . the Oaks grow quite down to the Beach, & . . . the Sea forms a number of Bays little & great, that appear glittering in the midst of thick Groves of them. add to this the Fleet (for I was at Portsmouth two days before it sailed) & the number of Vefsels always pafsing along, or sailing up Southampton-River (wch is the largest of these Bays I mention) and enters about 10 mile into the Land, & you will have a faint Idea of the <u>South</u>. from Fareham to Southampton, where you are upon a level with the coast, you have a thousand such Peeps & delightful Openings . . . I have been also at Titchfield, at Netly-Abbey, (a most beautiful ruin in as beautiful a situation) at Southampton, at Bevis-Mount, at Winchester &c . . .

That mid-century summer was the season of Netley's invention in the gothic imagination. 'On the arrival of a few fine days, the first we have had this summer', wrote Walpole, '. . . Mr Chute persuaded me to take a jaunt to Winchester and Netley Abbey, with the latter of which he is very justly enchanted.' Having spent the night in Southampton, they set out to explore Netley.

Walpole was ecstatic; its ruins seemed to fulfil his dreams. 'But how shall I describe Netley to you?' he rhapsodised to Bentley. 'I can only, by telling you it is the spot in the world for which Mr Chute and I wish':

The ruins are vast, and retain fragments of beautiful fretted roofs pendant in the air, with all the variety of Gothic patterns of windows, wrapped round and round with ivy – many trees are sprouted up against the walls, and only want to be increased with cypresses! A hill rises above the Abbey, encircled with wood; the fort, in which We would build a tower for habitation, remains with two small platforms. This little castle is buried from the Abbey in a wood, in the very centre, on the edge of the hill: on each side breaks in the view of the Southampton sea, deep blue, glistening with silver and vessels; on one side terminated by Southampton, on the other by Calshot Castle; and the Isle of Wight rising above the opposite hills. – In fact they are not the ruins of Netley, but of Paradise – Oh! the purple abbots, what a spot had they chosen to slumber in! The scene is so beautifully tranquil, yet so lively, that they seemed only to have <u>retired into</u> the world . . .

'. . . Gray has lately been here', added Walpole, acknowledging the poet's lyrical and romantic inspiration. Two months later Gray returned, drawn by Netley's mysterious spirit (and possibly by the area's 'lusty' boatmen). He wrote from Southampton, 'at Mr. Vining's, Plumber, in High-Street' to another friend, Reverend James Brown, with a description that competed with Walpole's to capture the dark romance of the ruins:

I received your letter before I left home, & sit down to write to you after the finest walk in the finest day, that ever shone, to Netley-Abbey, my old friend, with whom I long to renew my acquaintance . . . the sun was <u>all too glaring & too full of gauds</u> [Gray quoted from Shakespeare's *King*

56

John] for such a scene, wch ought to be visited only in the dusk of the evening. it stands in a little quiet valley, wch gradually rises behind the ruin into a half-circle crown'd with thick wood. before it on a descent is a thicket of oaks, that serves to veil it from the broad day & from profane eyes, only leaving a peep on both sides, where the sea appears glittering thro' the shade, & vefsels with their white sails, that glide acrofs & are lost again. concealed behind the thicket stands a little Castle (also in ruins) immediately on the shore, that commands a view over an expanse of sea clear & smooth as glafs (when I saw it) . . . & in front the deep shades of the New-Forest distinctly seen, because the water is no more than three miles over. the Abbey was never very large. the shell of its church is almost entire, but the pillars of the iles have gone, & the roof has tumbled in, yet some little of it is left in the transept, where the ivy has forced its way thro', & hangs flaunting down among the fretted ornaments & escutcheons of the Benefactors. much of the lodging & offices are also standing, but all is overgrown with trees & bushes, & mantled here & there with ivy, that mounts over the battlements.

To Thomas Gray's romantic imagination, such visits induced an almost trance-like state, the evocative ruins 'pregnant with poetry . . . One need not have a very fantastic imagination to see spirits at noon-day', and he visualised its abbot

bidding his beads for the souls of his Benefactors, interr'd in that venerable pile, that lies beneath him . . . Did you not observe how, as that white sail shot by and was lost, he turn'd and cross'd himself, to drive the Tempter from him, that had thrown that distraction in his way. I should tell you that the Ferryman, who row'd me, a lusty young Fellow, told me, that he would not for all the world pass a night at the Abbey, (there were such things seen near it,) tho' there was a power of money hid there.

Veiled in its ghost stories – 'Blind Peter' was said to guard the abbot's buried treasure (although such tales were also useful for smugglers using the ruins as a place to land contraband) – the reinvention of Netley was under way. Walpole and Gray's descriptions, rivalling each other in reverie, distilled the new spirit of the place. Over the next few years their refined taste would percolate through popular culture, spawning a new cult. Such descriptions, apparently private but written quite consciously for public consumption, would summon a host of artists, writers and gothic aficionados to this Hampshire shore, determined to commune with its ghostly spirits.

In 1761, the newly-rich Thomas Lee Dummer, William Chamberlayne's friend at Woolston House, acquired Netley Abbey and, fearless of Walter Taylor's fate, uprooted the entire north transept and transferred it to the grounds of his new home, Cranbury Park, near Winchester, where it was reassembled as an authentic gothic folly. Dummer's vandalism was a fashionable act of 'improvement': seven years later, Fountains Abbey, the great Cistercian foundation in Yorkshire, was bought by the local squire, who surrounded it with smooth lawns, subsuming it into his artificial landscape and 'providing its owner with an aesthetic object on the scale of the Roman Forum or the Colosseum'.

Yet despite Dummer's depradations, his eye for the picturesque was credited with the presentation of Netley's ruins as a sublime location – as though he himself had been directed by the Committee of Taste. Francis Gosse, the artist who recorded the still intact abbey in 1760 and 1761 for his *Antiquities of England and Wales*, praised Dummer for having 'greatly improved the beauty and solemnity of the scene by a judicious management of the trees which have spontaneously sprung up among the mouldering walls'. From its selection by the Cistercians as a wild site, through their civilisation and subsequent dissolution, Netley, recaptured by Nature, was now being subtly relandscaped, both physically and aesthetically, by the romantic

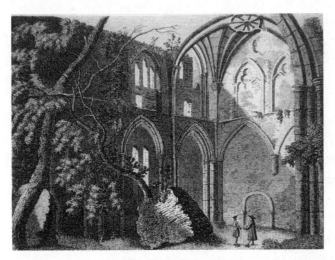

Netley Abbey, 1776

imagination, its stones 'so overgrown with ivy, and interspersed with trees, as to form a scene, inspiring the most pleasing melancholy'. The abbey's ruins were 'discovered' in the same way as were the classical remains of the ancient world. Engulfed by Nature and aged by Time, the abbey was like Rome, 'an immense garden ruin, a *hortus conclusus*, in which nature and civilisation had reached a kind of harmony'. It spoke of intangible eternities on an English shore, rising out of the vegetation like the Colosseum, or like an Egyptian temple emerging from the sands, a Hampshire version of the 'vast desolation' which greeted Shelley's traveller as he gazed on the lifeless works of Ozymandias.

With Continental unrest curtailing Grand Tours, the English imagination was turned in on itself and its own past. The search for the sublime had to be sated nearer to home, and Netley fulfilled this desire. By 1765 the effect of Thomas Gray's antiquary elegies was being felt in popular literature, with the publication of the pamphlet/tour guide, *THE RUINS OF NETLEY ABBEY A Poem in Blank Verse*, prefaced by a quote from Webster's *The Duchess of Malfi*:

I do love these ancient Ruins:
We never tread upon them, but we set
Our foot on some reverend History

And continuing anonymously,

High on the summit of yon verdant plain,
Beneath whose falling edge, the pebbled shore,
Swept by the billows of the Western flood,
Repels the rage of Neptune; there behold
The scattered heaps of Netley's ancient fane
Through many centuries in record fam'd:
At length her stately fabric is no more.

With Thomas Dummer's death, Netley's ruins passed, via his widow, to Sir Nathaniel Dance-Holland, himself an artist who, acknowledging the growing taste for the picturesque, allowed public access to the ruins. A flattering – if not obsequious – contemporary guide noted: 'It is fortunate for the lovers of antiquities that these beautiful ruins are now in the possession of a gentleman, whose regard for the arts, elegant taste, and practical as well as theoretic skill in picturesque matters, ensure to the public every care in the preservation of them.' Thus opened up and extolled, Netley's fortunes rose like the moon over its ruins by night, casting its medieval stones in a glamorous new light. In 1790, the poet William Sotheby, who lived nearby at Bevis Mount, just up the Itchen, produced his 'Ode, Netley Abbey; Midnight':

Within the sheltered centre of the aisle,
  Beneath the ash whose growth romantic spreads
Its foliage trembling o'er the funeral pile,
  And all around a deeper darkness sheds;
While through yon arch, where the thick ivy twines,
Bright on the silvered tower the moon-beam shines,
  And the grey cloister's roofless length illumines,

Upon the mossy stone I lie reclined,
And to a visionary world resigned
  Call the pale spectres forth from the forgotten tombs.

Such was its power that Netley Abbey began to acquire national status, admired even in the fashionable metropolis, seventy miles away. In 1794 William Shield staged his *Netley Abbey – A Comic Opera* at the Theatre Royal, Covent Garden. Its plot

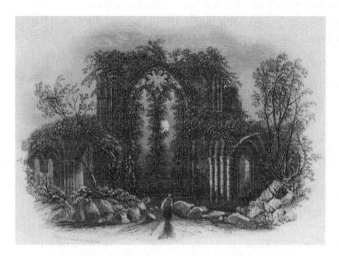

'Netley Abbey by Moonlight'

revolves around the Oakland and Woodbine families, representatives of the Georgian gentry who had settled on Southampton Water. Mr Oakland – played by Joseph Munden – is a modern man, and like William Chamberlayne seeks to capitalise on the nearby ruins, creating an improved landscape by clearing ancient woodland. In the first scene of act one, he is confronted by his daughter, Lucy, played by Miss Hopkins:

Lucy: Dear sir, in that case all the country about us, will appear desolate. I shall really fancy myself to be 'Zelinda in the Desart'.
Oakland: I know it will seem desolate – but you must be sensible 'tis done by way of improvement. How else can I

open the vista, to command a fuller view of Netley Abbey?

Lucy: And is the sweet embowered cottage belonging to Mrs Woodbine, where I used to read the 'Dear Recess,' indeed to come down?

Oakland: Yes, it is; for you must find some other nook to be miserable in ... How else are the improvements to go on? All to the Westward must immediately be cleared; and by the fall of the leaf, I hope not a tree will be left standing.

Lucy: Cruel as the office is, I must prepare Miss Woodbine for this event: the information may else come with a severity she cannot sustain. [*Exit*]

Oakland: That girl gathers all her absurd notions, from silly romances – and while I go on improving, she, as if in direct opposition, goes on reading ...

NETLEY ABBEY
an Operatic Farce in two acts,
as performed at the Theatre-Royal Covent Garden.

If Oakland is a vested member of the squirearchy, then it is equally evident that the passionate young Lucy is probably addicted to Mrs Radcliffe's gothic novels. Her proto-environmentalism is set against her father's use of the code-word of Whiggery – 'improvement'; they are also a symbol of the eighteenth-century generation gap. In the succeeding scenes Lucy's bosom friend, Ellen Woodbine, suffers a grievous loss when her family's cottage is burnt down and her fortune is lost, only for the hero – Lucy's brother, the dashing Captain Oakland (Charles Incledon) – to discover that Miss Woodbine's bonds were in fact stolen. In the final dramatic moonlit denouement, he uncovers them hidden in the ruins of the abbey. Even under these sublime stones, decency and rationality triumph.

The opera is also very much the product of Southampton's late eighteenth-century reputation as a spa resort, and the great influx of the fashionable who came to visit it and its tourist spots. Catering to that spa culture, the opera draws on sentimental whimsy and rousing patriotism, such Captain Oakland's stirring number:

> *Should dangers e'er approach our Coast*
> *The inbred Spirit of the land*
> *Would animate each heart*
> *Would animate each head*
> *Would bind, wou'd bind us in one general Host*
> *Would bind, wou'd bind us in one general Host*
> *ENGLAND ENGLAND ENGLAND*
> *... Our isles best rampart is the sea*
> *The midnight mark of Foes it braves*
> *And Heav'n that fenc'd us round*
> *That fenc'd us round with waves*
> *Ordain'd the people to be free*
> *Ordain'd the people to be free*
> *ENGLAND, &c*

Such robust sentiment, the eighteenth-century equivalent of a football chant, was hardly resonant with the fey subversiveness of gothic, although its fears of imminent (French) invasion concorded with Southampton's vulnerable position in the patriotic body and the dangers that might indeed approach its coast – a sense of insular adversity elsewhere represented in the recently-composed and equally stirring 'Rule Britannia'.

William Shield, born in County Durham in 1748, was a well-known and prolific composer, and his popular tune *Rosina* would become the melody for 'Auld Lang Syne'. A republican with 'sympathies with the Godwin circle', his opera-pantomime of 1784, *The Magic Cavern*, 'anticipated the Gothick Horrors of Mrs Radclyffe'; he died, presumably in London, in 1829. But *Netley Abbey* is also credited in contemporary texts to William Pearce, 'a pretty successful dramatist' working in the last quarter of the century, 'of whose life we have not been able to learn any particulars', as an early Victorian source notes. This intimate pair seem to have co-operated as composer and librettist – a list of

Pearce's works appears identical to those attributed to Shield: *The Nunnery*, 1785; *Arrival at Portsmouth*, 1794; *Windsor Castle*, 1795 – or perhaps they were one and the same, two sides of a prolific eighteenth-century Lloyd-Webber, teasing me with their identity down the years. On opening a bound collection of Shield's operas, the title page of his 'musical farce' *The Lock and Key* declared it to be 'Composed and Selected by Mr Shield. The Words by P. Hoare Esq.'

Displayed on the London stage in replica, Netley's ruins had become a gothic commodity. In 1795 the Reverend Richard Warner wrote his *Netley Abbey, a Gothic Story in Two Volumes*, another opportunist conflation, printed by the Minerva Press ('the most famous house of sensational fiction', publishers of Ann Radcliffe's gothic novels). Warner's morality tale – translated into both German and French editions – conflates Netley's myths in its medieval hero, Edward de Villars, who rescues an imprisoned nineteen-year-old girl, the beautiful, auburn-haired Agnes, from a cell in the abbey in which she was confined by the wicked Abbot Peter, in the pay of the yet more evil Sir Hildebrand Warren who has already murdered her father, and whose ghost comes back to haunt him. In the final scene both the Abbot and Sir Hildebrand meet a bloody end, allowing Agnes to be reunited with her brother and the author to draw his moral conclusion on 'persecuted virtue'.

As well as inspiring such sensational literature, Netley also prompted a healthy trade in cheap prints. Tourists could have the romantic ruins as seen through its woods, thrillingly overgrown, or from the shore, jauntily contrasted with the modern traffic of Southampton Water. Catering to the market, commercial artists provided visitors with a memento of their visit, a keepsake to take home with their guidebooks (after they had carefully cut their initials into the stones in eighteenth-century graffiti). But serious painters were also drawn to the site: the watercolourist Francis Towne made a series of pictures between 1798 and 1809; and in 1816 John Constable spent his honeymoon sketching at Netley, Weston Shore and Southampton. For the meteorologically-obsessed Constable, the sea-swept clouds and the abbey's setting below such changing skies were a large part of its appeal. The ruins seemed to evoke dark memories for the artist: after the death of his wife, Maria, from tuberculosis in 1828, he used a sepulchral sketch of the abbey for one of his nocturnal watercolours, issued as a popular engraving in 1829.

Directed by artistic and literary taste, a visit to Netley stirred deep passions. 'Few people, perhaps, who think at all', declared the 1796 pocket guide to Southampton,

> can visit the remains of these ancient religious fabrics, without expressing a sensation, which, as it arises from a combination of different emotions, is hardly to be described . . . the reflection that we are treading over ground peopled with the remains of our fellow-creatures, who were once young and vigorous like ourselves, inspires the awful idea of our own mortality – that we ere long must be like them, silent, neglected, and forgotten.

Such reveries were a symptom of the age. It was a century which began, as Isaiah Berlin wrote, 'by being calm and smooth . . . rationality is progressed, the Church is retreating, unreason is yielding . . .' But suddenly these clear skies were clouded by 'a violent eruption of emotion, enthusiasm. People become interested in gothic buildings, in introspection. People suddenly become neurotic and melancholy; they begin to admire the unaccountable flight of spontaneous genius.'

It was the Industrial Revolution that had darkened the horizon and produced the transition in which the goths of Netley, Cobbett's radicalism and Chamberlayne's Whiggish improvements were all caught up in their own ways. '. . . Under the surface of this apparently coherent, apparently elegant century there are all kinds of dark forces moving', wrote Berlin. The mystic necromancers, the experimenters in occult sciences, Dr Mesmer's 'animal magnetism', the *Illuminati* and William Blake's fantastic visions became the mysterious obverse to improved landscapes and scientific theorems. Superstition and alienation in a world of enclosure and transportation gathered in the clouds that gave gothic its darkness, and shaded the tourists' mock-pagan worship of Netley's Christian ruins with something more atavistic, something more than mere spectacle. It may have been a tourist site, but Netley also expressed a dissatisfaction with the age; its ancient stones spoke of modern concerns.

Like the plague culture of medieval times, gothic became almost entirely concerned with the grandeur of decay itself, obsessed with morbidity and decrepitude, passion and death. Its cult heroes were the heroes and creators of the sensational novels which the Reverend Warner's book imitated: Walpole's *The Castle of Otranto*, Ann Radcliffe's pulp fiction, Matthew Lewis's *The Monk*, with its pregnant nuns and rapist monks (followed by his *Crazy Jane*, a poetic encounter with a madman using material gathered from his visits to asylums). Its aficionados were drawn to extreme expression of their own self-questioning: young men such as Shelley, whose restless life, riven with disputed inheritance, suicidal lovers and psychological instability, seemed to live out gothic sensation. At eighteen, he wrote a gothic novel, *Zastrozzi*, in which the hero encounters a castle in the woods, 'a large and magnificent building, whose battlements rose above the lofty trees', just as Netley's ruins were hidden and revealed by its own verdure. And in 1818, his friend Thomas Love Peacock's *Nightmare Abbey* caricatured Shelley and his circle: the poet 'Scythrop Glowry' living in a mystical tower by the sea, like Netley, 'ruinous and full of owls', and Mr Flosky (based on Coleridge) for whom 'mystery was his mental element. He lived in the midst of that visionary world in which nothing is but what is not. He dreamed with his eyes open, and saw ghosts dancing round him at noontide.'

Netley had entered its most public phase, a spectacle as romantic, thrilling and sensational as any attraction in London's Oxford Street Pantheon. Tourists took the ferry from Southampton to Netley's shore to sample its sublime charms – the experience given a further piquance by the fact that their time there was proscribed by the tides upon which their return to civilisation depended. This special access made the abbey's ruins that much more wondrous and magical, as if it were a vision revealed at Nature's whim. And among the many who came across the water was one writer who had newly taken up residence in Southampton's fashionable spa: Jane Austen.

At the beginning of the eighteenth century, Southampton had been in decline, suffering the after-effects of the revisited plague of 1665, imported to the town when a misguided humanitarian gave sanctuary to an infected child from London. On his 1724 tour of the country, Daniel Defoe announced, 'Southampton is a truly antient town, for 'tis in a manner dying with age; the decay of the trade is the real decay of the town; and all the business of the moment that is transacted there, is the trade between us and the islands of Jersey and Guernsey, with a little of the wine trade, and much smuggling.' But like Netley's abbey, Southampton had reinvented itself, and within twenty years its fortunes had been turned around.

Fashionable eighteenth-century society demanded two particular nostrums: mineral waters and sea bathing; Southampton could supply both. Beyond the city walls a spring was discovered to produce chalybeate waters impregnated with iron salts, a homoeopathic pot pourri imbued with the power to cure all manner of ills, from leprosy to hydrophobia (although it didn't prevent an outbreak of the disease in 1807, whose rabid victims thirsted for water they could not bear to drink). For Southampton, as for Netley, water was its great advantage. 'Bathing has generally been attained with the best effect', the *Southampton Guide* informed its readers – affluent citizens most likely to suffer the nervous disorders of their station. For weak constitutions worn down by the stress of modern life, immersion in the sea was a celebrated cure. 'Relaxation is the common cause of complaints incident to the higher order of persons in England', the guide continued, 'and, except in the case of unsound viscera, the cold bath gently braces the solids and accelerates the blood's motion.'

Below the town's medieval walls, tidal sea-water baths were built, with elegantly-glazed 'Long Rooms' for 'interested spectators', and a promenade known as 'The Beach' along which, on their visit in the summer of 1755, Horace Walpole and John Chute had 'walked long by moonlight'. As Walpole noted, the town was already 'crowded; sea-bathers are established there too'. A month or so later their friend Thomas Gray was complaining,

> This place is still full of <u>Bathers</u>. I know not a Soul, nor have once been at the rooms. the walks all round it are delicious, & so is the weather. lodgings very dear & fish very cheap. here is no Coffeehouse, no Bookseller, no Pastry-Cook: but here is the Duke of Chandos . . .

As with any upwardly-mobile area, the facilities of a fashionable resort soon arrived. Mrs Remacle opened her coffee house in the High Street, and lending libraries and grander assembly rooms sprang up, the voyeuristic spa society and nexus for elaborate masked balls, although their proximity to the less salubrious parts of town encouraged dissent among 'the rougher elements of the poor, resentful of the amusements of the well-to-do and the fashionable visitors'. At one masque given in 1773, a young man leaving his lodgings dressed as a shepherd was set upon and 'tossed like a football for some time . . . [until] some humane persons intervened'.

The contrasts of privilege and deprivation which across the Channel were about to erupt in revolution were just as evident in Southampton's spa. The following year, 1774, a 'remarkably brilliant' masquerade made 'the mob so riotous that it was with difficulty the company got in and out of their carriages, and the streets were one continued scene of riot and confusion all evening'. As the balls grew more fantastic, so too did local opposition to such aristocratic decadence. One held at the new Polygon Hotel featured costumed revellers as 'a Jew pedlar, Tancreds, Spaniards, sailors, nosegay-girls and ballad-singers' – the kind of fancy dress hedonism in which the Bright Young People would engage two centuries later. On this occasion the event was marred by a large stone being lobbed through the window which narrowly missed the Duke of Gloucester.

However disgruntled the locals may have been at the excesses of their betters – against which behaviour their French colleagues *sans-culottes* would take direct action – the 'fashionable visitors' felt secure in the knowledge that Southampton's reputation as a genteel resort had been sealed by royal approval. In 1750 George II's son, Frederick Prince of Wales, had visited the town to bathe; by the 1760s, his two younger brothers had eschewed their now reigning brother's partiality for Weymouth – where the King went to soothe the onset of his madness – and had become Southampton's social patrons. By the 1780s, Southampton was enjoying the peak of its fashionability, confirmed by the arrival of Georgiana, Duchess of Devonshire, as *The Times*'s man on the spot informed its readers.

> *Extract of a letter from Southampton, Aug. 2*
> Fashion and taste have fixed their head quarters at this place, for the season. Dance and song succeed in merry round. The rooms crowded, which, by the bye, is not a little owing to the extreme attention and politeness of the Master of Ceremonies. Lodgings filled with fashionable belles and beaux – and, what is more decisively recommendatory, less extortion and imposition happen here, than at most sea-bathing places of summer resort.
>
> The beautiful Duchess, with her party, has just left Southampton; her return is expected in a few days.

Newspaper reports grew from single paragraphs listing various lords and ladies to spectacular two-column lists comprising a substantial muster of London's society. By 1788, the Southampton season was firmly in the social calendar, accompanied by the kind of hype that would be employed to advertise later resorts; the town had become the English equivalent of Antibes, yet more so in an era when European turmoil precluded foreign travel. The Beach and the Long Rooms thronged with dandified men and elegant women craning their necks and fluttering their fans. 'This place now boasts the most fashionable and numerous company of any of the watering places,' reported *The Times* in July 1788. The actor David Garrick had visited, it noted, 'the Duke of Gloucester will certainly be here, and the Duke of Orleans is so pleased, that he means to pass some weeks at this delightful spot'. The following year the King came with his Queen and Princess, entertained at breakfast by a dutiful, and doubtless grateful, Corporation.

It was the making of modern Southampton, bringing the kind of figures only the age of the ocean liner could entice back to the port. Indeed, not only were many introduced to the area's charms, some were persuaded to stay there, making it their country residence. 'If Southampton has decreased in trade, it has increased prodigiously in splendour and elegance', the 1781 *Guide to Southampton* could retort to Defoe's slur on an 'antient town', 'and many gentlemen of fortune have come to settle here, since it has become so polite a place'.

One of those gentlemen, James Dott, lived at Bitterne Grove, the building which was to become my school. Dott was an East India Company surgeon who, having served in the great new colonial acquisition of India, had ended up at Southampton, where his eccentric habits were supposed by local legend to have been the source of the adjective 'dotty'; in old age, Dott was to be seen being wheeled about town in a basket chair, as if staking his claim to his neologism. He was also remembered for the fact that he had employed as his gardener Touissant-Ambrose Talour de la Cartrie, the Comte de Villienière, an aristocratic casualty of Revolutionary France who had taken refuge in Southampton in 1796 after a series of miraculous escapades worthy of the Scarlet Pimpernel.

At school we were told that among the visitors to the eccentric James Dott were the Austens; legend even embroidered the scene to include Jane seated under the great oak tree on its lawn, writing, although there is nothing to substantiate such a romantic picture. The Austens lived in the leas of Lord Lansdowne's newly-built gothic folly, with the town walls at the end of their garden. 'We hear that we are envied our House by many people, & that the Garden is the best in Town', Jane told her sister, but she was scathing of Southampton's dressmakers, theatres, and 'young women without partners, & each of them with two ugly, naked shoulders!' The town featured just once in her fiction, in her youthful novel *Love and Friendship*, when it serves to remind her of 'stinking fish'.

Netley, however, presented a different prospect. She had completed *Northanger Abbey* four years previously, but it seems it is almost certain that Austen, born and brought up in Hampshire, an afternoon's ride from Netley, had drawn on its abbey – by now the stuff of novellas, odes and operas – for her gothic satire.

Austen the rationalist had parodied Mrs Radcliffe's books in her *fin-de-siècle* novel, in which her heroine Catherine Morland is a young girl who, like Lucy Oakland in Shield's opera, yearns for the romance she has read about in her gothic novels: 'As they drew near the end of their journey, her impatience for a sight of the abbey ... returned in full force, and every bend on the road was expected with solemn awe to afford a glimpse of its massy walls of grey stone, rising amidst a grove of ancient oaks, with the last beams of the sunset playing in beautiful splendour on its high Gothic windows.' The reality of the fictional Northanger is a house furnished in the modern taste, although Catherine discovers that, like Paulet's palace, it is partly housed in a medieval abbey:

> ... Northanger turned up an abbey, and she was to be its inhabitant. Its long, damp passages, its narrow cells and ruined chapel, were to be within her daily reach, and she could not entirely subdue the hope of some traditional legends, some awful memorials of an injured and ill-fated nun.

In September 1807 the Austens arrived on Netley's beach, clambered out of the ferry and set off to explore the site. Moving through the oak trees which still lined the shore, the sense of discovery and anticipation – and the limits of tidal access – made their expedition to this *laetus locus* yet more thrilling. Linger too long in this haunted, ruin-strewn wood, and they might end up having to spend the night there.

As the party came upon the abbey itself, the prospect of its grey stones and trees was almost too much for Jane's impressionable fourteen-year-old niece. Like Catherine Morland and Lucy Oakland, Fanny Austen was a girl of her time. Attempting to capture the effect Netley had upon her that afternoon, she wrote to her governess in the astonished, breathless tones of a gothic aficionado (which her aunt so excelled at parodying), her bosom all but heaving with the gushing tribute:

Never was there anything in the known world to be compared to that compound of everything that is striking, ancient and majestic: we were struck dumb with admiration, and I wish I could write anything that would come near to the sublimity of it, but that is utterly impossible as nothing I could say would give you a distant idea of its extreme beauty.

Carried away by reverie, Fanny could only sink into Netley's dream-like state, thrown into a medieval mystery, suspended from reality and Southampton's stinking fish.

Fanny Austen's reaction to the abbey ruins was characteristic of the day-trippers from spa-town Southampton. They sought the same kind of sensation from Netley as a modern audience would from a horror movie, and Netley catered to them with aplomb. It was a thrilling place. With its many chambers, galleries, arched windows and doors, some opening strangely into mid-air and all overhung with ivy in the shade of great trees, the very asymmetrical, twisting layout of the abbey and its outbuildings created an enchanted realm for visitors to explore, somewhere between an eighteenth-century theme park and a chamber of horrors. Around any crumbling arch might lurk the ghost of 'Blind Peter', jealously guarding the abbot's buried treasure.

Now the gothic thirst for sensation created a new Netley experience: the abbey by moonlight. Excited goths could set out, in keen anticipation of the abbey's morbid charms, on midnight tours accompanied by guides bearing flaming torches. Moving in procession through the dark trees and looming stone piles, startled by dancing shadows on ancient walls, young ladies in thin dresses clutched tightly to their gratified consorts' arms and affected to faint away at the thrill of it all.

Netley had become the equivalent of a night club, a fashionable venue for young people dressed in the extravagant spirit of the times, like their cousins across the Channel with their impossibly high collars, cutaway coats and sheer muslin dresses worn revealingly dampened. The French dandies wore thin red ribbons around their necks in a mocking gesture to the 'holy mother Guillotine'; their English counterparts sported black velvet collars in a similarly ironic gesture of mourning for their fellow aristocrats. While the unrest which threatened to import revolution to England required more troops to quell it than Wellington had under his command in the Peninsular War, their protest against industrialised society consisted of an obsession with neck ties and the latest gothic novel.

'The *reading public . . .*', *Nightmare Abbey*'s Mr Flosky complains, 'requires a perpetual adhibition of *sauce piquante* to the palate of its depraved imagination. It laid upon ghosts, goblins and skeletons . . . till even the devil himself . . . became too base, common, and popular for its surfeited appetite.' Like any other cult, gothic moved from creative originality to commercial exploitation. Soon unrestricted *fêtes champêtres* dispelled any notion of solitude at Netley's ruins. By 1815, when Mary Brunton visited the site, the proliferation of toy stalls, gingerbread sellers and common rabble of picnickers in the abbey's precincts had become an offence to the aesthetic eye, making romantic reverie all but impossible. Netley's popularity destroyed the very spirit that had generated it, and the gothic commodification begun by Walpole and his Committee of Taste became part of a popular culture to which its sexy sensationalism proved more appealing than Enlightenment rationalism.

By the time William Cobbett wrote his eulogy to Netley, Walpole's refined aesthetic had long been subsumed by its popularised version. On another 'rural ride', Cobbett encountered a certain Mr Montague's estate in north Hampshire, a man of new money who had enthusiastically decorated in the gothic fashion. 'Of all the ridiculous things I ever saw in my life this place is the most ridiculous', blustered Cobbett. 'The house looks like a sort of church . . . with *crosses* on the tops of different parts of the pile . . .' One gothic arch

was composed of Scotch fir wood, as rotten as a pear; nailed together in such a way as to make the thing appear, from a distance, like the remnant of a ruin! I wonder how long this sickly, this childish taste is to remain? I do not know who this gentleman is. I suppose he is some honest person from the 'Change or its neighbourhood; and that these *gothic arches* are to denote the *antiquity of his origin!*

Cobbett's polemic harked back to St Bernard of Clairvaux's pronouncements; the gothic style which had meant to replace excess had become imbued with it. As a reactionary refuge from a modern era of industrial unrest and protest, gothic was a symbol of conservatism, and rapidly becoming Britain's 'national style'. In the process, Netley became a place of common, if not uproarious entertainment. 'On Mondays, the Fountain Court presents a singular scene of gaiety', wrote an observer in the 1840s. 'It has long been the custom for people from Southampton and the neighbourhood to meet at the Abbey on that day, and to hold a kind of festival. Tea and other provisions are furnished by the inhabitants of a neighbouring cottage, and this is followed by music and dancing.'

The abbey had lost its edge. Its thrills debased, by 1840 Netley's reputation was such that it became a subject of Richard Harris Barham's satirical *Ingoldsby Legends*. A minor canon at St Paul's, and an eccentric figure himself (having been crippled as a young man in a carriage accident which left him with a twisted arm) Barham produced his ironic ode, 'Netley Abbey, A Legend of Hampshire' as a parody of all those verses that had gone before. His alter-ego 'Ingoldsby' imagines the abbey in its medieval heyday, with nuns winking at 'gardener lads' and consequently finding themselves 'Wall'd up in a hole with never a chink,/No light, – no air, – no victuals, – no drink!', and provides an antiquarian footnote to his tale: 'About the middle of the last century a human skeleton was discovered in a recess in the wall among the ruins of Netley. On examination the bones were pronounced to be those of a female. *Teste* James Harrison, a youthful but intelligent cab-driver of Southampton, who "well remembers to have heard his grandmother say that 'Somebody told her so'".' But the poet's reverie is broken by 'the popping of Ginger Beer!' dispensed to the modern crowds at Netley by 'a hag surrounded by crockery-ware', while chimney sweeps play 'pitch and toss', and

Two or three damsels, frank and free,
Are ogling, and smiling, and sipping Bohea.
Parties below, and parties above,
Some making tea, and some making love.

In a gentler echo of Cobbett's sardony, Barham ends his verse with a visitor

scandalized,
Finding these beautiful ruins so Vandalized,
And thus of their owner to speak began,
As he ordered you home in haste,
NO DOUBT HE'S A VERY RESPECTABLE MAN,
But – 'I can't say much for his taste.'

The term 'vandalized' was itself a witty play on words, as the original Vandals who ravaged Rome in 455 were a Teutonic tribe like the goths after whom the movement had been ironically named. The new barbarians had consigned Netley's gothic idyll to the fashions and taste of another time.

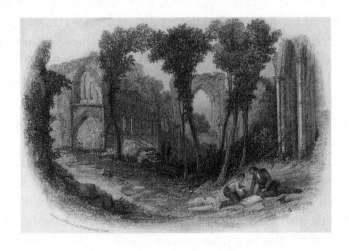

In Southampton, meanwhile, questions of taste were paramount, the barometer by which its fortunes could rise or fall. The island's waters still beckoned, but now the age of the spa had been superseded – in royal and aristocratic fashionability – by the age of the yacht, and attention had moved down Southampton Water to the Isle of Wight and Cowes, and eventually to Osborne, where Victoria would set up her holiday home. The 'gentry of the first rank and fashion' – that fickle bunch – were now only passing through the town en route for the island, hardly long enough for its tradespeople to make a profit, or its destitute to chuck a brick. By 1817 the Spa Gardens were virtually deserted, and by 1820 the town's tonic waters available only in bottles from local chemists. If it were to survive in the modern world, Southampton would have to change again. To this task its intrepid, waterside population proved equal. Once more its waters would rescue it, and within a generation, this geographically-blessed place – with its double high tides and safe harbour yet more accessible in the age of steamships and the railway line that now linked it to London – had entered a new period of success.

Like the rest of England, everything changed with the coming of the railways. Populations became mobile, and expanding towns were connected by this powerful new web of communication. As a result, Southampton had to cede its role as a 'retreat for retirement' to Bournemouth and Brighton, its decline as a seaside resort ironically sealed by the social mobility which elsewhere had made coastal towns accessible, but which in Southampton ran between the beach and the town, separating the citizens from their seaside with its iron rails and belching smoke. To the east, the line ploughed through Chamberlayne's improved landscape, gouging out its way with high embankments and brick viaducts, seeding the land with new suburbs like fireweed as it went.

In the process, it too, like Netley, grew a little commoner, as though it had been contaminated down the railway line with a Cockney accent. *The Whitehall Review* noted that in the town 'slowly, but surely, has been established the reign of Genteel Vulgarity' and that in the high street 'the talking is very loud, the laughter very loud, and the ladies' dresses for the most part to match. So, too, the garb of the Southampton youth is fearfully and wonderfully made, and he has a way of looking around him which seems to say, "See here – what a dog I am!".'

The railway also brought a new class of admirer to Netley. Picnickers now besported themselves in the ruins, as did their metropolitan counterparts at the Crystal Palace, where Paxton's gigantic greenhouse enclosed ancient elms growing in Hyde Park, just as mature trees grew up in the abbey's roofless nave. The Great Exhibition celebrated industry, progress and the future; Netley – with its own aspirations to being a crystal palace, its technologically innovative tracery windows having collapsed into decrepitude – represented the past. Gothic itself was turned from its effete, decadent eighteenth-century incarnation into a more rigorous, muscular nineteenth-century aesthetic. To Augustus Pugin, a Catholic convert, the championing of gothic was nothing less than 'an answer to current social and cultural crises'. From aesthetic spectacle gothic had returned to utilitarian function, although Pugin's crusade would culminate in suburban villas and terraces, their scaled-down gothic porches appealing to some atavistic sense of the mythic English past. It was a long way from Strawberry Hill's Committee of Taste, and even further from Abbot Suger's *opus modernum*.

Once more Netley's ruins would respond to the spirit of the times. Just as gothic changed its meaning, so did the abbey. In 1861, *Punch* noted that 'The place has been cleared and cleaned without having been Cockneyfied; it has been furnished with convenient and inconspicuous seats, and rendered permeable throughout.' At the same time it lamented the fact that when the Lady Chapel had been cleared of 'rubbish' and revealed 'a piece of encaustic tile pavement near the altar . . . several pieces have been stolen by some robbers who procured admission in the disguise of respectable-looking people'; the magazine called for police patrols of the area. Three years later, William Howitt noted the same reservations which Barham had satirised; the conflicting pressures of popu-larity and access with art and intellectual demands which the newly-mobile modern world had created:

> The visitors and tourists of to-day are just as much charmed with the ruins of Netley as the monks and Walpole were. They crowd there in summer to picnic amongst the ruined walls and lofty trees, and are not always careful to avoid desecrating these delightful spots with their relics of greasy paper, and of shrimps and sardine boxes. But the grounds are carefully kept, and these unsightly objects daily removed, to be only in fine weather daily left again; a strange desecration that one would think every lover of the picturesque would feel instinctively aware of.

These were egalitarian times, and romanticism – like the great unwashed – had to be kept in check. The rigours of Victorian technoculture had settled on the world, and fey imagination took a backseat. Howitt noted that 'Horace Walpole, in his days of gothic enthusiasm, was enchanted with Netley, and seems to have contemplated restoring at least enough of it for a house. What an escape it had of being Strawberry-hilled!' Sentimentalised on tinted postcards of picnic scenes and the ordinary people at play, Netley had lost its sense of subversion. Accepting their latest role, the abbey ruins gave up their sensational past and slipped back into sleepy indolence.

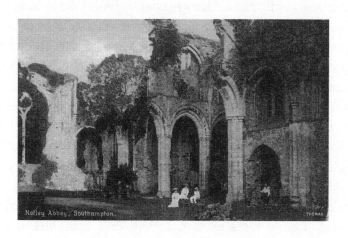

The sky looks as though someone has been dropping ink in it. At the beginning of the twenty-first century, rain-dark clouds seem almost to touch the trees around the ruins. Each year, the lowering stratosphere descends a little more, shrouding every horizon with an industrial gothic legacy.

In the 1880s, Ruskin, the champion of the Gothic Revival, lectured on *The Storm-Cloud of the Nineteenth Century* and his 'obsession with black skies and plague winds': 'I believe these swift and mocking clouds and colours are only between storms', he wrote. 'They are assuredly new in Heaven, so far as my life reaches. I never saw a single example of them till after 1870.' Edging nearer to madness – as though those clouds precipitated his insanity – Ruskin had become obsessed by the effect of industrialisation on the climate, writing in his diary, 'By the plague-winds every breath of air you draw is polluted, half round the world.' Like Pugin, who, overworked by his final commission to design the 'medieval court' for the Great Exhibition, had been admitted to Bedlam, Ruskin too became insane. After attacks of mania which left him remote from the world for his last ten years, Ruskin died in an influenza epidemic in 1900, watching the skies over his Lake District home.

Beauty had become a problem for the modern world. In his prose-poem 'A Phenomenon of the Future' – written in 1864, the same year as Howitt's antiquarian tribute to the abbey – the Decadent poet Stéphane Mallarmé envisaged 'A pale sky, over a world ending in decrepitude, will perhaps disappear with the clouds: faded purple shreds of sunsets dying in a sleeping river on a horizon submerged in light and water . . . in an age that has outlived beauty', *'une epoque qui survit à la beauté'*. Victorian champions of progress like T. H. Huxley, 'Darwin's bulldog' and coiner of the term 'agnostic', vigorously challenged such decadent romanticism. In 1886 Huxley rebuked the regressive aesthetics of the Wordsworthian 'Lake District Defence Society'. 'People's sense of beauty should be more robust', snorted the rationalist, 'I have had apocalyptic visions looking down Oxford Street at a sunset before now.'

Blakean revelation had little place in the reality of the new world, and Netley's romantic visitors – Walpole, Gray and all who came in their wake – could not have imagined the overcast world of their descendants, threatened by new storm clouds. Heavy rain floods the beach road, making it impassible, as if to revert Netley to the Cistercians' 'horrible' site. Passing the sign that marks the city's boundaries, you turn into the gateway beyond, where an older metal plate announces that 'Netley Abbey, the property of the Chamberlayne family, was placed in the guardianship of the Commissioners of Works under the Ancient Monuments Act 1913 by Tankerville Chamberlayne Esq. of Cranbury Park Winchester August 1922'.

The reforming, reconstructing twentieth century had a new use for Netley. It repaired the ruins, mowed the lawns, clipped the trees and imposed strict opening hours. The modern world had come to regard such places as educational, rather than emotional sites. The voice of authority and the lecturing texts of 1950s National Trust handbooks, rather than the florid romanticism of eighteenth-century prose, now dictated Netley's aesthetic. Clad in his grey suit and tie, the ascetic German émigré Nikolaus Pevsner arrived to survey the abbey in the early Sixties. 'In 1828 the ruins were embedded in trees', he noted. 'It must have been a wonderful site, but the Ministry of Public Works are rightly concerned with making the ruins instructive ... At Netley there is too much to learn, and intellectual pleasures have their privileges side by side with visual ones.'

The Buildings of England may have extolled the intellectual pleasures of ruins such as Netley, but few visit it with textbook in hand to be educated by these whalebone arches beached on Netley's shore. Its lawns are usually quiet and for the most part undisturbed, save for wedding parties using the stones as a photographic backdrop, and theatre companies taking advantage of a ready-made medieval set. Yet on one day each year its sanctity is revived on the Feast of the Assumption, the day the Blessed Virgin Mary ascended to Heaven, the moon and stars at her feet. On a summer's evening the ghostly procession of white-vestmented priests and altar-boys and the blue incense seem to retrieve the past, and placed on a pillar stump is a statue of its dedicatee, enshrined in flowers like a holy well.

A hundred years ago William Howitt could ignore the sight of discarded sardine cans: 'The visitor, seated on a fallen stone, still feels a forest silence around him; and the neighbourhood of the Southampton Water seems to complete the feeling of the monastic tranquility which for ages brooded over the spot.' It is still possible to access that spirit: the Cistercian monk's austere regime, the aesthete's rarefied contemplation, the Regency adolescent's bosom heaving with delighted horror. Arches frame dark yews, crows caw in tall beeches, and an ancient, blowsy oak which survived the Commissioner of Works' cull might still be modelling for Constable's sketchbook. In dank chambers, cold clear water runs through the ferny channels which were once monks' latrines. Above, buddleia sprouts in lofty cracks, and the red-brick traces of Paulet's palace pock the grey stone like ruddy lesions, their manmade clay crumbling faster than the spiritual granite.

Like some coastal cliff, the strata of brick, tile and stone reveal the abbey as a gigantic fossil, a great gothic ammonite. The abbey's story is carved on these walls, from its foundation stone cut with Henry III's name to the initials of nineteenth-century tourists and now the hieroglyphic felt-tip of modern taggers. Walking in the grassy gap where the north transept once stood, my foot hits a piece of rubble: a fragment of encaustic floor tile which escaped those nineteenth-century robbers disguised as respectable-looking people. Decorated with a fleur-de-lys, its colours imbedded in the ceramic, it weighs heavy in my hand. How much longer will this building stand, these towering chunks of stone that seem only tentatively held together by medieval mortar? For all its tribulations, Netley's abbey endures. Sanctified and plundered, hymned and neglected, it is still a mysterious, elusive place. Like some forgotten countess sequestered in a bosky lair, it draws the romantic past around itself, and leaves the modern world behind.

Never quite making up its mind to be a village, Netley spreads fitfully along the shore, shadowing the low cliffs buttressed by furze and pine. Hidden by rhododendron and laurel from the road, the fort built by Paulet also became a house,* gothicised by Sedding, the prolific nineteenth-century architect, for the

---

* On 17 March 1627, the fort's personnel consisted of a captain, two soldiers, a porter and six gunners, 'the whole yearly cost of the establishment being computed at 103l.8s.4d'. Cromwell's Parliamentary forces had bombarded the castle – only to repair it in anticipation of a Jacobite invasion. In the early nineteenth century the castle was owned by the Chamberlaynes, who leased it to a Southampton brewer and property speculator, George Hunt who in the 1830s commissioned George Guillaume to build an asymmetrical gothic tower and further additions.

Crichton family. Here they entertained their friends Robert Baden Powell – who spent his honeymoon at the castle – and Queen Victoria's grand-daughter Princess Alice, whose lady-in-waiting married their son. But their genteel life of garden parties, yacht races and local munificence had long since faded by the 1970s, when Netley Castle became a nursing home where Peter and I visited our ailing deputy headmaster, attending his bedside in a dark-panelled room as he sipped his whisky, still fearful of his leather girlfriends.

On Friday nights, dressed up to look as old as we could, Peter and I would walk through the village, past its tiny, disused 1930s cinema, its working men's club and its little garage and shops to the pub at the end, the Prince Consort, where, in our Oxford bags, we aspired to decadent sophistication by drinking acid-yellow Pernod and crimson Campari. A new subversion had arrived in my bedroom, a flame-haired alien in a red telephone box. I played *Ziggy Stardust* over and over again on my primitive one-speaker cassette recorder with the volume wheel pushed as far as it would go, headphones on, miming in the mirror to the apocalyptic fantasy of 'Five Years'.

Alongside my pin-ups of Bowie, with his kohl'd eyes, ice-blue satin suit and lamé ties, were pictures of Roxy Music, fellow time travellers in an alternative universe of decadence. One morning Peter brought the first Roxy album to school, and before class we stood by our desks admiring the gatefold sleeve. Inside was Bryan Ferry in tigerskin bomber jacket and blue-black quiff, and Eno in leopardskin and eye-liner, denizens of a fantastic night club, while splayed on the front cover was a kitsch goddess in a white Fifties swim suit with pink and blue satin edging, all pout and décolletage, her teeth bared in a cerise come-on, an ironic gold disc at her silver-platformed feet.

It was this vision of Sodom and Gomorrah that our maths master saw as he marched past the corridor, looking in through his round NHS spectacles and over the half-glazed wall. He dashed into the classroom and knocked the record sleeve from our hands. 'I'm a man', he hissed like a pressure cooker, a characteristic of his desperate but doomed attempts to control his temper. 'I don't need to look at pictures of women.' The irony, of which neither he nor we had been conscious, was that in fact our sin was much greater: the object of our admiration was a gallery of men in satin and mascara.

Three years later, we left school. Peter went to university for two terms, but was lured away by North Sea oil, diving in murky waters to earn thousands of pounds. I was steered away from art school to study for a proper degree at a college which my uncle had attended – yet another Catholic establishment, also called St Mary's, and run by religious in the suburbs of London. It was surreal to attend seminars on *Women in Love* in which one's fellow students were nuns in habits and wimples. But then, St Mary's former owner would have appreciated this particular scene: the college occupied the building that had been Horace Walpole's Strawberry Hill.

At night, after the bar closed and emboldened by the decadent fumes of Pernod, I'd steal into the eighteenth-century house, which was connected to the halls of residence by a brown lino passageway. It was as though I'd emerged from a semi-detached villa into a bit of Windsor Castle. At one end of a great gilt and mirrored chamber, a curved door opened into a round turret room opulently hung in swags of blue velvet, where Lady Elizabeth Waldegrave, Victorian chatelaine of Strawberry Hill, supposed mistress to Edward VII and a dabbler in the occult (like the Duchess of Devonshire before her) was said to have conducted seances. Lady Elizabeth had married her cousin, the 4th Earl Waldegrave, while her mother was the love child of Sir Edward Walpole, second son of the Earl of Orford, Horace Walpole's heir. By strange synchronicity, her family had owned Mayfield, the Weston estate they had acquired in 1854 from the Chamberlaynes.

It wasn't difficult to bring *The Castle of Otranto* to life here, in its birthplace. Even the men's halls of residence, constructed when, like my old school, the house had become a Catholic seminary, had been built by the firm of Pugin and Pugin. The rooms were consequently narrow and cell-like, designed to contain the passions of a would-be priest, and across the corridor was a communal shower room with its thick dividing walls apparently made of dark, institutional stone, its taps dripping, the odd item of clothing – a pair of football shorts, socks or a towel – left behind on the benches.

Outside the window, wide lawns insulated Walpole's fantastic creation from the suburbia beyond, and in my cubbyhole I read *Gormenghast*, conflating Peake's 1940s gothic with the lapidiary prose of Denton Welch, whose *Voice Through a Cloud* I'd found in a jumble sale. Steerpike's pinched cheekbones and Satanic stare anticipated another cult hero, Johnny Rotten, and in a world of three-day strikes and power-cuts, the present promised no future. Yet there was still the past to deal with. On visits home to Southampton – often coinciding with Peter's return from Aberdeen, his pockets bulging with money – I'd return to Netley. Now it was not the abbey which preoccupied me, but the building which seemed to have inherited its gothic spirit: the Royal Victoria Military Hospital.

PART

II

Pray Stop All Work

You might as well take 1,100 men every year out upon Salisbury Plain and shoot them.

FLORENCE NIGHTINGALE

On 19 May 1856, Queen Victoria sailed across the Solent from her island retreat at Osborne in the Royal Yacht *Victoria and Albert*, accompanied by a grand flotilla of a frigate and twelve gun boats. She had come to lay the hospital's foundation stone, her first public engagement since the end of the folly and bravado that had been the Crimean War. The time was right for a new symbol of national pride. With the country's focus on Netley, the local press was particularly excited about the event and the building it was to bring to the county's shore: 'It will be one of the greatest national schemes which, of the kind, has been yet undertaken', declared the *Hampshire Independent*, 'and will, we think, completely eclipse the asylum at Chelsea, both in extent and beauty.'

A 300 foot jetty stretching out into Southampton Water had been constructed for the occasion, and was decorated by an archway of evergreens surmounted by a crown, its length covered with scarlet cloth to await the Queen's arrival. It was said that she could have landed perfectly easily at Southampton but had conceived a dislike for the town, having been heard to say that it had 'snubbed' her on a previous occasion. Perhaps South-ampton and its climate decided to ruffle her feathers again, for the day was windy and the sea too rough for the Queen, who took refuge below deck during the crossing. Meanwhile, local shipping had been warned to keep clear of the area, 'to prevent any confusion or accident which might otherwise be occasioned' – a warning which proved all too prescient.

That day 11,000 people and 400 vehicles crossed by the Itchen Floating Bridge, and Netley Abbey was packed with picnickers. In the evening it was proposed to 'light up the Ruins ... with variegated lamps at the rate of eight pounds per thousand for no less than six thousand lamps', and the daytrippers were looking forward to a grand fireworks display. Down at Netley Hard, crowds eagerly awaited their monarch and her consort. These were glorious times, and it seemed the whole country was *en fête*. Basking in the mid-century glow of empire, England was the cynosure of the civilised world, its imperial progress epitom-ised by the recent success of the Great Exhibition, with its myriad of souvenirs decorated with the images of the glamorous young Queen and Prince.

Some of that glamour was about to arrive on Netley's shore. The royal party included the young Prince of Wales and Princess Royal, and all the men of the entourage were in uniform, a panoply of gold braid, silk and cockades. It was a state occasion by any other name, and the party was to be met at the pierhead by Lord Panmure, the Secretary of State for War, 'Lord Winchester (Ld. Lieut of Hampshire), the Admiral, General, & the authorities &c.', as Victoria noted in her journal. But when the Royal Yacht arrived, the waves were washing over the jetty and *Fairy*, its tender, had to be unceremoniously beached on the shingle. 'A considerable and rather amusing confusion was caused by this sudden change in the Royal movements', noted the *Hampshire Independent*:

There was, of course, no scarlet cloth laid on the beach, and though it was torn up piecemeal from the jetty the moment

Her Majesty's intention was perceived, yet she landed before it could be transferred. Then a rush was made to the obstructive hoarding which excluded Her Majesty from the presence of the corporate and other officials assembled on the platform to receive her, and, amid the hearty laughter of the Queen, the planks were torn away, and Her Majesty was admitted within the enclosure, having in the interim been kept back among the crowds at this part of the shore, who never anticipated so good a view of the Royal party.

After this hilarious and somewhat embarrassing scene of flummoxed dignitaries, Victoria replied to a welcoming address from Southampton's Deputy Mayor – his superior having been taken ill at the last moment. 'We then walked a short way up to where the ceremony was to take place . . . troops lining the way'. Arriving at a large marquee, she examined the plans of the hospital. Then, in a copper casket, the Queen placed coins of her realm, a Crimean Medal and an early Victoria Cross, made from Russian guns captured at Sebastopol (although it was later discovered that the Russians had actually captured them from the Chinese), along with documents signed by herself and Albert.

This Victorian time capsule was then sealed and set in a trench, there to remain for the marvel of some future generation. Six hundred years after Henry III's name had appeared on the foundation stone of the abbey, his successor watched as, with due ceremony, the two-and-a-half-ton Welsh granite foundation stone of the hospital was lowered by pulleys on to the prepared mortar bed. Dwarfed by the great system of wooden block-and-tackle which loomed above her as though it were about to lower the royal visitor into the earth's core, the Queen 'tried the stone with the plummet and level, and tapped it in the usual form, taking counsel with Lord Panmure as to the correct and truly masonic method of doing so'. The Secretary of State then declared, 'I am directed by Her Majesty that the first stone of the Military Hospital has been laid, and that Her Majesty has been pleased to sanction its being called the Royal Victoria Hospital.'

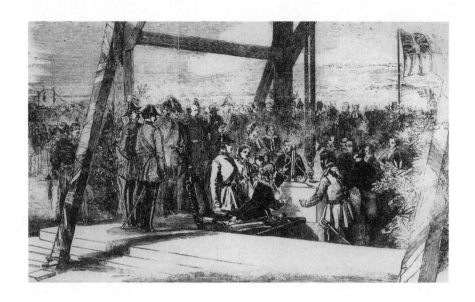

At that moment, the gunboats assembled out on Southampton Water fired a salute in the Queen's honour. But on one of the boats, the *Hardy*, she was told of 'a gun exploding & 2 poor men being blown to pieces. So sad, & so grievous, just on such an occasion!' In fact the *Hardy*'s gun had gone off prematurely, casting into eternity the mortal remains of Ordinary Seaman Michael Deran and AB Cornelius Flannigan, and wounding several other sailors. Meanwhile, on Netley's shore, oblivious of the carnage precipitated by the thunder of the guns, the Bishop of Winchester offered a blessing and the choir sang Psalm One Hundred: 'Enter his gates with thanksgiving,/ And his courts with praise!'

'... After which we went into a large tent, specially prepared for us, where we conversed with the different Gentlemen there', wrote the Queen. The man from the *Hampshire Independent* rivalled his metropolitan peers with his description of the scene, 'one of the most imposing and exhilarating character'.

The long 'red lines' of the troops, bending out into a spacious circle, contrasting with the black robes of the Corporation, the black gowns of the Clergy present, the white scarfs [sic] of the Cathedral choir, and the many-coloured hues of the gay dresses in which the ladies, who graced the stand, were arrayed – the masses of people and carriages assembled all around – flags floating in all directions – the water in the river dancing and sparkling in the sunbeams, and covered with the various vessels and gunboats, all dressed in colours, and jetting forth their white curls of smoke as the salutes were fired – the whole, combined, made up as pretty a picture as can well be imagined, whilst the ear was gratified by the performance of the National Anthem by the military bands.

Among all this uproarious splendour processed their Sovereign, the centre of attention, and of the civilised world. Having seen 'the soldiers at their dinner' – where the reporter noted that when the men were ordered to continue with their meal, 'Her Majesty smilingly observed the zest with which they appeared to obey' – the party 'returned at once on board the Royal yacht, and immediately left for Osborne'. It was another rough crossing, and Victoria was glad to be back on dry land in time for lunch and an afternoon drive, as 'nightingales sing charmingly in the woods'.

From her newly-built seaside villa – a Victorian version of the Brighton Pavilion, designed by Prince Albert, painted bright yellow and set like a great stately ship on the verdant slopes of the Isle of Wight – the Queen had made plain her concern for her troops serving in the Crimean War – a war in which for every one of the 1,700 who died of their wounds, another nine would die of disease.

The previous year Victoria had twice visited the wounded and afflicted at the General Hospital at Fort Pitt, Chatham, a former Napoleonic fortification. With straw mattresses, no toilets, no exercise space and the kind of 'malodorous sewers' which had created the diseases of the barrack hospital at Scutari, conditions at Fort Pitt were cold, damp and unhealthy. On the Queen's second visit, in June 1855, she declared the facilities wanting, according to a reported conversation which had the air of a caption to an engraving in a Victorian history book: 'Are these really the barrack rooms of these invalids?' asked the Queen, to which her Consort replied, 'Well, it seems very extraordinary that there should be no difficulty in obtaining money to erect a magnificent building like that for convicts, and that it should be impossible to find the means for building a commonly comfortable building for our convalescent soldiers.'*

A society which appeared to treat its convicts better than its soldiers was a source of concern for Victoria. On 5 March 1855 Lord Panmure, her Secretary of State for War, received a letter bearing the royal crest:

> The Queen is very anxious to bring before Lord Panmure the subjects which she mentioned to him the other night, viz. that of providing hospital for our sick and wounded soldiers. This is <u>absolutely</u> necessary and <u>now</u> is the moment to have them built, for no doubt there would be no difficulty in obtaining the money requisite for this purpose from the strong feeling existing in the public mind for improvements of all kinds connected with the Army and the well-being and comfort of the soldiers.
>
> Nothing can exceed the attention paid to the poor men in the Barracks at Chatham, and they are in <u>that</u> respect very comfortable: but the buildings are bad, the wards more like prisons than hospitals, with the windows so high that no one can look out of them, and the generality of the wards are small rooms, with hardly space for you to walk between

---

* The prison to which Albert referred was a product of a new penitentiary system set up to cater for criminals who could no longer be transported. Set on St Mary's Island, 'a dreary piece of swamp land' in the Thames Estuary, six years after the Queen's first visit, the inmates of its 'magnificent' gaol rioted, and the army was sent in to quell their rebellion 'with but little loss of blood', according to the *Illustrated London News*.

the beds; there is no dining room or hall, so that the poor men must have their dinners in the same room in which they sleep, and in which some may be dying, and at any rate suffering, while others are eating their meals.

The proposition of having hulks prepared for their reception will do very well at first, but it would not, the Queen thinks, do for any length of time. A hulk is a very gloomy place, and these poor men require their spirits to be cheered as much as their physical suffering to be attended to ...

The Queen's critique had the influence of her Consort, and that of the pioneering efforts of Florence Nightingale, behind it. Panmure's equally weighted reply agreed 'the necessity of one or more general hospitals for the Army', and proposed 'an immediate survey to be made for a proper site or sites, which shall combine all considerations for the health of the patients and the facility of access to invalids'. Panmure thought 'it would be for the advantage of the public service' if the hospital were built 'within a moderate distance of either of the great ports of Portsmouth or of Plymouth'. The next man in the chain of responsibility, the Director-General of the Army Medical Department, Dr Andrew Smith, agreed with the minister that the new establishment should be 'on the coast, or on some large inlet of the sea, so that invalids from abroad could be landed immediately, and marched into their Barracks, and the sick, without injury, be placed in Hospital'. And so the search began.

With the Crimean War already drawing to a close, the new hospital would come too late to help most of its victims. Yet there was still a sense of urgency to find a site (more especially with the impetus of the Queen's wishes behind the project), and just as the Bishop of Winchester had commissioned the Cistercian abbots to investigate a location for Netley's abbey 600 years before, so Dr Andrew Smith now charged the Deputy Inspector-General of Fortifications, Captain R. M. Laffan, to find a suitable place on the south coast.

Captain Laffan reported back on potential locations near the naval hospital of Haslar, Gosport and on the Roman remains of Porchester Castle – both on Portsmouth Harbour – along with possibilities at Herstmonceux in Sussex and Appuldurcombe on the Isle of Wight, but none of these proved practicable. Then the Queen's Physician, Sir James Clark, suggested a spot on Southampton Water which he had presumably passed on his journeys to Osborne. Clark informed Captain Laffan of its 'numerous advantages, as a site for a great Military Hospital, presented by the sloping ground on the eastern side of Southampton Water, a little below Netley Abbey; that the ground there seemed to be gravelly, and to slope upwards from the water, while there was a high ridge behind it, which sheltered it from the cold northern and eastern winds'. 'Sir James handed me a strip cut from the Ordnance Survey of Hampshire, upon which he had marked the place he wished Dr Mapleton [Laffan's colleague] and myself more particularly to examine . . .'

Yet questions were already being raised about the salubriousness of the proposed site, prompted by reports of 'exhalations' of gases in the area. During the Napoleonic Wars, soldiers stationed on the commons of Netley and Sholing had suffered outbreaks of cholera, and it was feared that there was something unpropitious about this desultory peninsula; that the afflictions of Scutari might manifest themselves on Hampshire's shore. Southampton had been trumpeted in the eighteenth century as a healthy watering hole; Netley was now seen as quite the opposite, and the *British Medical Journal* went so far as to call the place a swamp whose tidal mud would make the site 'a pestiferous marsh for twelve hours out of twenty-four'. Any hospital built there could not only subject its patients to cholera, but possibly even malaria.

A subsequent report detailed the problems: 'Three miles above the site of the Hospital the sewage of the town of Southampton flows into the estuary. Its population in 1851 was 34,000 and it is rapidly increasing.' The location was 'of a soft and relaxing climate and opposite a large mud bank. No site on the banks of a tidal estuary with soft mud banks, large quantities of rotting matter giving off gases and offensive smells during warm weather and having the discharge of sewage from a large town, should be entertained.' Far from benefiting from the sea breezes and healthy ozone, this shoreline was now seen as inimical to health, polluted by a modern town, with a belt of brackish mud, exposed at low tide, believed to emit noxious gases. It was hardly a site for a hospital, still less one intended to serve an empire and its wars.

The intrepid Captain Laffan, who had seen service in South Africa and Mauritius, set off to investigate, with Dr Mapleton in tow. They discovered a small brig, *Partridge*, permanently moored and embedded in the mud off Netley's shore. This Dickensian vessel functioned as a home for members of the Preventative Service – coast guards – and their wives and families. At low water, *Partridge* was 'entirely surrounded by the wide expanse of mud', noted Laffan, 'and we thought, therefore, that the men and women and children living on board would be good witnesses to examine as to the healthiness of the place, and as to any inconvenience which might arise from the vicinity of the land'. Interviewed, the brig-dwellers were found to be

unanimous in declaring that their dwelling was healthy; that at all times, at low water, a slight smell might be perceived from the mud, but that it was not at all offensive, or injurious to health. Their statements were borne out by their appearance; all looked healthy, particularly the children.

From this happy scene of naval mudlarks, the pair drew positive conclusions about the site, noting clear drinking water from wells and freshwater percolating through gravel resting 'on beds of brick earth'. Laffan and Mapleton also recorded 'the concurrent testimony of all the people living near the spot [who] declared the neighbourhood to be eminently healthy', and visited the local churchyard, where they noted the advanced ages on the tombstones. Finally, having engaged in wayside conversation a sprightly pair of eighty-year-old furze-cutters harvesting the area's characteristic wild crop of gorse, they were convinced. Captain Laffan triumphantly reported back to his superiors that they had found nothing at Netley to deter the building of the hospital (although ironically, when another report was ordered on the site, Laffan was unavailable for further research as he had fallen ill).

On 21 August 1855, negotiations began with the landowner, Thomas Chamberlayne, William's son, to purchase '109 acres, 1 rood and 32 perches of land', for which £15,000 was authorised in payment; the deal, for five fields, was concluded under the new Defence Act in January 1856. Meanwhile, the building plans were being hurriedly drawn up by Mennie's office – possibly to designs by the great Sir Charles Barry, the architect, with Pugin, of the new Palace of Westminster.* The Queen, prompted by her architecturally-aware husband, reminded Panmure that she was 'very anxious' to see the results, and so a delicate watercolour of the plans was made, each room carefully labelled with its function, and the proposed site embellished with decorative parterres.

This four foot long parchment was signed by the relevant parties and laid before Her Majesty, who was 'graciously pleased'

––––––––

* The Lancet's critical 'Visit to Netley Hospital', published on 9 May 1868, noted: 'It possesses a bold façade as seen from the water, though the original design by Barry was marred by a piece of economy on the part of the authorities which necessitated the curtailing of the central dome and clock tower, which is therefore out of proportion to the rest of the elevation.' Given the grandeur of the project, it seems possible that Barry, who worked in both gothic and Italianate manner, provided the initial designs: its style certainly concords with his later work. Barry died suddenly in 1860, and his work on Westminster was carried on by his son. The furore which would greet the Netley project, and the architectural emendations by the military authorities, may have been the reason for Barry's apparent withdrawal from it. There are no records of any original designs for the hospital by Barry.

to approve the proposals, and added her signature in black ink. Victoria's cipher was the royal imprimatur for the project, both physically and spiritually. The proposed building would indeed appear 'as though a Venetian palace had been erected on the scale of Versailles with traditional English materials', as one contemporary report speculated, and the Queen would declare, 'I am only too glad to think, if indeed it be the case, that my poor brave soldiers will be more comfortably lodged than I am myself', while Prince Albert remarked that it was a source of 'deep gratification' to them to know that the sick and wounded would be treated near to their own home at Osborne. As a further indulgence, the Queen asked to be allowed to lay the foundation stone herself, 'when we are in the Isle of Wight during the Whitsuntide holidays'.

The project was hastened along, with contractors given just one month to tender and two years to complete the building. Matters seemed on course, but when the plans made it necessary to expand the proposed site to accommodate a military asylum, Thomas Chamberlayne proved reluctant to sell the extra land. He was probably holding out for a better price, but his hesitancy was also evidence of the continuing doubts about the site – not least among a local gentry suspicious of the hospital, and still more so of its proposed asylum. It was in the interest of such nineteenth-century nimbys to encourage rumours about the unhealthy gases, and they may have played on Victorian fears of 'effluvia' and pervasive miasmas, a fearful memory of plague-ridden times; but in an industrialised country already polluting itself and its waterways, some of these fears were well founded, and for all Captain Laffan's evidence to the contrary, their shadow hung over the wooden scaffolding going up on Netley's shore.

The fact that the bricks used to construct the hospital were made from clay dug for its foundations – the building growing organically from its terrain – seemed to invest its very fabric with the germs of the land, or its spiritual malaise. Just as the abbey's stones were cursed, so the land appeared imbued with a dark gothic spirit about to be passed on to this new institution. Far from being removed from such concerns, the nineteenth-century's response to these superstitions – the scientific assessment of the site's suitability – was an echo of the 'enormous importance' the philosopher Montesquieu 'attached to soil, climate and political institutions'. At Netley, the clash of rationality versus the romanticism of gothic decay was set to run over again, as if it were caught in a cycle that would continue for generations to come, 'that great drama in a hundred acts reserved for Europe in the next two centuries, the most terrible, most dubious drama but perhaps also the one most rich in hope . . .' as another philosophical exponent of blood and soil, Friedrich Nietzsche, would write.

If the *Hardy*'s exploding gun at the hospital's foundation had been an omen, it was one to which many critics were already attuned – not least in the wake of the disastrous losses in the Crimea. As the Queen's letter to Panmure indicated, public opinion had been sensitised to the plight of its troops – largely by the very public campaign of one woman. Florence Nightingale was determined to learn by the war's lessons and not let British hospitals replicate the hellish conditions of the Scutari Barracks. 'I stand at the altar of the murdered men and while I live I shall fight their cause', she pledged, and having visited Chatham, declared, 'This is one more symptom of the system which, in the Crimea, put to death 16,000 men.' Just as her inspiration underlay the building of Netley's new hospital, so Nightingale's animus – a weapon quite as mighty as the guns of Sebastopol – would now be directed against it.

Tall, dark haired and rather more beautiful than some portraits suggest, Nightingale's sharp, ascetic features betrayed an even sharper intelligence, driven by a sense of religious duty which gave her the moral right to challenge even the highest authority. As a sixteen-year-old girl, she had recorded, quite precisely, that on 7 February 1837, 'God spoke and called me to His service.' Part nun, part nurse, part reformer, her passionate zeal was both shared and sponsored by her friend Sydney Herbert, then Secretary of State at War, who had sent her to the Crimea as 'Superintendent of the Female Nursing Establishment'. She returned as a national heroine, openly compared to Joan of Arc. 'What a comfort it was to see her pass even', wrote one wounded veteran. 'We lay there by hundreds, but we could kiss her shadow as it fell, and lay our heads on the pillow again, content.' The Lady with the Lamp became a cult, nightly revived in stage tableaux. The image of a saintly miracle worker was one with which she was not comfortable; nonetheless she would use it, adeptly, in order to pursue her campaign.

Thanks to Nightingale and her fellow nurses, soldiers were no longer regarded as cannon fodder, but in Lord Panmure, Herbert's successor, she found another example of bureaucratic lassitude which had so frustrated her in the Crimea. Nicknamed 'the Bison' on account of his large head which he moved slowly from side to side as he spoke, Panmure, Herbert wrote, was adept at avoiding both trouble and work, which 'he found easy through the simple process of never attempting to do it'.

Lord Panmure was at Balmoral in September 1856 when Nightingale was introduced by Sir James Clark to the Queen. Here the two great female figures of the age – each the subject of iconographic imagery and china statues – came face to face in the middle of a century they represented; two women who would assert their will, in varying degrees, over Netley's hospital. 'She put before us all the defects of our present military hospital system', noted Albert in his diary that evening, 'and the reforms that are needed. We are much pleased with her; she is extremely modest.' As a result of the meeting – and the appearance of Nightingale's exhaustive *Notes Affecting the Health, Efficiency, and Hospital Administration of the British Army* – it was agreed to set up a Royal Commission on the subject. Its chairman – as she had engineered – was to be Sydney Herbert; her suggestion of setting up an Army Medical School was also to be acted upon. And Panmure agreed to show her the plans for Netley's hospital.

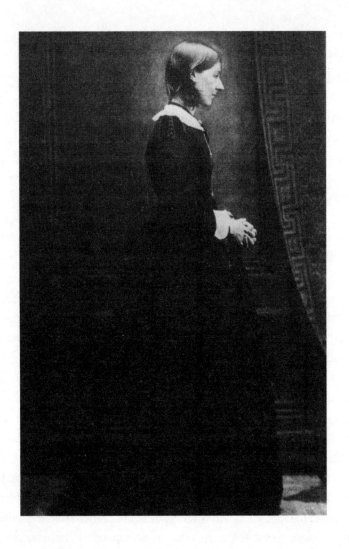

It was a decision he would come to regret. For the indolent Secretary of State, the effect was as though he had 'accidentally released a genie from a bottle', wrote Nightingale's biographer, Cecil Woodham Smith. 'The accumulated experience of fourteen years was suddenly put at his disposal; the fruit of her researches in France, Germany, Italy, London and Switzerland; of the endless miles she had tramped down the corridors of hospitals, prisons, asylums, orphanages; of the endless questions she had asked; the endless figures she had tabulated.' Such research had led her to the conclusion that the future of hospital design lay in 'pavilion' schemes which separated medical, surgical and convalescent cases in large airy wards to dispel 'miasma'. But at Netley she discovered small wards separated by corridors from the healthy sea air and sun of the south-western aspect, while their windows looked on to the north-eastern back yard, overshadowed by the long service wings at the rear. Far from the large wards she favoured, Netley's rooms were designed to accommodate as few as fourteen, twelve, nine and even two persons. They were little more than medical cells.

Not only did this go against progressive practice, it appeared to be a completely topsy-turvy manner of treating the inmates for whom the place was supposedly being built. The technical experts appeared to agree. In the September of 1856, as the Queen and Nightingale were meeting at Balmoral and only months after the foundation stone had been laid, Godwin of *The Builder* magazine criticised the site, drawing on the authority of a Manchester surgeon, John Roberton (who held similar views to Nightingale on the ventilation, sanitation and planning of hospitals), to declare that 'whenever the hospital shall be full of patients more disease will be generated there than cured' and, later, that each corridor would act as 'a pipe to conduct the contaminated atmosphere of one ward to the comparatively pure air of its neighbour'.

When Panmure's response to Nightingale's objections pointed out the 'susceptibilities' to be considered, her reaction was to set off from her home at Embley Park to nearby Broadlands, Romsey, there to lobby her family friend Lord Palmerston, former Hampshire Member of Parliament for the Liberals, and now Prime Minister. She may have been a woman, but she was a social peer of these men and, as Lytton Strachey wrote in his Bloomsbury version of her life, that made her doubly hard to dismiss: 'She knew her power, and she used it.' The result was a letter, dated 17 January 1857, written by Palmerston to his Secretary of State, full of indignation and Victorian melodrama:

It seems to me that at Netley all consideration of what would best tend to the comfort and recovery of the patients has been sacrificed to the vanity of the architect, whose sole object has been to make a building which should cut a dash when looked at from the Southampton river ... Pray therefore stop all progress in the work until the matter can be duly considered.

Panmure was taken aback when this prime ministerial imprecation landed on his desk. Nightmare scenarios arose before him: 'Rupture of extensive contracts'; 'reflections cast on all concerned in the planning of the designs'; even Questions in the House. Whether out of fear of greater consequences, or from an extraordinary degree of *laissez-faire*, Panmure was reluctant to accede to the Prime Minister's wishes. Palmerston's self-dramatising, even petulant response was to declare that he would 'rather pay himself for throwing away every brick and stone laid here than be a party to completing a building likely to send thousands upon thousands to a premature grave'.

On 28 February 1857 a 'memorial' was presented to Panmure by the physicians and surgeons of the Middlesex Hospital. Like Nightingale (whose own school of nursing was founded at St Thomas's Hospital), the London doctors could not approve of the perverse arrangements of the design. Its signature long corridor was 'highly objectionable as it forms a permanent receptacle for contaminated effluence which will escape from the wards into it and will pass from ward to ward', while the 'lateral ventilation' of the wards opened on to sculleries or latrines. As a result, work on Netley's hospital would halt. The questions Panmure had feared were asked in Parliament, and on 12 March another, yet more weighty critical report (as historians have pointed out, the Victorians were inordinately fond of reports) was submitted by the Royal Commission to the Sanitary Condition of the Army – led by Sydney Herbert.

In a wide-ranging, analytical text filled with graphs and diagrams, the Commission itemised the drawbacks of the site, the problems which were already holding up the hospital's construction. It considered the '*clay*, or rather *brick earth*' which might complicate the digging of the hospital's foundations; it worried that the 'admixture' of salt and freshwater off the shore might lead to malarial conditions; and it found that 'the mud contains sulphuretted hydrogen in combination' similar to other sites

> to which the sea-coast malaria of tropical climates have been attributed, and that though the air disengaged from the mud, at the time the samples were collected, was apparently atmospheric air, it affords *no reasons* for supposing that noxious gases are *not generated* during the summer, as is known to be the case with the Thames.

For Parliamentarians who had endured the 'Great Stink' of the sewage-polluted Thames – so great that the curtains of the newly-built gothic Palace of Westminster had to be drenched in disinfectant – these were serious considerations of which they had personal and unpleasant experience.

The Commission also protested at the size of the wards shown on the hospital plans, made deliberately too small, they said, so as to enable the disciplining of the patients rather than to cure them. Calling Nightingale as a witness-in-writing, Herbert's committee heard her evidence of the European 'pavilion' hospitals: she cited two modern French hospitals – L'Hôpital Lariboisière and the Military Hospital at Vincennes – as diminishing the risk of fire, facilitating administration and discipline, and most importantly, circulating light and air, although in her mind this had more to do with morale and sanitation than with actual fear of infection.* The report noted Nightingale's reply to 'question 10,025': 'In the event of a death taking place in the ward, the survivors, when they are

----

* Although suspected, the scientific nature of bacteriological infection was as yet unproven; the discovery that cholera and typhoid were carried in water was made in 1860. Nightingale would remain sceptical on the subject, even after Pasteur and Lister's work on infection: 'she had never seen it, therefore it did not exist', as Strachey wrote.

few in number, are far more likely to be affected by it than a larger number.' Furthermore, the Commission noted that 'a Hospital should be capable of easy extension by addition of parts – Netley Hospital is incapable of extension without injury either to its sanitary state or to its means of communication'. Such inability to cope with future states of emergency would severely compromise Netley in its capacity to serve an expanding empire. The Commission concluded that as £70,000 had already been spent on the building, it ought to be completed – not as a hospital, but as 'a gigantic barrack' – and a more modern pavilion-style hospital built elsewhere on the site.

In the light of such professional and considered objections, on 25 May 1857 a new report appeared, this time from the committee headed by Colonel Terence O'Brien, the Assistant Quartermaster-General, and Colonel Laffan. Submitted to the Secretary of State for War, it conceded 'that the means of affording light and air, both to the wards and corridor, might be increased with advantage' and recommended 'that along the whole front of the building the windows in the corridors be replaced by wide-arched openings, capable of being kept entirely open in fine weather, but provided with sashes that can be closed when necessary'. Artificial ventilation was to be introduced, different uses found for twenty or so internal two-bed wards which lacked proper ventilation, and better toilet layouts designed.

O'Brien's committee also allowed that 'military medical education was in a more advanced state' across the Channel, and sent an officer to Rotterdam to examine a state-of-the-art hospital which had just been built there. But the besieged Panmure and his department decided against such foreign innovations: a hospital of Netley's size would require at least thirty 'pavilions', and the result would be a sprawling, inefficient site, difficult to administer, and nothing like as neat, or as grand, as the edifice which was to grace the shores of Southampton Water. And so the hospital's overall design remained largely unaltered: even fifty years later, many of the two-bed rooms were still in use as wards.

Down at Netley, the monumental, problematic project lurched back into motion; and as it did so, new tales began to circulate in its wake, fomenting dissent like a subversive yeast. Now the rumours claimed that Mennie's plans (themselves rapidly becoming mythic documents, invested with all manner of portents and doom) actually drew on those made for a similar establishment in India, and that the open arches in its long corridors were originally designed as a gigantic verandah (the grandson of its first Professor of Surgery would even maintain 'that one of the first problems which confronted my grandfather on taking command ... was having to glass in the open verandahs ... which were open to the south west gales!') That which would have suited a subtropical climate – reserving wards to the cooler aspect, away from the sun – would in chillier Hampshire prove disastrous. It was even said that the hospital was built the wrong way round. Like the legends of Spike Island and the tales of tunnels under Netley Abbey, these stories had the air of urban myths, the kind of folklore that grew up around such grandiose undertakings and the mistakes of a faceless bureaucracy. But the truth was that imperial hubris had taken precedence over humane function: good intentions had been compromised by political intransigence and the pursuit of an imperial ideal – an empire which Netley would service, and in which its very bricks were complicit.

As the more rational voice of public concern, Nightingale's warnings continued to hang over the gargantuan building steadily rising on the shore, and in October 1857 the government decided it was time to settle the matter once and for all, lest the growing array of criticism should sabotage the project before it was even finished. One last report was commissioned on the hospital, a Parliamentary commission charged by a self-justifying Panmure to look at 'the authority for, and the evidence on which rested, the choice of site'. In a spirit of democratic zeal, scientific rationality and a certain political bias, the report dismissed the objections – from human mortality to climatic conditions – felling them point by point like so many trees.

107

Entabulated, paragraphed and calculated, the facts were laid down in a manner which would brook no further dissent. The report stated unequivocally that Southampton, being on a peninsula proper, was subject to increased rainfall on all sides, 'as compared with Netley, which is situated on a higher level, and with water only on one side'. The three miles between them – the timeslip of Weston Shore – made all the difference: 'the climate of Netley is mild, moderately bracing, and as favourable for the generality of those cases which the Royal Victoria Hospital is intended to receive as any to be met with on the southern coast of England'. Far from being unsalubrious, Netley was portrayed as a veritable English Baden Baden.

In didactic Victorian text and page after page of tables, facts and figures, the arguments were marshalled to defend the authorities' decision. There were detailed cross-sections, looking rather like 1950s abstract paintings, of the composition of '*brick earth*'; mathematical tables of the flow of sewage from Southampton and verifications of the purity of the air; observations on the access to the site by water and the ventilation and construction of the building; all addressed in exhaustive detail, as if, by the sheer accumulation of facts, the critical enemy would be defeated. Triumphantly bound and presented to the Commons in April 1858, the Report was a *fait accompli*. There was no going back now.

The construction of the much-delayed hospital continued, serviced by workers living in ships moored out in Southampton Water – albeit with new interruptions, this time from industrial unrest as the stone masons went on strike. Police were called in to supervise the dispute and escort blacklegs on to the site. Two striking masons were arrested for intimidation: the Southampton court heard that one of them had threatened the strike-breakers: 'You are all right, you — blacks, when the Bobby is with you, but we will wait for you till half-past five to-morrow night. We will learn you better than to go and work in our places.' The offenders were bound over to keep the peace, and threatened with imprisonment. The authorities would brook no such proletarian disruptions to the now-inexorable rise of the great building from its foundations – just as later that year, at Christmas 1861, it was announced that a military camp of 300 to 400 soldiers was being settled near the site, 'and the occupiers of the shanties have been given notice to quit'. Like the abbey, and like William Chamberlayne, the hospital was clearing the way for its own wilderness, its own improved landscape. Meanwhile, deteriorating relations with America seemed to threaten a new war, and a new urgency for the hospital rising on the shore.

At night it presented an eerie sight as the half-built structure stood in the moonlight, a mirror to the gothic ruins of the abbey, now in the contrary process of deconstruction. For many, the coming of the hospital promised great things. Exultant imperialists saw a triumph of technology and dominion; contractors saw an excellent source of income; and locals saw a guarantee of future employment for them and their families. But Florence Nightingale saw only a building as gross and cavernous and as ill suited to its purpose as the notorious Scutari Barracks. 'The patient', as she ironically referred to it, was a hopeless case: 'With the sick and dying mixed up in the same wards with Convalescents and men in health, a principle contrary to all humanity as well as to all discipline, [Dr Andrew Smith] would have committed an atrocity and an extravagance he could never have contemplated . . . The Country has been landed in an irretrievable mistake. And a Very expensive mistake for its pocket too.'

Although local legend would continue to associate Nightingale with Netley, there is evidence of only one visit, in a postscript to one of her fervently-written letters, dated 4 June 1857: 'I have been down at Netley inspecting.' Yet it was held that she worshipped in its chapel and even had her own carriage there; indeed, her mythic presence at Netley is still remembered in the names of houses and streets – evidence both of her iconographic status, and her admonishing spirit. In 1861, Nightingale published her *Notes on Hospitals*, which included a ground plan of Netley, and her comments on the place, the most favourable

109

being reserved for the washing machines which were being installed in the building.* Time would vindicate her attempts to alter or even completely reconfigure the building; as a much later report would note, 'to avoid the fulfilment of its critics' prophecies', the hospital was 'reserved largely for convalescent cases'. But for Nightingale, Netley was 'a notable defeat', proof that 'no single person concerned had had the faintest idea that any special importance ought to be attached to the way in which a hospital was designed'. It was an ignorance for which its planners were responsible, and for which its inmates would pay.

The hospital was finished in 1863, at a cost of over £350,000 (around £24 million today) rather than the estimated £150,000, and having taken seven rather than the two years expected to complete it. 'The entire staff of officers and other officials' at Fort Pitt, along with their patients, were transported to Netley that spring, to be settled into their new home. At 480 yards – one quarter of a mile – in length, it was proclaimed the largest building of its kind ever constructed, able to accommodate, in its 138 wards, one thousand men.

Accommodate, but not cheer; it was ironic that it had been a prison which had spurred Victoria and Albert to lobby for the building of a hospital which came to resemble little more than a prison itself, another Spike Island. Indeed, to its inmates, it became known as 'The Workhouse', the Spike. The relative isolation that had attracted the Cistercians to the 'horrible site' was an advantage to military discipline: its geography dissuaded disaf-

---

* She would have less impressed with its other amenities. On its 1868 visit to the hospital, *The Lancet* would note that 'to each ward is attached a watercloset, urinal and bath, which latter looks very comfortable and clean, but has this peculiarity – that it is never used! It appears that all these baths are made of slabs of enamelled slate set in metal fittings, and the admission of hot water within them in many cases cracked the sides, so that an order has been issued that the baths *are not to be used*.'

fected soldiers from desertion, and its dark and disciplined wards discouraged malingerers. No one would want to stay there for longer than necessary.

As its museums with their glass cases of dead snakes and mummified skulls indicated, the hospital seemed to embody a morbid strain of Victorian culture, an essential darkness derived from the contradiction, in intent and purpose, of the words 'military hospital': a place built to make men better so that they could return to battle, just as asylums sought to cure the mad by shutting them up with other mad people. Netley was also resonant with other paradoxes. The age of exploration had given way to the age of exploitation – of scientific processes, foreign resources or native peoples – at a cost partly paid by the future inmates of Netley. The hospital was an expression of the culture of sacrifice, a monument to the glory of Queen and Country. To die that others might live was an article of faith to which the building's very bricks bore testament.

Yet as an example of the Victorian preoccupation with progress, science, medicine and death – the rational markers of the age – Netley's hospital also battled, psychically, with the darker, romantic undercurrents of the era, never quite free of the deeper fears which the new rationalists tried to keep at bay: the myths invested in it and the land on which it stood. It was as if by its sheer superhuman scale the building sought to suppress such fears; as if its millions of bricks rooted it in reality and conquered mortality – the sort of will-to-power of which Nietzsche was writing. And just as its presiding ethos and the technologies which implemented it led to a new century of war, so those same processes, that same progress, would keep the great brick monster alive, supplying it with ever more willing – or unwilling – victims.

In the Very Best Style

Standing in the midst of beautiful grounds, and over-looking the Southampton Water, from which its noble frontage of nearly 480 yards can be seen to the best advantage, it proves to the world that faithful service is not forgotten by Queen or country. What a contrast it presents to the recent surroundings of its worn and wounded inmates! Here there are peace and quietness, lovely scenery by land and water, the best nursing, and the most skilful medical care.

The Navy and Army Illustrated

———

That visitor arriving at Netley for the first time could be forgiven for thinking he had strayed into the grounds of some extraordinary new palace. From its domed and turreted centrepiece, the hospital processed across its site in a pattern of arches and pillars set in walls sometimes four feet thick, as solid as any Solent fort built by Sir William Paulet. If it was not quite the Versailles which earlier plans and illustrations had made it out to be, it was certainly an impressive statement, and would be more so when its sapling trees had grown to maturity along the gravel drives.

Behind the gracious façade of this brick Crystal Palace, the great corridors coursed the hospital's body like major arteries,

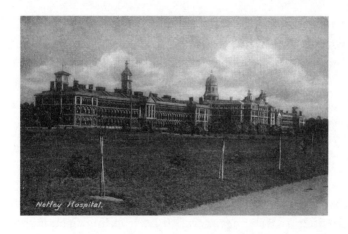
Netley Hospital.

running spectacularly from one end to the other – so long that, later, postmen would ride their bicycles along them to deliver the mail. But these were medical carriageways, and their traffic more usually consisted of marching officer doctors and hurrying nurses, or patients on stretchers and in wheelchairs pushed towards the windows for a tantalising view of the sea, the watery light of winter falling on their legs. As the visitor stood within the building's dead centre, it seemed as though he was reflected in a pair of mirrors facing themselves, endlessly repeating on its three floors. The effect was to underline the inescapability of the hospital, and one's place within it. For staff or patient, to walk these corridors was to be permanently on parade, caught in an unreal eternity of polished floors and arched windows which gave only intermittent glimpses of the outside world.

If the architecture of the building was the equivalent of a military drill, its hundreds of rooms functioned as a lesson in social hierarchy. The great projecting centrepiece, designated 'C' block, was reserved for administration and for 'sick and invalided officers', with nurses accommodated in the upper storeys. All other ranks were kept to the extended 554 foot arms of 'A' and 'B' blocks, the medical and surgical wards respectively, with the ground floor reserved for operating theatres and consulting rooms. Each block was virtually a separate hospital, with its own kitchens, dining rooms and offices; in a building this long, these were not luxuries but a physical necessity. Behind them stretched two-storeys of offices, wards and stores, with their stable-like sheds and first-floor galleries, their featureless quads a stark contrast to the Palladian pilasters, Doric columns and ornate architraves of the hospital's façade. They contained such facilities as the 'Dead Room', 'Post Mortem', 'Dirty Clothes Store', and the 'Itch Wards' (used for treating patients with scabies, then known as 'the itch').

Unlike civilian hospitals, Netley's was a contained space under military discipline; permission was required to leave or enter the site (in 1862, a Parliamentary Bill had 'extinguished' two public footpaths passing through its grounds). Sealed off from public scrutiny, there was little need to leave the place; it provided for every contingency. As Netley's abbey before it, so the hospital was a self-sufficient community, a colony on the shore, a world unto itself.

Like the estates on which it bordered, the hospital too could boast idyllic grounds. They had been planted by William Bridgewater Page, the Southampton nurseryman whose own arboretum 'we are sure', the *Gardener's Magazine* had noted, 'will be of immense service to this part of the country, by showing to the resident gentlemen those sylvan treasures hitherto known only to botanists and landscape-gardeners'. Page's nurseries supplied all manner of exotic and native trees to create an Eden carved out of the Hampshire shore.

And like Eden, it was envisaged that its inhabitants should want for nothing. This was a town in its own right, complete with its own water supply from three artesian wells and a reservoir which held three million gallons and powered one of the hospital's few design successes, its hydraulic lifts – although in the great drought of 1870 the reservoir dried up completely, thereby putting the lifts out of action. There were gas works (including a gasometer) and later an electricity generating station, post office and railway; a laundry, school, fire station and bakery; shops, stables, storehouses and brickworks. There was even a swimming pool, filled with seawater by a windmill 'pump' by the shore – although this was replaced by a steam engine – and which could be covered with planks for conversion into a theatre.

Just as the hospital catered to its inmates' every need, so it also exerted its power over the outlying areas. It created its own satellite village of Netley, and the tradespeople of Woolston and the market gardens of Sholing came to depend on the hospital's business. It became a microcosm of the rational, ordered Victorian world where everything was under control; there was even an observatory to keep track of the weather and the stars above, as if Netley existed in its own universe. There was no need, nor excuse, for anyone to leave the site; indeed, many never would.

The great brick hospital on the shore had become an imperial processing plant, its raw material – its patients – arriving by sea to be admitted into its interior, like the red-brick buildings of Ellis Island in New York Harbour, to which it bore both stylistic and functional similarities. Both were insular buildings invested with hope and fear, fraught with medical and bureaucratic decisions on human destinies; individuals catalogued and assessed as they arrived from foreign lands. And like Ellis Island, the hospital also had its own pier to receive its intake, although this too was an example of official miscalculation.

Netley's first patients had arrived by steamer at 'the Queen's stairs', the landing place used during the hospital's foundation ceremony. The Commanding Officer, Inspector General A. Anderson, reported in 1863 that, having disembarked, the soldiers 'have been moved in stretchers if unable to walk, or marched up, if in tolerable health, to the hospital'. But within a year the temporary jetty had rotted away, to be replaced in 1864 by a cast-iron 'screwpile' construction, 'one of the earliest of its kind', designed by the Shoreditch-born engineer Eugenius Birch who would build the piers at Brighton and Bournemouth. At 560 feet it was half the length originally planned and largely useless to hospital ships arriving from the colonies as it could not reach deep enough water – thereby undermining the convenience of Netley's waterside position. A purpose-built vessel, named *Florence Nightingale*, was devised to access the pier even at low tide, but with the coming of the railway line in 1866 most patients would arrive via Southampton Docks and Netley station, and from there by carriage – an uncomfortable journey 'down a steep hill and up a steep hill', recalled one veteran, 'they had four horses and they galloped them down the cobbled road and quite a number of the patients died from the vibration and shaking'.

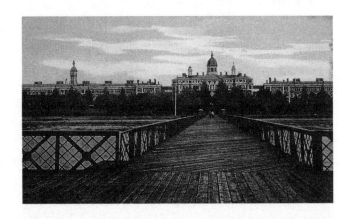

From the pier, 'The Avenue', the hospital's tree-lined grand promenade, led directly into the centre of the building, through its gruesome museum and into its spiritual heart. Here, below the mausoleum-like dome, lay the Royal Chapel, named in honour of the hospital's patron and around which it revolved: a physical embodiment both of Her Majesty's presiding spirit – not least in her role as the Defender of the Faith – and of the era's Christian ethics. Part parish church, part barrack chapel, it would in time be lined with commemorative plaques to the deeds of its officer doctors. In an era when belief in God was almost as compulsory as obedience to the Monarch, this centrepiece had been constructed to hold the entire population of the hospital. 'At Divine Service it contains a uniquely picturesque congregation', reported one later article.

In the Chancel is the white surpliced choir, some thirty men and boys, while the front pews on the left are occupied by the pensioners in their scarlet coats, and behind them are rows of khaki-clad orderlies. On the other side of the aisle, behind pews reserved for the officers of the hospital and their families, sit the matron and her nursing staff, whose grey uniform, white caps and scarlet capes, form a pleasing contrast to the blue suits and red ties of the patients who sit behind them. Other pews are occupied by families connected with the Hospital and by civilians.

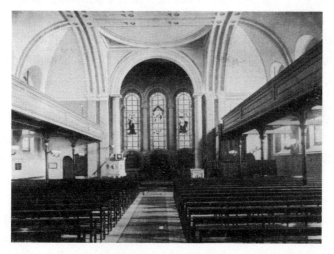

The Hospital Chapel

Here they would kneel, gazing up at the nave's stained glass and its triumphant Christ, resurgent on a heavenborne cloud and surrounded by radiant light, a Victorian *lux nova*. On Sunday, as on every other day, everyone at Netley was in their place, and knew their place. In this respect – as in many others – the hospital reflected the rest of Her Majesty's kingdom.

Meanwhile, at the other end of the building, great vats of food were being prepared for the church-goers in a clatter of pots and pans and clouds of steam that might have been supervised by Gormenghast's Swelter. On the receiving end few other ranks in 'the workhouse' would have risked a protest about the products of the hospital kitchens, although there were certainly

117

complaints from the officers in their mess. Barely three years after the hospital opened, their grandly-designed quarters – constructed as an after-thought to the main building – were the subject of 'severe censure'. Discovered by the tenants to be 'very damp and ill-ventilated', they were actually making the healers ill. 'Nothing more unwholesome can well be imagined', reported the latest investigation into Netley's shortcomings: one doctor had to be given sick leave when it was found that on 'one of the finest days of the season when all the windows were open, the front walls of the stairs leading up to his quarter, his sitting room and bedroom, were damp, weather-stained and mouldy and a noisome smell like a cellar'; his wallpaper was mouldy, and his rooms covered with fungi.

Such problems would not have surprised Florence Nightingale. Her biographer wrote of a 'difficult, depressing and unsatisfactory hospital', while the newly-arrived doctors, faced with the reality of the building's design, confirmed her reservations: 'A corridor passes from end to end, and the wards are mostly on the northern side. The majority of them have no lateral ventilation, and the vitiated air of each finds its way across the beds into the corridor. This is a faulty arrangement, and in winter the ventilation of the wards is very defective.' In those wards, men lay on thin metal beds standing on bare wooden floors, tight-tucked with coarse woollen blankets as if to prevent them from escaping. Everything was wood, wool, glass and metal, rough or polished, their unyielding textures revealed in the tantalising light that managed to penetrate the gloomy wards from beyond the corridors.

Set on its grandstand site, the hospital's very situation emphasised its importance. In an era in which scarlet British uniforms were being exported around the world to administer the spreading blush of pink on the map, Netley's graphic façade entered the national consciousness. Where Netley had been known for its abbey, now it was synonymous with its hospital.

Press coverage, from its foundation ceremony through its disputatious construction to its final completion, had installed the image of the hospital in the public imagination. Netley became part of the fabric of British life, an entry in nineteenth-century encyclopaedias and the columns of *The Times*. Just as the abbey had become part of popular culture in operas, prints and gothic tales, so the hospital would appear in newspaper and magazine articles, and on countless postcard views produced by local photographers of every aspect of the building. There were aerial views and views from the sea; the hospital by bright hand-tinted day, all turquoise skies and vivid green grass; or ghostly and dark, silhouetted by moonlit night. Scenes printed on silver card and or picked out in a dusting of glitter; shots of neat wards with shiny floors and soldier-patients comforted by prim, caring nurses. Mundane scenes of the stables and their firemen, the boilers and their stokers, the skittle alleys and the swimming pool; intimidating scenes of the operating rooms and their surgeons, their instruments neatly laid out and ready for action. And perhaps most characteristic of all, shots of its signature corridors, their dizzying *Alice in Wonderland* perspective drawing the viewer into the interior of the building and the lives that were lived within it. Other artefacts bore the hospital's image, too: delicate embroidery samples and German-made transfer prints on teapots were all stamped with Netley's aesthetic, the repeating motif of its arched windows as a recurring symbol of itself, fixing it in the English psyche as part of the national, and now imperial, identity.

And like the abbey, the hospital would enter the realms of fiction: as defining a period text as Arthur Conan Doyle's Sherlock Holmes series begins at Netley. *A Study in Scarlet* – the first in a line of stories which would reinforce imperial stereotypes with its foreign opium dens, criminal masterminds, and a clinically-brilliant, cocaine-taking hero – opens with John Watson, MD declaring: 'In the year 1878 I took my degree of Doctor of Medicine of the University of London, and proceeded to Netley to go through the course prescribed for surgeons with the Army . . .' Conan Doyle had written the story when practising as a doctor in Southsea, just along the coast from Netley; the author of *The Lost World* and later fervent spiritualist would also serve as a physician in the South African War. He therefore had ample opportunity to come into contact with Netley and the doctors who trained there.

If the hospital represented a part of unwavering Victorian culture, then the coming of the Army Medical School, with its pioneering aims, was a confident expression of that surety. The school was the brainchild of Sydney Herbert, Nightingale's ally who had become Secretary of State for War in Palmerston's government of 1859, and was intended to provide medical specialists in the military field and prevent the recurrence of the disasters of the Crimean War. More than that, it was to become a positive contribution to the progress of science, actively seeking cures for the ills that beset an imperial army. Netley was eminently suited to this experimental role. As the Empire's main military hospital with a ready supply of guinea pigs from actions around the globe, Netley became one great medical laboratory. The presence of the Army Medical School would make the hospital more than just somewhere to patch up wounds, amputate limbs or tend to fevers.

When it moved in on 1 April 1863, the school colonised part of the building, taking over wards and offices, converting one large ward into a lecture room and another into an operating theatre. Its professors were accommodated in the central C block, along with their secretaries, and their museum; the young student officers were housed in the quarters across the way. A later report itemised their rigorous timetable of medical instruction and military discipline:

Drill before breakfast; hospital work and clinical instruction thereafter. Each man was placed in responsible charge of one or more wards in the medical and surgical division, under the supervision of the professor and assistant professor. Instruction in the hygienic and pathological laboratories followed, and a systematic lecture given by the professors in turn in their several subjects closed the day's work about 1 o'clock. Attendance at operations and *post-mortem* examinations was required according to opportunity. A tour of twenty-four hours' orderly duty was taken in turn. The laboratories were open in the afternoon for voluntary and special work, and an evening visit to the wards was imperative. Instruction in lunacy was given at the asylum on Saturdays.

Even spare time seemed under orders: 'Ample time remained for recreation, and sports, boating, sailing, cricket, football, hockey, and golf were actively resorted to', noted the report. 'Social entertainments and amusements were not wanting' – although this stress on Netley's other amenities may have been an attempt to encourage recruits, as figures would drop appreciably during the 1870s, partly as a result of mistrust between army doctors and the rest of the service. There was also a danger that in this whirl of duty and leisure the patient himself could become a mere adjunct to medical progress and the next round of golf. Such concerns certainly troubled the conscience of Thomas Longmore, Netley's Professor of Military Surgery.

Longmore was one of a procession of great Victorian figures, resplendent in their uniforms and austere air, who worked in the hospital. Loyal servants of the state, they yet retained an individuality which the vastness of the hospital indulged and even encouraged, as if its many rooms gave free reign to their eccentricities, their triumphs and their mistakes. Born in 1816, Thomas Longmore was the son of a Royal Navy surgeon, and served in the Crimea, where he was 'present at the Battles of Alma, Inkerman and Balaclava', and on whose 'bloody fields his surgical skill was in constant requisition'. A colleague of Florence Nightingale's, on 8 November 1854 Longmore had written to *The Times* describing the appalling conditions around Sebastopol, and it was partly through Nightingale that he was nominated as Professor of Military Surgery at Fort Pitt. Three years later, Longmore arrived to assume the same post at Netley.

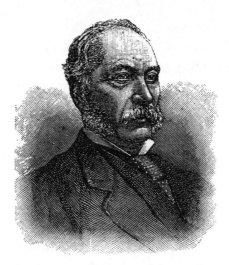

The late Surgeon-General, Sir T. Longmore

From his house in Woolston, the professor would take the train from Sholing to Netley, accompanied by his secretary who would carry his bags and bundles of papers. It would have been he who trained Dr Watson; and not unlike a Conan Doyle character himself – recalling the eccentric and brilliant Dr Joseph Bell, the Edinburgh surgeon on whom the writer had based Sherlock Holmes – Longmore was 'clear, precise, and methodical'. His experience made him the leading authority on gunshot wounds: his 1861 publication, *Gunshot Wounds*, was required reading for surgeons in the new, mechanised conflagration across the Atlantic, the American Civil War. He was also a humanitarian: in 1864 Longmore had been the British Representative at the first Geneva Convention, when the tradition of neutrality for army medical services, and the potent symbol of the Red Cross, was adopted.

Behind his formidable whiskers and stern exterior, Longmore had an 'amiable disposition', and his was a progressive influence on the hospital, as borne out by his address to the real-life Watsons beginning their probation at Netley:

I sometimes meet with surgeons who do not consider the pain inflicted [by digital pressure on an inflamed eye] as being of any moment. They regard the shrinking from the approaching touch as a mere act of exaggerated sensitiveness or timidity on the part of the patient that does not deserve attention. Might it not be regarded, however, with more justice as an instinctive defence against threatened injury?

The mere fact that Longmore considered such a caveat necessary was indicative of nineteenth-century medical care, especially in a hospital which when it opened had no military anaesthetists and relied on chloroform alone for surgical procedures. Some doctors tended to treat patients as subjects for the advancement of science (even the phrases 'medical practitioner' and 'patient' implied the notion of compliant bodies on which to rehearse techniques); in the medical school of a military hospital this was an even greater danger. But the techniques which had relied on the speed and skill of the surgeon's saw were changing rapidly, and it is to the credit of Longmore and his peers that they positively applied their humanity to the practice of their duties. And nowhere was Professor Longmore's care for his patients better illustrated than in the extraordinary case of Major Hackett.

Robert Hackett was a prime example of a Victorian career soldier: a decent man, as devoted to the service of his country and his profession as Longmore was to his. Born in 1839 at Riverstown, King's County, Ireland, into the landed gentry (George Bernard Shaw was a distant cousin), Hackett had enlisted in the 90th Foot Regiment during the Crimean War, and had served in the East Indies and the Cape. Both his brothers were distinguished soldiers: the eldest, Thomas, had served as a lieutenant in the 23rd Regiment in the Indian Mutiny in 1857, where he won the Victoria Cross for his action in rescuing a wounded corporal under enemy fire at Lucknow. By 1879, their younger brother, now a major, was stationed in South Africa during the Zulu War. Earlier that year, the Zulu army commanded by Cetshwayo (who only two years previously had declared, 'I love the English. I am the child of Queen Victoria.

But I am also king in my own country. I shall not bear dictation. I shall perish first') had killed 800 British troops at Isandlwana. It was a humiliating defeat for the Empire, and reinforcements were sent to restore order in the colony.

What followed was a fierce campaign, a proving ground for imperial heroes; indeed, that June it would claim the life of the French Prince Imperial, Louis Napoleon, a slight, reckless boy with hooded, sad-looking eyes who was in love with Queen Victoria's daughter Princess Beatrice, and who had pleaded with his parents (the French emperor and empress, now exiled, somewhat incongruously, to Chislehurst, Kent) to be allowed to fight. On patrol in what was known as Zululand, the prince fell from his horse during a skirmish. Revolver in hand, he ran at the enemy, and tripped; as he fell, eighteen assegais pierced his body. The heroic scene was rendered in oil as a colonial parable, the red coat of civilisation versus the noble savage: the grassy undulating Land of a Thousand Hills hiding the naked Africans, dark and muscular as they advance on the prince who lunges, wild-eyed, with his revolver as his horse and the rest of the patrol flee into the distance. When it was brought home to Chislehurst, his body was so mutilated that it had to be identified from a gold filling. With the Zulus as brave and worthy opponents ('My, how they do come on', said a British officer as wave after wave of *impis* launched themselves on the Queen's troops), Major Hackett's action in a similar skirmish with Cetshwayo's army was equally heroic and nearly as deadly as that of the French prince; with the example of his VC brother before him, he had a personal precedent to follow. His may have been a foolhardy and potentially fatal action; the remarkable thing was that it did not prove so.

The news of Major Hackett's wounding unfolded in a series of reports, written on the blue-tinted stationery of Her Majesty's Service. The first, from the field hospital at Utrecht in the Drakensberg Mountains, recorded that the officer had been wounded in the battle of Kambula Hill on 29 March – an action in which the Zulus were comprehensively defeated, with 2,000 of them killed and just twenty-eight British dead. The British troops were set up in a fortified camp, which Cetshwayo's warriors, armed with captured guns, attacked, shooting only at close range; to warriors otherwise used to knobkerries and assegais, 'the concept of killing at a distance – the very basis of modern warfare – remained alien'. But one far-sighted *impi* took aim, and from a range of thirty yards, shot Hackett through the head. The bullet passed clean through one temple and out of the other. No one who witnessed it could have expected the wound to be anything other than instantaneously fatal. Yet amazingly Major Hackett was still alive. The officer was rushed to a field hospital, where the Surgeon Major of the 'Flying Column' reported on what must have seemed little short of a miracle:

The projectile, a spherical bullet, entered the right temporal fossa, passed through both orbits, causing protrusion of the eyeballs and complete loss of sight, [and] was extracted from the left temporal fossa. He was transferred to the Base Field Hospital Utrecht on the 7th April 1879. Slight discharge issued from both temporal wounds. Both sclerotics were freely incised to relieve tension and subsequently both eyeballs were extirpated as fully at least as the injured and disorganised mass would allow. The right lower lid which was drooping was drawn up towards the upper by means of islinglass plaster and the eyes touched with oil to prevent adhesion. Small spicula of bone came away from time to time from wounds in temporal fossa, and several pieces can be felt grating along a probe passed in the direction of the wound. There is no symptom indicating any injury to the brain except that the memory seems much impaired and a total indifference to everything seems to exist. Major Hackett does not appear to suffer constitutionally as much as might be expected from such a grave injury. The bodily functions are comparatively speaking normal and on most days of late he is able to engage in conversation with his friends for a short time. He seems however to have no recollection of the battle in which he sustained this severe wound. I recommend that he be sent to Pietermaritzburg with a view of being invalided to England and that his soldier servant be allowed to accompany him to England.

On the reverse of the paper was a second report, which noted that Hackett had been brought before an invaliding board at Pietermaritzburg and was 'recommended to proceed to England on six months leave of absence'. The idea of 'leave of absence' for a man who had received a bullet through his head appeared to encourage the casualty – who seemed to have little real idea of what had actually happened to him – in the notion that his wound was not so serious. It was a cruel deception.

On 5 July Hackett left the officers' hospital for Durban, where he embarked on HMS *Euphrates*, transferring to HMS *Jumna* at Simon's Bay at the Cape on 21 July. Dudley, the surgeon on board ship, contributed the next instalment in the story – as if it were a Holmes mystery in the *Strand* magazine – in a third report:

During the voyage to England he improved in general health, gaining weight & strength. But on the morning of 18th August he was most suddenly seized with a fit, closely resembling epilepsy. His breathing during the fit was stertorous & very laboured. The fit lasted for 10 minutes – He remembered nothing of it. His servant, who has been with him 15 years, says he never had a fit before. Slight discharge of pus . . . from the wound & between the eyelids all thro' the voyage – there is a stiffness of the lower jaw preventing the opening of his mouth farther apart than to admit the tip of his little finger.

Meanwhile, back in Netley, Professor Longmore, the world expert in gunshot wounds, was alerted to the arrival of this notable patient by a friend serving at a military camp on the Kent coast:

Shorncliffe, 28 July 1879

Dear Mr Longmore,

Major Hackett, 90th regiment, is on his way home, badly wounded & deprived of sight, to go to Netley, to be under your kind care & able treatment.

His sisters who are friends of ours wish to be near him while at Netley & will take apartments in the village.

I told them that might be sure of receiving from you every consideration. I am persuaded that you will say that I was right in telling them this from all that I know of your kindness & true sympathy.

I hope that you & Mrs Longmore & the children are all well . . . I have lingering affection for Netley. But there have been many changes since my time . . .

Yours sincerely,
W. Ponsford.

PS One of Major Hackett's sisters is married to a Chaplain: Mr Crooke now at Cork

At the end of his long journey up the African coast to Southampton Water, Hackett arrived at Netley in early August, where, armed with his case reports, Professor Longmore finally met his new patient and was able to make his own deductions. The professor's 'Observations at Netley', once again written on the calm, cool blue of official stationery and couched in medical terminology, nonetheless exhibits his sympathy for his patient's injuries and the tragedy that accompanied them. Longmore realised, to his dismay, that his patient had been cruelly deceived:

The nature of the injury inflicted on the two eyes excludes all possibility of any degree of visual power whatever being recovered. Unfortunately this does not appear to have been made clear to the patient, so that on his arrival at Netley he still had a hope that he might recover the sight of one eye. It has been explained to Major Hackett how baseless this hope is & he has received the information, which it has been painful to communicate to him, with composure.

The sense of smell is much impaired. Major Hackett can smell a flower for example, but he cannot distinguish between the odour of a rose & a carnation. The sense of hearing remains perfect on both sides as does also that of taste. Neither does there appear to be any degree of paralysis of sensation or motion . . .

Major Hackett does not suffer from headache or giddiness. No mental faculty appears to be impaired except memory, & that only as regards circumstances which have occurred since the date of his wound. I was in the same regiment with Major Hackett in India in 1857 & 1858, & every incident of that time Major Hackett remembers perfectly, more minutely, indeed, than I do myself. He remembered about the fight in which he was engaged up to the time he was wounded, but he neither remembers receiving the wound, nor anything that occurred subsequently until the time he was in hospital at Maritzburg, & his recollections of this period are very imperfect, neither does his memory appear to be very tenacious of circumstances which are now occurring from day to day.

Fortunately Major Hackett's general health & spirits are good, & conversation pleases him. Two of his brothers, Colonel Hackett formerly of the 23rd regt. & Capt. Hackett of the 5th Fusiliers, are at present staying with him.

Thomas Longmore, Surgeon General H.P.

There was little Longmore or Netley could do for Hackett beyond record the remarkable fact of his survival, but the surgeon retained his scientific and personal interest in the patient long after the officer had returned home to Ireland. The fact that Longmore kept and neatly filed the regular reports from the local doctor, Hogstead, as well as those from Hackett's sisters, who had taken up the task of nursing their brother, indicates a certain emotional as well as professional investment in the case.

Sending his accounts on black-edged stationery, as if to stress the sombreness of the situation, Dr Hogstead described the incidence of more fits, a regrettable consequence, 'but he may perhaps have been living a little more freely than usual and having too many visitors. Major Hackett & his friends are fully aware of the importance of quiet and freedom from excitement of any sort . . . A sister of his had certainly the severe epileptic fit but there is further family history of the disease . . .' Longmore's replies, drafted from his home in Woolston, offered Hogstead detailed medical advice – including a recommendation of 'saline before breakfast'. Hackett's carers were determined to look after him, whatever the intimacies that demanded. His sister told Longmore:

> Of course I can not know much but still I can not but think that the fit was caused by bowels being neglected & that he did not like to tell me they were not acting properly but I trust the plan I intend adopting tomorrow will enable me to know daily whether he is right in that way or not. He is still cheerful & would send his compliments . . . if only he knew I was writing to you . . .

But the last letter in the file, dated 9 October 1880, tells of another tragedy to hit the family. 'I suppose you have seen something in the papers of the bad accident Colonel Hackett met with last Monday out shooting', wrote Dr Hogstead.

> In lifting his gun from the ground by the muzzle one barrel exploded and the contents penetrated the epigastrium & lodged. He was taken into a farm house about 7 miles off, and died in about 33 hours after the injury – I was not sent for to see him, but I understand the stomach & liver were extensively lacerated & both himself & two civilian surgeons at once recognised the fatal nature of the wound. It has been a terrible shock to his brother Robert, and to his poor

widow, both are deeply afflicted – but they have also both been most mercifully sustained by Providence. I feared much for [Major] Hackett but he has gone through everything without any manifest injury – has had no epileptic attacks ... His mind is evenly balanced, and while he has obviously suffered much, I have every reason to hope that no injury will now result to him.

The courageous Thomas Hackett, VC, had survived the Indian Mutiny and all that colonial service had in store, only to perish by his own gun. Sustained by Providence, Robert Hackett, a luckier survivor, lived on in Ireland until his death, on 30 December 1893, his fortitude an example to his family, whose sons, far from being deterred, would continue to produce soldiers – among them General Sir John Hackett, the much decorated veteran of the Second World War.

In his papers, Professor Longmore preserved other case histories as instructive, living versions of the specimens in Netley's museum vitrines:

Case of Capt. Strange, 10th Hussars, upper ½ of humerus removed. Interesting to watch results after so extensive a removal of parts ... Accidentally received a charge of shot from a fowling piece near Muttra 22 July '75 ... When he came to Netley, he could not do this nor indeed bear it to hang down loosely. He wore a leather cup for the elbow ... since then ... he has been practising difft. kinds of movements with much benefit ...

Captain Strange, Longmore's notes added, 'lives at Hounslow – mother – expects to go into Commissionaires ...' Stitched up like Frankenstein's monster, these beneficiaries of Netley's operating theatres were specimens of the modern surgeon's skill. But as the few surviving pathology reports from the early years of the hospital show, even twenty years after the Crimea's mis-

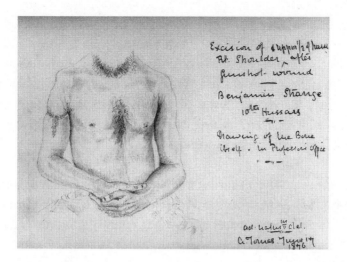

takes most soldiers died from disease rather than their wounds. Laid out in the hospital's post-mortem room, their emaciated bodies were dissected in the cause of medical science, and every detail noted on pre-printed forms.

Tuberculosis, or phthisis, was the biggest cause of death, as it would remain for generations to come. Its myth would create the 'white death' as a romantic poetic disease with a decadent association ('phthisis' came from the Greek for 'decay'), but in reality it was a classless and cruel killer, caused in part by the overcrowded conditions of modern living. Its bacillus would not be discovered until 1882 by Dr Robert Koch in Berlin, proving – against Miss Nightingale's judgement – its infectious nature; but the discovery came too late for Private William Hearen, aged thirty-three, who had contracted the disease in Madras. Admitted to Netley on 22 April 1879, he died at 3 pm on 5 May. His case was dutifully entered in Netley's pathology book, which required a 'History of Disease or Injury which has proved fatal, and state on admission. NB – Note especially a History or not of *Syphilis*, and of *Hereditary Disease*':

Habits intemperate (formerly) . . . Nothing could be eluci-dated from this man concerning his previous history. In Netley he was 'vacant' in his manner . . . The patient

131

complained of not being able to see & constantly called out in a purposeless manner. He became more & more unconscious until he died ... NB It is noted that 'when fighting with another man at Bellany in Jan '77, he being drunk at the time, he was thrown down and sustained concussion followed by inflammation of the brain – since then he suffered from headache & vertigo ...'

Like shorthand obituaries, the post-mortems seemed to delight in their arcane, pathological narratives; in elegant copperplate script, they tell sometimes heroic but usually pathetic tales. Corporal Charles Heppleton had caught a fever in Cyprus; he died three weeks after being admitted to Netley. The dissection of his body sounded more like the assessment of livestock at market rather than the final audit of a human being:

Head: An <u>excessive</u> amount of arachnoid effusion. Brain firm – small & rather dense.
Mouth and Throat: Teeth tolerably good.

But Heppleton's liver, like most of the patients', was 'considerably enlarged', a testament to endemic alcohol abuse among long-serving soldiers. Fred Roule, still a private at forty-four, had contracted tuberculosis in Lucknow:

On admission to Netley he was in a state of emaciation ... On the morning of his death expectoration was rust coloured, breathing quick and laborious. He was conscious up to the moment that he died.
  Pathological Summary or Epicrisis ... A case of an 'old soldier' worn out from long tropical service and malarial cachaemia. I find further that he was thrice in hospital in India for sec. syphilis (74 days) ...

Private Patrick MacCormac, twenty-six, had also arrived from India: 'On admission into Netley he was very ill, in fact he died

132

in a few days', noted the report. 'His expression was noticed to be anxious – lips pallid – pulse 136 – finger ends livid. Resp. very laboured ...' Like so many of his comrades, MacCormac had contracted syphilis in India, for which the only treatment was poisonous 'mercurials', and which, if the victim lived long enough for the disease to enter its tertiary stage, would send him to the lunatic asylum. The incidence of syphilis was so common that, as the post-mortem forms indicated, it was presumed that soldiers were more likely to be suffering from it than not.*

Dysentry, tuberculosis, typhoid and cholera were everyday causes of death, and few of their victims were regarded 'of interest or importance' enough for anything more than 'partial examination' in Netley's post-mortem rooms. Their symptoms were lumbered together with the paltry possessions left by these men, recorded in the hospital's casualty lists: 'two rupees', '6 photographs', 'small packet of papers'. The case of Private William Miller, aged twenty-nine, who had contracted 'Paralysis' in the West Indies, was an exception: 'When admitted to Netley Hospital his intellect was so impaired he was placed in the insane wards. No record of commencement of paralysis – he was helpless face void of expression ...' On dissection his brain was found to contain 'a soft yellowish ... deposit the size of a nutmeg (Deposit preserved)'. Under Netley's Professor of Pathology, Sir William Aitken, the hospital museum grew apace with such exhibits, a gruesome cabinet of scientific curiosities:

1171: Three sections of liver substance ... from Joseph O'Loughlan, aged 32 ... admitted to Netley 18 Nov 1862

---

* A report on venereal disease in the army noted that in 1873 'the constantly sick from this cause stood at the relatively low figure of 170 per 1,000', but that this rose to 511 per 1,000 in 1895 – in other words, one in two soldiers, 'the maximum on record'. Later Netley's William Leishman and Sir Alfred Keogh would co-operate on *A Manual of Venereal Disease*, published for army use in 1907.

... died in a typhoid condition on 15th December, 1862. There was a sloughing of the penis ... and also of the point of the nose ...

787b: Six pieces of crude opium, which were swallowed with intention of suicide, and brought off the stomach by emetics of sulphate of zinc.

788: One hundred and eighty-two pebbles, and two pieces of flint, which had been swallowed with a suicidal object, by an insane patient, in the Military Lunatic Asylum, and passed by stool without prejudice to his health.

Throughout the century, the Empire continued to deliver its wounded and diseased up Southampton Water to Netley. 'Our troopships every year bring home from foreign stations hundreds of invalids, many of them, alas! only to die', noted one Victorian essayist. 'But it is something to know that their last hours are soothed by womanly sympathy and tenderness ...'

In a building constructed by and for men, a place had been found for women: a role uniquely within the male-dominated military machine. It was ironic, given her vehement objections to the hospital, that Netley should have seen the introduction of Florence Nightingale's nurses into the military. Here the image of the Lady with the Lamp became reality; but it was a reality riven with issues of class and sex, and played out in a melodrama which veered from the comic to the tragic.

A Remarkable
Improvement

We look down the ward and we see in imagination the
great British Empire stretching out north, east, south and
west. It is like having a map before us. That poor fellow
in the corner contracted his illness in Barbados. The man
in the next bed to him was injured in an accidental
explosion in Halifax. The chappie in the wheelchair in the
verandah lost his leg by a charge of 'pot-leg' fired into it
at close quarters in the African bush ... And so they
come, from all corners of the globe, some to be more-or-
less invalids for life, some to become once more hale and
sound, some to have paid to them the only honours we
can give to the dead brave – the roll of the muffled drums
and the sharp retort of the volley firing.

———

Even as it was being planned, it was envisaged that Netley
should be the first British hospital to employ nurses in military service; it was another aspect of Florence Nightingale's
influence on the building. Given the problems over the hospital's
design, it was inevitable that in such arrangements the forces of
reform – as represented by Nightingale – would again clash with
the exigencies of military bureaucracy. Only this time, it would
be Miss Nightingale's own nurses who would be held to blame.

In the winter of 1856, after Queen Victoria had laid Netley's foundation stone, Nightingale had written to her colleague Lady Cranworth that her old adversary in the Army Medical Department, Dr Andrew Smith, 'tells me he wishes to see female nursing in the Victoria Hospital near Southampton done by *Nuns*!!! (He is a Roman Catholic convert).' To Nightingale, for whom nursing itself was a vocation, this was anathema, and a retrogressive step. As the man responsible for the misconceived hospital, Nightingale disagreed with Dr Smith (more especially suspicious for his Popish faith) on most things. Lady Cranworth concurred that this was an appalling prospect, and pledged herself to 'keeping all thought of these dreadful Nuns out of even Dr A. Smith's head'.

Nuns and monks had for centuries been regarded as fit carers, partly because they saw themselves as ministers in Christ's image, as had Netley's Cistercians of the abbey. But like many others, Dr Smith considered nuns particularly preferable for such tasks because they were incorruptible by the temptations of the flesh. It was a time when 'It was *preferred* that the nurses should be women who had lost their characters, i.e. should have had one child', as Nightingale noted; up to that point, some surgeons had considered sex with the nursing staff as a perk of the job. It is ironic, given the religious connotations, that Nightingale suggested the nurses should be called 'Sisters', 'to discourage the men thinking of them as potential wives' (other commentators would cite Nightingale's attraction to such sorority as evidence of her lesbianism).

Questions of morality were uppermost in the minds of those overseeing the female staffing of Netley. Dr Smith's assistant, Deputy Inspector General Mouat, had stated that 'women, as a rule, can only make good and useful nurses when led to the adoption of this most trying and disagreeable of occupations from strong moral feelings', and that if 'adopted from sheer necessity or for mere mercenary considerations, as will in all probability be the case in a great majority of candidates, the risk of failure will be great'. He declared that a 'great moral change must come over this class, and Protestant Sisters must form an

136

integral portion of the community . . .' A high moral tone was required because women were being brought into unusual and intimate physical contact with the opposite sex; it was therefore decided that female nurses should care for only the most severely sick men as they were least likely to invite sexual misconduct. At Netley even the building had been designed to contain possible passions: the nurses' rooms were left deliberately unheated, and with 'no *door*, because, if capable of being closed, irregularities are more likely to take place . . .'. They may not have been nuns, but they were expected to behave as such, and many felt cloistered by the hospital's corridors and walls and Cistercian-like isolation. It was a sensibility which would stay with the place: a later hospital chaplain, the Reverend C. J. Hardy, would note in the 1880s, Netley's nurses 'cannot and do not enter much into general society'.

To avoid the hospital regressing to the medieval state of Netley's abbey under Dr Smith's Catholic tendencies, Jane Shaw Stewart, the aristocratic daughter of a Scottish landowner and MP, and friend and colleague to Florence Nightingale, agreed to lead the first nurses to Netley. She arrived promptly on its opening in spring 1863, together with five trainees, leading her nurses down the corridors, ready to do their duty in their sensible brown dresses and starched aprons. With the reputation of their predecessors to live down, the stakes were high: their leader, Miss Shaw Stewart, officially designated 'Superintendent-General of Female Nurses at the General Hospital at Netley (not commissioned)', was the first woman – after the Queen – to appear on the British Army List.

Like Florence Nightingale, Jane Shaw Stewart saw nursing as a holy mission. She had readily cast herself in the role of female subservience, professing her dedication to the 'coarse, repulsive, servile, noble' service of her calling (and proving herself as ready with a vivid phrase as her colleague). A martyr, like Nightingale, in the Greek meaning of the word – a witness – she too was a Crimean veteran. The strident imperative of her letters from Scutari Barracks detailing problems with hospital diets and

French cooks (and a particularly bitter argument with Dr John Hall, responsible for army medical services in the Crimea, over the making of toast for officers), indicates both her passion for nursing, and her frustration with its military commandant, Lord William Paulet, descendant of Netley Abbey's owner and a man whom Nightingale accused of seeing the barracks' evils, but who then 'shuts his eyes and hopes when he opens them he shall see something else'.

Nightingale acclaimed her colleague's work at Scutari: 'Without her, our Crimean work would have come to grief – without her judgement, her devotion, her unselfish, consistent looking to the one great end ... her accuracy in all trusts and accounts, her truth, her faithfulness.' Yet she also wrote: 'What a twelvemonth of dirt it has been, of experience which would sadden not a life but eternity. Who ever had a sadder experience. Christ was betrayed by one, but my cause has been betrayed by everyone – ruined, destroyed, betrayed by everyone alas one may truly say excepting ... Mrs Stewart ... And Mrs Stewart is more than half mad. A cause which is supported by a mad woman and twenty fools must be a falling house.'

Suffering the after-effects of her work in the Crimea which had permanently compromised her health, Nightingale was now a semi-invalid, confined to her bed or couch from where she would receive visitors and send out streams of letters, dashed off in her almost unreadable handwriting as if trying to keep up with her own thoughts. Her melodramatic prose took up the offensive for campaigns directed from behind the front lines; the 'half-mad' Jane Shaw Stewart was her woman in the field, fired with the same determination. But her persistence would come to plague Nightingale – so much so that by 1859, Nightingale's Aunt Mai, who acted as her protector, instructed Shaw Stewart that she was neither to write to Miss Nightingale or hear from her again except through her aunt. Yet Shaw Stewart continued to write ever more disputatious letters. For all Nightingale's early praise, Shaw Stewart became increasingly idiosyncratic, and her imperious rule over Netley's wards would do much to discredit the fledgling service she had helped to pioneer. Indeed, Shaw Stewart's 'horror of publicity' conspired to cover up what was a badly-bungled attempt to introduce female nurses to military service, and within five years of her arrival at Netley, she would have to resign her post.

In making plans for the hospital it had been established that all sisters joining the Army Nursing Service should serve a probationary period of six months at Netley. But barely a month after Shaw Stewart was installed there, medical officers were refusing to allow her nurses to accompany them on their rounds. This reluctance had much to do with male chauvinism, but the evidence also indicates that the staff had good reason to be sceptical of the newly-fledged angels. The poor quality of nursing probationers and the inadequacy of their training were such that one sister was discovered to have nearly poisoned a patient by dosing him with liniment instead of castor oil. Later the same nurse was ordered to apply an 'Ether Spray' to a patient suffering from quinsy, an inflammation of the tonsils; instead of 'silently receiving the order and asking information' as her superior expected, she told Dr MacLean that 'she did not know how to do it'. Another nurse, 'Sister L', when requested to take a patient's temperature, admitted she didn't know how. A third errant carer, Sister Clarke, 'made a sad mistake in the application of leeches to the eye of a patient', applying one so close to the inside of the eye 'as to cause hemorrhage [sic]...' The Ward Orderly remarked: 'If Sister C had used the Eye-glass such a thing could not have happened. These glasses are always used here but Sister C had never seen them.'

Such ignorance was bad enough, but it was not just her nurses who proved amateur and dangerously inefficient: Shaw Stewart's imperious management – characterised by interminable memos and intemperate outbursts – was itself brought into question. Ill-trained, dispirited, and perilously close to doing more harm than good, the women under her care suffered the further indignity of being publicly abused and even struck by their own superior: in 1866 the Superintendent-General would admit to having beaten one of her nurses. Shaw Stewart's attitude to her patients was even more disastrously arrogant, and was to prove her downfall – although paradoxically this came as a result of her strict adherence to the rules of the system which, like the building itself, seemed to care more for structure and order than care and comfort. Eventually Shaw Stewart would have to take responsibility for her actions and the inadequacy of her staff.

In May 1868 the War Office set up a 'Committee of Inquiry' at Netley, charging Lieutenant General C. Hay with the official investigation into the 'state of the nursing service' and the conduct of its haughty Superintendent-General. With its cast of characters and passionate exchanges, it was a set-piece of theatre, another scene in Netley's Victorian melodrama.

Professor Longmore was the first witness to give evidence to the enquiry. '. . . My impression is, I am sorry to say, decidedly that the nursing system has failed', he declared. '. . . Nurses are no sooner acquainted with their duties than they leave, not for any reasons emanating from the medical officers, but, according to the nurses' own statements, because they cannot continue to serve under the Superintendent-General.'

> There cannot be a stronger illustration of this statement than the simple fact that about a fortnight ago, on the occasion of some slight operation being performed in the surgical division, neither of the nurses in the division, as recorded officially by the Superintendent-General herself, had ever seen a surgical operation performed, and that she could therefore not be accountable for their nerve and manner of conducting the duty if they did attend, this being the sixth year of training nurses for this very work . . . As far as the nurses themselves are concerned I have no complaints to make . . . but very strong objections have occasionally been made by the patients to the Superintendent-General of Nurses coming to them, on account of her temper and manner.

The next witness was Sergeant-Major Ward: 'On the evening of the day that Corporal Galbraith's leg was taken off', he reported,

> the Superintendent-General informed me that the ward-master and orderly and nurse had given Galbraith an egg against the doctor's orders. She appeared very excited, so much so that I could scarcely understand all that was said ... the Superintendent-General then spoke [to Private Reid, the orderly attending Galbraith] ... in a very loud and excited tone, making such a disturbance that the patients in the wards on either side ... came to the doors to see the cause of the noise. Some short time afterwards the Superintendent-General went into the ward (43) and spoke to the orderly officer and also Private Looby. She was still very excited, and spoke in a very loud voice. On returning out of the ward the door was pulled too violently. Private Reid was in such a nervous state that I ordered him to go away for an hour from the patients, until he (Reid) was more collected.

Dr Fyffe was then called to prove his testimony: 'The manner of the Superintendent-General has been frequently to me extremely unpleasant and disagreeble', he told the enquiry; 'on one occasion, I consider that it was insulting'. Fyffe was attending one of Shaw Stewart's nurses, Anne, who was 'very seriously ill ...'

> I conversed with her regarding this nurse, and gave her directions respecting the treatment of the case. While I was doing so I half leant, half sat, against the table, and wrote a prescription in that attitude; as soon as I had done the Superintendent-General said to me in an unpleasant manner, 'I'll thank you, Sir, not to sit upon that table again.' I bowed and withdrew.
> The next day I went again to see nurse Anne. The Super-intendent-General admitted me, and walked with me down

the corridor, and as I was entering the nurses' dormitory, she turned round and said to me, 'The Director-General would take off his cap, Sir, if he came in here.' I am not in the habit of taking off my cap when in uniform in the corridors of the hospital. I said to the Superintendent-General that I declined to receive instructions from her in matters of this kind, and I went immediately to the Inspector-General and asked him to relieve me from the duty of attending the nurses; he instructed me to continue my attendance on nurse Anne until the matter was referred to the Director-General.

In the meantime the Superintendent-General of Nurses reported me in an official letter, in which she used language which I consider to have been wholly unjustifiable. She stated that I had been guilty of excessive roughness and conduct unbecoming an officer and a gentleman in the presence of honest women, or words to that effect. I consider that had I not possessed the good opinion of the Director-General such a charge might have been destructive to my character, and I determined that nothing short of a written order from the Commandant or the Inspector-General in Netley should ever induce me to enter the nurses' quarters again unless accompanied by another officer.

Shaw Stewart, defending herself, was allowed to cross-examine her witnesses, and asked Fyffe,

Did you not on several occasions about the time you were attending nurse Anne sit on the table with your feet in the chair in the nurses' common room?

To which the doctor replied,

It is quite possible that, in a moment of absence I may, when considering anxiously what was best to be done for my patient, who was seriously ill, have sat for a moment on the edge of the table, but I never absolutely sat upon the table with my feet upon a chair in the American fashion to which the Superintendent-General refers.

Such incidents may have verged on the ridiculous, a comic clash of ego and petty manners, but more damning was a letter written by Fyffe and produced in evidence to the enquiry. Addressed to G. S. Beatson, the Inspector-General, and dated 18 April 1864, it noted:

I have the honour to inform you that the following report was made to me this morning by Private J. Jackson, 48th regiment, a patient, in the last stage of phthisis, in ward 27.

He states that for some time past he has felt very cold at night, and that especially he suffered from cold since he was placed on a water bed, a proceeding found necessary on account of the formation of bedsores, under these circumstances medical candidate in charge of the case ordered an extra blanket to be placed immediately under him, over the sheet.

The man informed that the Superintendent-General of Nurses came to his bedside last evening and removed this blanket, and that in consequence he passed a very comfortless night.

I refrain from offering any comment upon this matter, leaving you to judge of the propriety of it. I would merely remark that this man is in a dying state, and hardly, I think, a subject from whom the strict letter of regulation is to be exacted.

Private Jackson died two days later.
From these scenes Jane Shaw Stewart emerged as a theatrical anti-heroine, the darker side to the myth of the Lady with the Lamp. Another soldier witnessed one incident in which 'she flew in a violent manner, snapped her fingers in Dr Anderson's face, and said, "Why, what are you but a mere medical candidate!"', while Nurse Frances Johnson took the stand to say,

143

I have been very abominably treated by the Superintendent-General; I have had to sit at the side-table away from the nurses, and before I could hardly finish my dinner I have been sent into my sleeping compartment, where we are not allowed to speak, and the other nurses were forbidden to go out walking with me. I am not allowed to go into prayers night or morning ... She has accused me, because I have been attentive to [Private] Danel, that I was making love to him, and that I was too kind to my patients, and ought to treat them as soldiers.

In self-defence, Shaw Stewart told the hearing that she was applying the higher standards of civilian hospitals, while admitting regret for her loss of temper 'which was beyond her control' (implying that there may have been 'physical reasons' for her outbursts). But in response to these protestations, the Commandant of Netley, Major General Wilbraham, issued an ultimatum. In it he stated that it would be 'impossible for any commandant to discharge his duties with satisfaction to himself, or with due justice to the public service, so long as the nursing service continues under Mrs Shaw Stewart's management'. The Superintendent-General had no alternative but to tender her resignation.

To some extent Shaw Stewart had been a casualty of male prejudices about women in authority, although her personal manner had been abrasive and high-handed, and her character perhaps even unstable. The Netley experiment in nursing required her resignation as a sacrifice for the betterment of the greater whole, and as a result of the enquiry new regulations were issued. No superintendent would be allowed to continue in service after the age of sixty; all nurses must be able to read and write, and would be paid £30 a year. 'Sisters are required to take frequent exercise in the fresh air', and were not allowed to receive presents from patients. Most importantly, nurses should receive training in a civil hospital before joining the Army, and that year, the Nightingale Fund Council, which ran the training school at St Thomas's, agreed to undertake this training. Probationers now 'had to provide evidence of good health and character and be aged between twenty-five and thirty-five, with preference being given to widows and daughters of army officers'.

In an essay appended to the new regulations, Florence Nightingale wrote that, 'Hospitals were made for patients – not patients for hospitals', adding, 'Nothing can be less unwholesome than the "breezes" ... which occasionally sweep through the best regulated hospital – the free air which freshes all the atmosphere – the good-humoured rubs between administrative, medical, and nursing heads of staffs ... It makes the difference between a prison and a public school. But we must not expect if we sow the "wind" not to reap the "whirlwind". And "whirlwinds" are indeed unwholesome and destructive.' It was plain that she had one particular whirlwind in mind – her erstwhile companion, Jane Shaw Stewart.

After the departure of their Superintendent-General, the nurses at Netley were accused of having fallen into 'impropriety' with the male staff, and when one of the nurses married an orderly, Nightingale declared that the place had become 'a bear garden'. Mrs Wardroper, Matron of St Thomas's and Superintendent of the Nightingale Training School, was sent to inspect Netley and declared the nurses' quarters quite unsuitable: the Superintendent and her staff were expected to sleep in an open dormitory, separated only by a curtain, and they had to provide their own furniture. Wardroper recommended that the Superintendent ought to have three rooms, and each nurse a room to herself – along with footbaths to soothe corridor-weary feet.

The following year the School dispatched Mrs Jane Deeble and six new ward sisters to Netley. Mrs Deeble was an entirely different sort of woman from her aristocratic namesake – short, plump and comfortable-looking, a widow with four children, and therefore fulfilling at least one of the requirements for a good nurse (although Nightingale was doubtful at first, declaring that Deeble 'will be engaged in planning a nice tea for the nurses'

145

and would let the 'nursing go anyhow'). After Shaw Stewart's turbulent reign, Mrs Deeble's time at Netley was a marked success, and the army trusted her well enough to send her, with fourteen nurses, for service in the Zulu War of 1879, caring for the likes of Major Hackett in field hospitals. Visiting Netley that year, Queen Victoria noted that Mrs Deeble 'with 8 nurses, [sic] [has] gone out to S.Africa & onto the front. One of the nurses, a Mrs Wedden, is acting as Lady Superintendent for the time.' The Queen was particularly impressed with the neat – and rather nun-like – appearance of Netley's nurses: 'They wear a nice practical dress, grey woollen stuff with white aprons & a little scarlet cape, – on their heads a long sort of white handkerchief, tied at the back, & hanging right over the hair.'

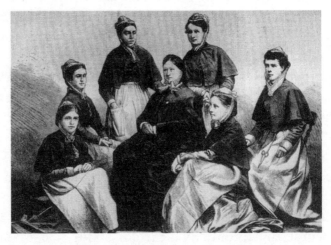

Mrs Deeble and nurses, 1879

In contrast to their predecessors, these woman were decidedly professional, dedicated to their cause and to acquiring experience both at home and in the field. Mrs Deeble would become one of the first – after Miss Nightingale herself – to receive the Red Cross Medal, and in 1883 she and an expanded team of twenty-four sisters would be sent to the Egyptian Campaign. Nightingale exhorted her nurses on their departure:

Remember when you are far away up country, possibly the only Englishwoman there, that those men will note and remember your every action, not only as a nurse but as a woman your life to them will be as rings a pebble makes when thrown into a pond – reaching far and reaching wide, each ripple gone beyond our grasp, yet remembered almost to exaggeration by those soldiers lying helpless in their sickness. See that your every word and act is worthy of your profession and your womanhood. God guard you in His safekeeping and make you worthy of His trust – our soldiers.

With the romantic image of the military nurse lodged in the popular imagination, and thanks to Shaw Stewart's distaste for vulgar publicity, few were aware of the reality of the kind of work they were required to undertake in a military hospital. It was not a question of drifting angelically up and down a ward, soothing the brows of wounded men, but of changing stinking dressings and bedpans, and getting shouted at for their efforts. Netley's bureaucratic and overwhelmingly masculine culture seemed to conspire against them. As one of Mrs Deeble's nurses, Mrs Rebecca Strong, noted, 'each sister had from six to eight of these wards under her charge, and speedily found that the nursing must be done by herself' without reliable help from ward orderlies, who 'were often taken away for relief work such as coal carrying, etc... A special orderly could be had in emergencies, but the nursing was minimal.'

But to the outside world, all issues of sex and class, and the pragmatic difficulties of their day-to-day duties, were forgotten in the encompassing myth of the Lady with the Lamp. Indeed, the place of women in the military hospitals and the grand imperial scheme was emboldened, if not empowered, by the fact of the sex of its reigning monarch. When the Victorian essayist wrote rhapsodically of the idealised carers at Netley, 'so much prized "when anguish wrings the brow"', he might have been referring to the hospital's ultimate ministering angel, 'our gracious Queen' herself.

*   *   *

Of all the Victorian personalities associated with Netley – its surgeons, doctors and nurses, the subfusc-clad, stern and sometimes eccentric characters who populated its wards and corridors – none could be more eminent or, in her own way, more intimately involved with the hospital than its founding matriarch, the woman for whom the building, and the era, were named.

Victoria was particularly attached to her hospital at Netley, perhaps because her mourning spirit felt at home in this example of her beloved Consort's philanthropy. After Albert's early death in 1861 (ironically from typhoid, the disease for which Netley would produce a cure), the Queen felt her every move should be determined by what he would have said or done. For a clinically depressed queen cloaked in widow's weeds, 'her' military hospital in Hampshire, so close to the now memory-filled Osborne, was a fitting memorial to her departed consort, one long brick monument to his physical loss.

It is a measure of Victoria's emotional devotion to Netley that her visits to the hospital constituted the few public appearances of the monarch during a time when she was seen to be ever more remote from her subjects, isolated by grief, power, family and memory. When she did appear, her figure glittered not with the diamonds of her royal ascendancy, mined from her South African and Indian colonies, but with shiny, polished jet of deepest black dug from the fossilised strata of Whitby. They were the accoutrements of the cult of death of which she became the age's paradigm – a culture epitomised by the disembodied models of her children's hands and feet that lay on black velvet under glass domes at Osborne; a reminder of her two children and several grandchildren who predeceased her, and of lost, innocent angels in an era of infant mortality. To Victoria, Netley's stricken young men could have been multiple reflections of her already enormous family, to be blessed by royal benediction as her own shadow passed down the wards like a regal version of Florence Nightingale at Scutari. In her public image of grief and solemnity, her visitations at Netley took on the air of a dark angel in black

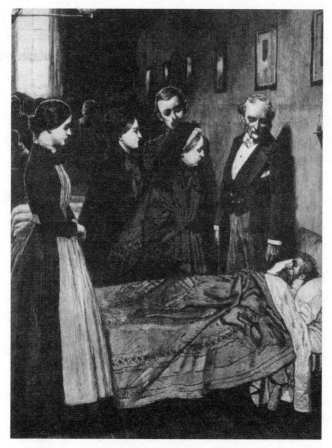

'I thank God that He has allowed me to live long enough to see Your Majesty with my own eyes'

taffeta; a remote, royal nurse dispensing grace and favour, the conduit of a nation's pity.

The Queen and her Consort had visited Netley no less than three times after the foundation ceremony in 1856, with Albert landing to eagerly inspect the construction site of the building. Now, two years after his death, came Victoria's first official visit to the completed hospital on 8 May 1863, a month after its opening, sailing once again from Osborne to Netley Hard. It is a testament to the importance of Netley to the Queen that, just as the foundation ceremony had been her first public appearance after the traumatic end of the Crimean War, so this was her first public engagement after Albert's death. (Indeed, it seems likely that it was the Prince Consort's sudden death which had curtailed any notion of a grand opening for the building in which he had been so interested.)

Accompanied by the eminent scientist and her Lord in Waiting, Dr Lyon Playfair – who had been summoned to Osborne to discuss plans for a memorial to Prince Albert – and without her Consort by her side, the Queen admitted to her diary that she was 'nervous at the thought of going to the Netley Hospital which I felt however was a sacred duty'. The visit was purposefully kept low key, and only afterwards did *The Lancet* report that 'The first public act of the Queen after her bereavement has been a characteristic one ... Her Majesty expressed a wish to visit first the foundation stone. She stayed here a few minutes, but it was evidently a painful reminiscence. She bore it, however, firmly, and then entered the hospital.'

Having presented portraits of herself and Albert to the Surgeon-General, the Queen progressed to the Army Medical School, another example of the age's faith in the progress of civilisation. Here she exhibited the same sort of interest in its science as Albert would have done. Touring its laboratories with Dr Playfair – who had been an adviser to the Prince and was an ambassador of technology (during the Crimean War he had suggested that phosphorous- and cyanide-filled shells should be deployed on the Russians, thereby prefiguring chemical warfare by seventy years) – the Queen was entertained by the courtier-scientist with amazing facts, such as the current belief that 'without doubt the moon was uninhabited', and that 'with the telescopes they were able to discern things as small as Westminster Abbey'. Technology made anything possible, and the omnipotence of science underlay the hospital's function.

More emotional – and therefore more touching to the grieving Queen – were scenes of devotion from the men who risked their lives for her. While among the sick, one patient was reported to have told her, 'I thank God that He has allowed me to live long enough to see Your Majesty with my own eyes.' The popular press played their part by relaying such incidents with sentimental alacrity, complicit in the creation of Netley's legend. It was a necessary myth. The ever-expanding Empire demanded such unquestioning loyalty; it was the glue that held it together, and there was as yet no poetic irony in statements of *dulce et decorum est pro patria mori*, an implacable faith in the morality of the age.

It was, accordingly, an age which liked to mark its progress in brick and stone. In August 1864 the Prince of Wales arrived to lay another foundation stone, that of the thirty-five-foot high roadside Memorial Cross dedicated to the fallen doctors of the Crimea, resembling a smaller version of the great gothic memorial to Albert, then being built by George Gilbert Scott in London. Two weeks later Victoria was back at Netley, moving through the wards' and along 'one of the corridors [where] 15 wounded from New Zealand, were drawn up . . .'

It pleased the Queen to meet the men from around her empire, especially fine, upstanding figures of Victorian manhood. On a subsequent visit, in April 1874, medical students and soldiers from the Gold Coast lined Netley's avenue and pier to greet her: visiting the wards, 'one young good looking man', she noted, 'was badly wounded in the thigh'. In August 1879, with the casualties arriving from the Zulu War – among them, Major Hackett – the Queen landed at Netley Pier for another summer tour, noting it was 'very hot going through the Wards'. While she was there she presented her greatest honour, the Victoria Cross, to a Private Hitch, another 'tall good looking young man' who had served gallantly at Rorke's Drift, where a handful of red-coats, eleven of whom received VCs, held out against 4,000 of Cetshwayo's warriors.

The Queen was not ignorant of the sacrifices made in her service: her sympathy, and her own loss, connected the monarch to her people. '. . . It was very touching to bend over the beds of these brave, noble, uncomplaining men . . .' she wrote. In August

1881, she bemoaned, 'It is really very wrong to send out poor boys like that.' Whether the Queen meant this as an implicit criticism of the wars being fought in her honour, or whether it was an indulgence in characteristic sentimentality, almost did not matter: the sentiment was there. Public opinion of the monarchy, and Victoria's remote and apparently reclusive rule, had recently grown to a vocal disaffection; as a result her visits to Netley became in part a public relations exercise. In a world increasingly aware of the power of appearance and opinion, the monarch's words were published to fit the engraved images of her visits in the newspapers, pictures which reflected the iconography around the Lady with the Lamp.

'Her Majesty's visit to Netley on Friday of last week was one of those kindly and gracious acts which do so much to make our sovereign beloved by the least of her subjects, by the most insignificant unit in her Army and Navy', detailed a later press report.

> Her Majesty was wheeled in her bath-chair round the wards in which her soldiers lay wounded, convalescing from injuries received in wars on the Indian frontier, or from the malarial fevers of the Gold Coast. At the side of this bed or that the Indian attendant stopped wheeling the chair, and her Majesty asked a few questions of the patient, adding a hearty wish for his recovery. To say that her visit was greatly appreciated is to say the obvious; and it is but a little stretch to prophesy that the presence of her Majesty did more good to the poor invalids than would tons of drug-stuff. It put heart in them, and that drugs would never do.

Victoria's sympathy was nonetheless genuine for being the professional care of a monarch for her children, encompassing even – as her Indian attendant indicated – the darker skins of her imperial progeny. And as with her genetic children and grandchildren, she often found favourites among the patients, to the point of requesting photographs of men she had visited, with descriptions of their cases to be written on the back; a gallery of keepsakes as though they were children of her own, as though she were there to tuck them into bed at night. Indeed, one of her gifts to the hospital – after a portrait of herself and Prince Albert – was a pink and white woollen shawl she had lovingly knitted, and which she stipulated should be used by the most valiant of her wounded troops.

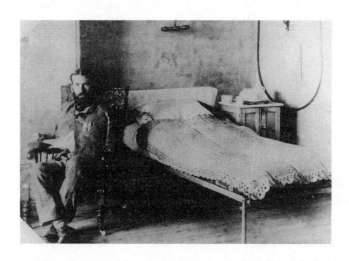

A forlorn veteran was photographed sitting by his bare metal bed which is covered, ceremoniously, by the shawl. The Queen's gift was a munificent, even intimate gesture, but one which was equivocally received, as the local newspaper noted: 'Heroism often went hand in hand with fatal injuries, and the honour of using the blanket soon became morbidly linked with death.' Soon, 'what had once been a sought-after symbol became more like a grisly shroud that no one was keen to wear'. Eventually one trooper declared, 'Oh, not that ruddy Shawl for me, no thank you, it means I'm a gonna'; and with this the dark angel's gift was relegated to a display case in the museum. A group of nurses who later inspected it there were not impressed. 'I'm afraid I do not think the examiner would have been very pleased to see it,' said Nurse Kneebone. 'It was thick, heavy wool . . . [and] there were many knitting mistakes in it.'

Towards the end of her long reign, the Queen's attention turned increasingly to her beloved hospital and its men. It was as if, in old age, she was ready to remember the events of the distant rather than the recent past in which her empire seemed to be becoming more restive, its conflicts more internecine, and her progeny ever more disputatious. In 1898, in her seventy-ninth year (and her sixty-first on the British throne), Victoria made no less than three trips to Netley.

On 11 February 1898, accompanied by her daughter, 'assisted by her Scotch servant, and leaning on the arm of an Indian attendant', the Queen was escorted into the 'roomy hydraulic lift, draped with Union Jacks and lighted with lamps' and up to the top floor and its surgical wards. Her Majesty had come to see men wounded on the Indian frontier, but 'entered every ward in which patients are to be found'. She was presented with Private Clow 'who is minus his left leg'; Davis, a 'bright young fellow, crippled at the age of twenty-one, having just put in three years of service'; and a boy from the Duke of York's School with necrosis of the jaw 'brought forward', from whom the Queen 'ascertained . . . his age' – which the *Daily Telegraph* forbore to communicate, perhaps in respect for its readers' sensibilities. One adult soldier introduced to the sovereign, it noted, was Corporal Grey of the 11th Hussars, 'quite the pet of the establishment, for he has been three years at Netley fearfully paralysed. He occupies a corner bed, and on a table at his side and on the window-sill are arranged Christmas cards and portraits, conspicuous among which is a photograph of the Queen.'

'There is no more cheerful fellow in the whole hospital', claimed the *Telegraph*, 'and, though his affliction made his story rather difficult to catch, it was with infinite glee he repeated her Majesty's questions to him, and his answers.' When asked how he had been paralysed, 'I told her "sunstroke in India; in a march from Rawal Pindi to Barraco – sixteen miles".' Such was his tale. As the paper reported, 'no distinction whatever is made between sick and wounded at Netley – both classes of invalids are rightly held to be equally deserving of honour. A man coming from a campaign with no scar of battle may yet, in the service of his country, have permanently injured his constitution ... Yet the one-armed, one-legged, robust old soldier will always command the greater sympathy.' That evening, back in Osborne, Victoria instructed her man Fleetwood J. Edwards to write to Netley's Surgeon-General Nash informing him that she wished to 'present all the patients at Netley ... who have had the misfortune to lose their legs and arms an artificial limb with all the latest improvements ... and in due course send the account to me ... You may be glad to hear that our Queen was much pleased with her visit today ...'

Victoria's arrivals and processions through Netley were models of her greater rule, local manifestations of the pomp that had accompanied her London processions on her Diamond Jubilee in 1897 when her subjects had gathered to catch a rare glimpse of their black-bonneted monarch passing through the great classical thoroughfares of the Empire's hub. The following May, cheering crowds lined the decidedly parochial streets of Netley as the Queen arrived by Royal Train from Windsor and, taking the arm of her turbaned attendant, Abdul Karim, walked across the red carpet and into her carriage. At the hospital she was met by braided and plumed officers, the panoplies of empire, and yards of bunting. Netley was *en fête*, ready to honour its heroes in a public, semi-state occasion which once again the press were invited to witness.

The Queen was to award two more Victoria Crosses, even now being carved and moulded from the same Russian guns captured in the Crimea. The dull bronze medal with its imperial purple ribbon was a marker of the wars of her age, just as its recipients' exploits told the romantic story of those wars in heroic acts of derring-do to inspire new generations. That the reporters were there to record the occasion was a crucial factor in the creation of such legendary acts of bravery, the last in a sequence of photogravure deeds accomplished in foreign lands.

One hero was Private Sam Vickery of the Dorset Regiment. Like Major Hackett's brother, he had distinguished himself by

155

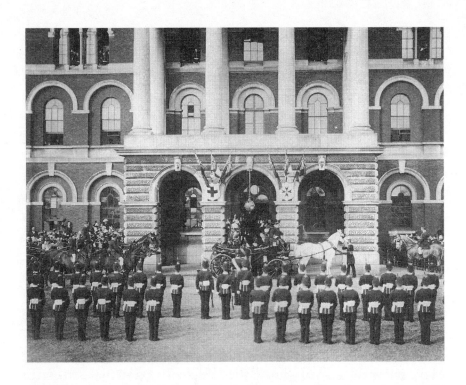

rescuing a wounded comrade under fire, this time during the attack by Indian rebels on the Dargai Heights at the North-West Frontier, an action which had already joined Rorke's Drift in Victorian military myth. A pugilistic-faced, moustachioed former farm labourer, Vickery was a true soldier of the Queen: when he left Netley, he re-enlisted for the South African War and was severely wounded at Nooitgedacht, near Pretoria. Fourteen years later, he enlisted once again, and having survived the Great War, worked in the GPO in Cardiff, where his portrait still hangs in the sorting office – as tough-looking in middle age as he was as a boy.

The second VC went to Piper George Findlater of the Gordon Highlanders for his actions at Dargai Heights. Faced with hordes of 'marauding tribesmen', his company officer had made a speech in 'words that thrilled the entire Empire': 'The general says this hill must be taken at all costs. The Gordon Highlanders will take it.' As if conscious of his part in the historic scene, the kilted Piper Findlater, a bluff, stocky, sandy-haired Scotsman, carried on playing 'Cock of the North' on his bagpipes even though he had been shot through both feet and had to prop himself up against a boulder to do it, his bravery encouraging the regiment's advance under heavy fire.

When the Queen awarded the piper his medal and exclaimed in appreciation, 'Oh, another Aberdeenshire man!', the scene was complete. 'Findlater was quite overcome,' observed the *Hampshire Chronicle*, 'and burst into tears.' Having left the hospital, Findlater, however, took the theatricality of his role a step further, and, in an era eager for both showmanship and assertions of the imperial will, went on to re-enact his moment of bravery for the benefit of enthusiastic music hall audiences. Findlater's astute self-marketing was censured by the military authorities for having brought the award into disrepute, but he was doing little more than profiting by the same sort of myth-making which had recreated Florence Nightingale in Crimean tableaux enacted on the same stages (although the portrayal of living figures on the public stage had recently been proscribed, too). And unlike his critics, or indeed Miss Nightingale, Findlater had no private income on which to fall back upon; only the one provable, and perhaps profitable fact – by virtue of his royally-bestowed bronze and purple emblem – of an heroic act. Only after questions were asked in Parliament was it acknowledged that some VC holders like Findlater had become so destitute that they were driven to such lengths, and an increased pension of £50 was awarded to forestall future degradations of the Empire's ultimate award.

Having bestowed these honours and performed her tour of the wards, 'I was on the point of going away', wrote the Queen, 'when Miss Norman, the Lady Superintendent, begged me to go into a ward, where there were some poor men, dangerously ill, not likely to recover. I also saw the poor paralytic man [the cheerful Corporal Grey], who was really better. Before I left, I saw an Officer, who had been wounded in the leg. We were ¾ of an hour late & only got back at 8.20. It had been a very fine afternoon & the country was looking lovely.'

* * *

Back at Osborne, Victoria – who in 1876 had become Empress of a sub-continent which she would never see – had recently ordered the construction of a Durbar Hall, a place of foreign declarations and state receptions. If she could not go to India, the jewel in her imperial crown, then India would come to her. In 1890 Bhai Ram Singh, supervised by John Lockwood Kipling (director of the Lahore School of Art and father of Rudyard Kipling), was brought to England to hang Osborne's ceilings and walls with Indian gothic plasterwork, great white icing-sugar stalactites as ornate as any medieval cloister roof. Later the room would be filled with the plunder of empire: intricately-carved ivories, illustrated manuscripts, wrought and beaten silver and brass, jubilee tributes from far-flung colonies arriving at Southampton's docks – the same docks which also received the casualties of the Empire's wars.

In 1894 Southampton had become headquarters of the Indian troop service, with the ships *Nubia, Jumna, Dilware* and *Dunera* using the newly-christened Empress Dock and bringing more wounded from the North-West Frontier and the Sudan. Candidates for the Indian Medical Service were trained at Netley, exporting its reputation to the sub-continent: so much so that my sister's mother-in-law – who would sail past the hospital's dome as she arrived at Southampton Docks from Colombo in the 1960s – was trained as a nurse in Ceylon to Netley's standards, with Nightingale's *Notes on Nursing* as her bible. In the engulfing arms of the great mother hospital itself, the sound of the sitar and the rule of the Raj seemed to reverberate in the high-ceilinged corridors with their potted palms and cane furniture set out as though on the verandah of a massive bungalow. Soon they would be thronged with foreign faces as well as those of Britons; the colonies come to the mother country, precursors of a multi-cultural century yet to come.

'What a contrast it presents to the recent surroundings of its worn and wounded inmates!' declared Lieutenant-Colonel John Graham in an article written to celebrate the Queen's Diamond

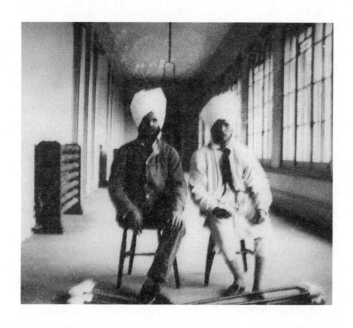

Jubilee and extolling her hospital's charms as though it were a spa. 'Here there are peace and quietness, lovely scenery by land and water, the best nursing, and the most skilful medical care. These blessings are enjoyed by invalids who arrive from India by hundreds at a time, and who are placed under the care of the Principal Medical Officer of the Royal Victoria Hospital.' But Graham could not deny that forty years after it was built, the hospital was outmoded. 'It is ... thought that for some classes of patients the site is not all that could be desired. There is insufficient shade and shelter, and although the corridors are warmed with hot water pipes, and protected by glass from the full force of the blasts that come from the sea, the place is said by some medical authorities to be rather more exposed than is desirable for invalids who have just returned from a long sojourn in India ...'

Lieutenant-Colonel Graham's piece was published in *The Navy and Army Illustrated*, and illustrated on still-shiny paper alongside other articles on 'The Divers of the Navy', showing men in baggy diving suits and brass helmets about to plunge into the murky depths. With its grainy grey images of bewhiskered

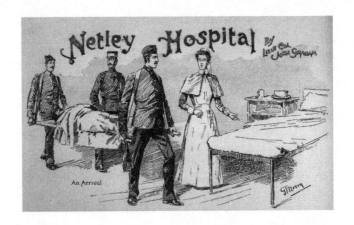

An Arrival

officers and stern nurses, Graham's was an account of a self-secure world in which 'Tommy Atkins, unless fatally smitten, has an irrepressible vitality that is bound to come to the front in one form or another'. Rendered in patrician, state-avuncular terms, the soldier-patient became an errant schoolboy, likely to take off 'his splints when unobserved, even if he has soon to expend utmost pains in replacing them to avoid detection'; or, 'so consumed with thirst', willing to risk 'health and freedom for a good drink of beer' by disguising himself and walking, 'with impunity, the two and a half miles into Southampton, to have what he considers a proper drink for once'. Such transgressions would be met with strict admonition.

Even those inmates that died seemed victims of their own infantile wilfulness, extended casualties in an era of high mortality and low habits – as Netley's pathology reports would indicate. But the predations of bad sanitation and loose sexual conduct were hardly suitable subjects for the Lieutenant-Colonel's report. 'It falls to the lot of some to pine and die, notwithstanding the care bestowed on them', Graham noted, a little euphemistically, of these unlucky souls. 'When Netley patients are invalided from the Army, and are too ill to be passed out of the Hospital, they are allowed to remain on a free list until they die, or are sufficiently restored to travel. This is a fact that ought to be more widely known than it is', wrote Graham. 'Paragraphists' – that is, uninformed civilian reporters – 'are so

160

apt to pounce on cases of seeming hardship, as if our methods of dealing with old soldiers were totally unfeeling. Such is not the case. Our regulations may be rather wooden occasionally, but they are not conceived in any spirit of harshness.'

As an employee of the hospital (and moonlighting as a paragraphist himself), Graham's is a vivid insider's view of the daily workings of the great medical-military machine. For the other ranks, reveille was sounded at 6 am in winter – 5.30 in summer. Breakfast was served at 7.30 am, 'dinner at half-past twelve, and tea at half-past five' (a regime which my own family still followed religiously two generations later); the repast-less *longueur* from 5.30 in the afternoon till 7.30 the following morning accounted 'for some of the voracity with which the convalescents are credited', admitted the author. 'Lights out' was called at 10.15 pm.

Officers had a more genteel regimen – breakfast at 9 am, dinner at 2 pm, supper at 7 pm – but even they were forbidden alcohol 'except when ordered by the medical officer in charge'. In a world divided by rank, the hospital was demarcated in ascending order of need, in a reflection of the Victorian hierarchy: its ground floor reserved for ambulant, convalescent patients; the first for bed-ridden 'medical cases'; and the second for newly-operated surgical ones. Yet the regime had lightened a little since the strict early days of disciplined wards designed to contain men who were often seen as little better than convicts. This was a more professional army of trained men, an investment deserving of better care, as the hospital menus bore witness, apparently aspiring to those of a grand hotel crossed with the healthiness of a Bavarian spa.

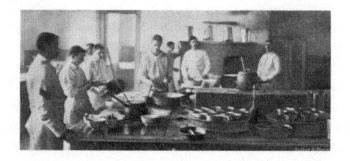

'The diets vary according to the cases. Grilled chop, grilled steak, stewed steak, roast beef, soup, chicken cooked in various ways, fish, beef tea, are the most common features in a menu to which there is practically no limit' – although the accompanying picture showed patients sitting on benches, presided over by a uniformed man standing at the end of the table, and there was still the formidable presence of military policemen to impose martial order.

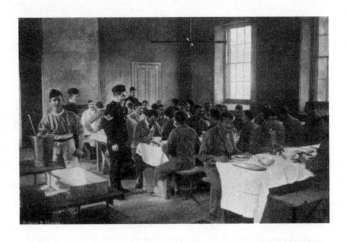

'The Corporal of the Medical Staff Corps is the Assistant Wardmaster, and is inquiring whether there are any complaints.'

Throughout these years of imperial sway, the hospital had settled down to a regular timetable, taking casualties (sometimes as many as 3,000 a year) in the campaigning season from October to May, and training doctors and nurses. But with continuing unrest in India and the stirrings of new wars in South Africa and closer to home, the troubled years ahead would see the hospital put to the test of modern warfare.

It was an irony of military medicine that it developed because the conditions it was required to treat also evolved. The South African War would bring new wounds to Netley, inflicted by machine guns and high-velocity shells. In a handsome, green-

162

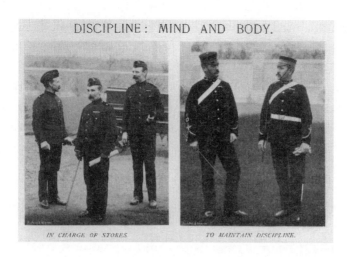

DISCIPLINE: MIND AND BODY.

IN CHARGE OF STORES   *TO MAINTAIN DISCIPLINE.*

leather-bound album embossed, *Literary Notes*, Lieutenant-Colonel William Dick, Professor Longmore's successor as Professor of Military Surgery, preserved photographs, press cuttings, and reports 'on operations performed at Netley', case histories stuck into his thick card pages as ghoulish mementoes. Dick's records indicate both the extraordinary variety of afflictions, and the adept skill of the surgeons in treating them. The unfortunate 'Private B. A., Royal Lancaster Regiment' was wounded by a Boer shell at Spion Kop on 24 January 1900; on his return to England his wound was found to be full of 'putrid pus' with a 'necrosed humerus'. 'This was removed, and the man made an excellent recovery,' the report noted breezily, 'although, of course, the lower end of the humerus and the forearm hang from the shoulder like a flail.' Another casualty of Spion Kop – many of them Liverpudlians, in whose memory a stand of their football ground would be nicknamed 'the Kop' – was Lance Corporal 'C' of the Royal Lancasters, who had borne the brunt of the explosion of a shrapnel shell:

Fragments entered his right cheek, upper eyelid, and external canthus. Another portion of the shell had entered his orbit and had caused blindness of his right eye, which at times became congested and painful. The fragments were removed,

163

but he declined to have the useless eye enucleated. He was sent on furlough.

The columns of diagnoses and schemata of treatments recorded for the benefit of the healers necessarily excluded graphs of human pain; for all Professor Longmore's efforts, that was still immeasurable, as were the traumatised, marred lives of the sufferers.

A large number of amputations have come home from South Africa, and in nearly all of them the stumps are most excellent. In no case where the limb has been conserved at the front has it been necessary to amputate after arrival home. After all it is much more satisfactory to the surgeon to conserve a limb, however ugly it may be, than to lop it off, however satisfactory the resulting stump might be.

Such instructions sound more like advice for the pruning of fruit trees rather than medical techniques.

Sometimes the surgeons were frustrated by their subjects' intransigence; one sceptical Australian soldier declined further operations on a tumour on his face which began when, he said, he was scratched on the nose in South Africa. The suspicious tribe of soldiers had long memories – and fears – of pre-anaesthetic surgery, and many remained loath to submit to the surgeon's knife, no matter what progress medical science might have made.

The South African War had once again proved how much of a problem disease continued to be in foreign campaigns. The need for a cure for diseases such as typhoid was greater than ever, and at Netley valuable research would be carried out into a vaccine for typhoid by another of the hospital's idiosyncratic doctors. Almroth Wright would extend the reach of modern science from Netley's laboratories into the glamorous world of medical discovery, and the less certain areas of human experimentation.

Born the son of an Irish clergyman in Yorkshire in 1861, Wright was educated at Trinity College, Dublin, where he won a gold

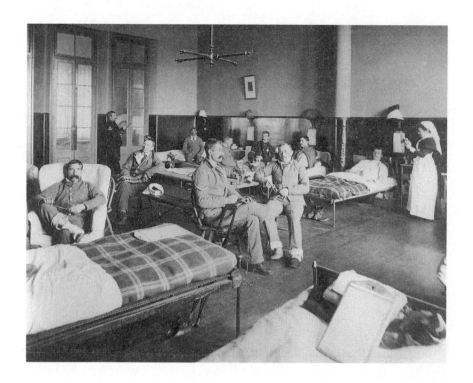

medal for English Literature and collected degrees in literature and medicine; he studied physiological chemistry in Germany, read law in London and took a clerkship at the Admiralty. This impressive portfolio secured him a series of posts at Leipzig, Sydney and Cambridge universities before succeeding Sir William Aitken as Professor of Pathology at the Army Medical School in 1892, aged just thirty-one.

Like Thomas Longmore, Almroth Wright was a character worthy of fiction, and duly provided another celebrated writer with the inspiration for one of his dramatic works. A 'colourful and mercurial character of tremendous ability', Wright was a man of the modern age, too dynamic to be confined by Netley's Victorian wards (or over-sensitive liberal ideals: like Dr Lyon Playfair, he supported vivisection and compulsory vaccination). Wiry, bespectacled, possessed of a nervous energy, Wright was not only extraordinarily learned (he read Nietzsche in the original German, and would learn Eskimo at the age of eighty), he

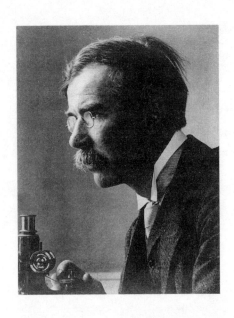

was also well-connected with an acquaintance that ranged from the politician Arthur Balfour and the actor-manager Granville Barker, to the spiritualist Sir Oliver Lodge. Passionately interested in ethics and philosophy, he wrote many theses, with intriguing if vaguely baffling chapter abstracts, such as 'On the different forms of graphic representation which have followed each other from the "Schematogram" of the cave-man onward to the "Retinograms" and "Para-Retinograms" of the modern artist'. In his 'Discursus on the vocabulary of pleasure and pain', Wright explored the 'neuronic pleasures' of sex and evacuation and quoted from the works of Pavlov. His controversial theories – which acknowledged Nietzsche, Darwin and Freud – were both revolutionary and reactionary at the same time. Wright claimed that the 'feminine mind' was 'inferior and irrational' and that 'a woman who shows any of the higher gifts of the mind should straight off be naturalized as a man'. He also opposed the bill for women's votes, publishing newspaper articles on the subject and expanding on his view in *The Unexpurgated Case against Woman Suffrage* (1913). As a result, the redoubtable (and rather mannish) composer Dame Ethel Smyth announced her intention to throw a brick through his window. Unfortunately she overslept, and arrived to find her intended target surrounded by policemen.

But it was at Netley that Wright instigated the research into parasitic disease and the protective power of blood against bacteria which would make him a scientific celebrity. Wright's experiments, conducted on his own body in the hospital's laboratories, were manifestations of Victorian science as caricatured in literature: the eccentric scientist, working obsessively among his test tubes like Dr Jekyll, using himself as a petri dish. In the wake of Koch's discovery of the TB bacillus, Wright would also experiment on inoculations for that disease, too; but it was his discovery of a vaccine to treat typhoid, the pernicious curse of foreign campaigns, which made him famous.

Unfortunately, his discovery was met with suspicion, perhaps because of his very eccentricity. Having conducted his experiments on himself and his students, Wright suggested all soldiers should be given his anti-typhoid inoculation, but the army did not agree (the scientist had already made plain his exasperation with military authority: when one of his laboratory technicians had been taken off to perform routine drill, Wright had marched out on to the parade ground and 'plucked' him out of the ranks). Even when Wright did persuade some doctors to carry his vaccine out to South Africa, their colleagues dumped the consignments overboard in Southampton Water, from where they were salvaged and returned to Wright by the local coastguards. Of the 328,244 men who went out to South Africa, Wright managed to have only 14,000 – four per cent – inoculated.

As a result of British losses, the Army Medical Corps – based at Netley – were generally (and unfairly) blamed for the war's heavy death total: of the 22,000 British and colonial troops who died, 16,000 perished from disease, not wounds. With disastrous epidemics of typhoid in camps such as that at Bloemfontein, it seemed to be a rerun of the ineptitudes of the Crimea (still more so for the 120,000 Boer civilians in British concentration camps, of whom 28,000, the vast majority children, died of disease or malnutrition, while of the 115,000 blacks held in the camps, an estimated 20,000 perished). Practically none of these benefited from Wright's innovation; or indeed from the lessons learned by Florence Nightingale nearly fifty years earlier. On 27 June 1900, Mr W. Burdett-Coutts, MP, wrote to *The Times*, vehemently criticising 'the medical arrangements in South Africa, more especially as regards the severe outbreak of enteric fever at Bloemfontein and Kroonstadt'.

In this sorry state of affairs, Netley and its doctors became the scapegoat. A Parliamentary debate and yet another report followed, which discovered that 'the condition of the Royal Army Medical Corps had been known to be unsatisfactory for years. It was unpopular and unmanned, and . . . had experienced the greatest difficulty in obtaining officers and men for service in South Africa.' It was the death knell for the Army Medical School at Netley. The school was moved to Millbank in London (although candidates for the Army Medical Service continued to be trained at Netley), where it was hoped that proximity with non-military hospitals (such as the pavilion-built St Thomas's where Nightingale's nurses trained and where her statue now stood) would have a better effect on its medical evolution than the relative isolation of Netley.

Irritated by bureaucratic and military intransigence, Almroth Wright also left the hospital in 1902, likewise seeking more progressive surroundings, although his work in Netley's laboratories inspired his assistant professor, Leishman, to identify the parasite which caused kala-azar, a tropical disease which left its victims literally bloodless. Wright became Head of Pathology at St Mary's, Paddington, where his cultured profile combined with his pioneering work to make him a sort of medical superstar. Interested parties would gather in Wright's laboratory, which became an 'at home' for men of science and literature. In 1904 Wright sent his pamphlet on tuberculosis inoculation to George Bernard Shaw, and an intrigued playwright came to one of Wright's 'late night tea-parties' among the test tubes. Shaw asked Wright what would happen if more people applied for his help than he could deal with: 'We should have to consider which life was worth saving', replied Wright, with more than a touch of Nietzsche about him.

This extraordinary notion – which seemed to define the problems of medical progress – inspired Shaw to write *The Doctor's Dilemma*. The play was 'conceived in Wright's laboratory', admitted Shaw, who sent it to the scientist for his comments, but as Michael Holroyd, Shaw's biographer, notes, Wright was irked by his portrayal on stage and walked out on the first night of the play. Wright and Shaw disagreed on many issues – notably on female suffrage – and when Shaw was invited by Wright to lecture at St Mary's on the link between science and art, the scientist stood up and declared impatiently, 'I believe that the effect of sanitation is aesthetic.'

Others saw Wright's attitudes as underlying notions of racial superiority, citing his subsequent experiments with pneumonia vaccines on black miners in South Africa. His colleague Leonard Colebrook described how they had gone to Pretoria 'to carry out a mass inoculation of the natives at the Premier Diamond Mine one Sunday morning'.

> Some thousands of them, in a wonderful variety of garments, from beads to bowler hats, were assembled in the compound, and the stage was all set for proceedings to begin, when all of a sudden the 'victims' went shy and a great clamour of dissent arose. To some of us the situation looked a little alarming, but Wright was quite unperturbed. He could not, of course, talk to the natives directly, but his benign smile and his quiet demonstration of the inoculation procedure . . . gradually won their confidence, and all was well.

To Colebrook, it was 'a triumph of personality'; to others, it was a triumph of will.

In 1906, the War Office, now persuaded of the efficacy of his anti-typhoid injection, somewhat cynically had Wright knighted 'and then used his knighthood as evidence of the unassailability of his theories'. Yet he had also acquired the nickname of 'Sir Almost Wright', and in the First World War, when he served as Consultant Physician in France (and wrote a paper 'On those who have the conscientious objector type of mind'), Wright would be criticised by the British Union for the Abolition of Vivisection, which published a pamphlet accusing him of having 'cooked' the statistics regarding his anti-typhoid inoculation used on the troops. Nor would Wright's celebrity status outlive him, eclipsed as it was in the public imagination by the discoveries of his pupil Alexander Fleming and his wonder-drug of penicillin – ironically funded by the money raised by the use of Wright's vaccine.

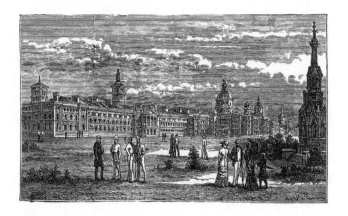

The latter half of Victoria's reign saw many changes in England: a second Industrial Revolution, bringing telephones and typewriters, bicycles and motor cars; technologies which had even reached this far shore, and the wards and yards and corridors of Netley's hospital. On 3 December 1898, Victoria made her final visit of the century, accompanied from Windsor by Lord Kitchener, the moustachioed imperialist ennobled for his service in the Sudan, and soon to distinguish himself in South Africa.

As she was wheeled along the corridors in her chair, the Queen expressed particular interest in the experimental use of x-rays in the operating room. Here stood an example of Wilhelm Röntgen's newly-invented apparatus, an extraordinary contraption laced with leather and with metal arms holding a small rectangle of glass in front of it like a Victorian VDU, 'as if a magic lantern threw the nerves in patterns on a screen'. Although it looked more like a particularly ingenious instrument of torture worthy of Kafka's penal settlement, this latest technological development made for exciting medicine, as one newspaper cutting, proudly preserved by William Dick, reported:

> Of the scientific attainments brought to bear in treating the wounded here, I had an opportunity to form a judgement from personal observations. Colonel Stevenson and Major Dick, professors of surgery in the school, were engaged in experiments with the latest appliances for locating bullets by Röntgen rays ... What bungling and haphazard work all former methods seem to be by comparison with this!

The ghostly glow of these back-lit images, photographs of the interior, illuminated the dark rooms like radium, the dangerous new discovery which had created them. For a century Man had been examining the outside world; now he was looking into his own body, to discover its secrets and, perhaps, his soul.

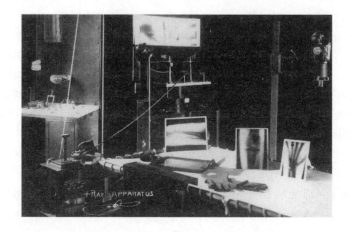

Now, before the aged black-clad Queen, moving slowly through Netley's wards and laboratories in her wheelchair pushed by her Indian attendant, the modern world was in sight, predicted by the progress of science. Analysed, dissected and experimented upon by the men of rational progress, by Thomas Longmore, Almroth Wright and William Leishman, it seemed Man's very spiritual existence, x-rayed and examined, was about to be empirically proved, and all the advances of the century vindicated; as though the old faith in God had been replaced by faith in humanity itself. This progressive history, of which everyone felt themselves a part, would conclude in a *fin-de-siècle* assertion of imperial power on the South African veldt.

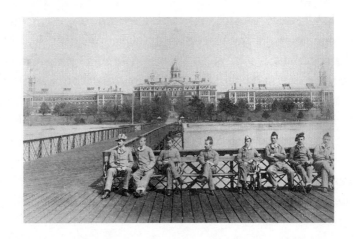

Another turn-of-the-century photograph, taken at the end of the hospital pier, shows a group of Boer War veterans, among them one particularly insouciant figure, handsome in an English manner, moustachioed, his cavalry hat turned up on one side. The pier on which he and his fellows lounge has long since proved useless for landing troops, and is now given over to recreation, as though to echo the resorts of Bournemouth and Brighton. Victorian piers were built for pleasure and health – to allow the inhalation of health-giving ozone from the sea – and as its usefulness as a landing place was limited, Netley's promenade had become a therapeutic amenity, a welcome escape from the rigours, duties and demands of the great building behind it.

With its glazed shelters and viewing bays for promenading convalescents, the pier presented an idyllic prospect, as though admission to the hospital were akin to going on holiday. In this resort scene the soldiers relax as they take the air dressed in their blue 'pyjama' uniforms, known as 'hospital undress'. They might as well be sporting striped blazers and straw boaters, waiting for the band to strike up, winking at the girls who pass by with their parasols and bustles. Their duties are behind them – for a while, at least. Their world has no reason to doubt itself, and out on Netley's pier they bathe optimistically in the glories of an imperial sun.

On 16 May 1900, Victoria made her last trip to her hospital. The great corridors were lined for the occasion with 100 men of the Royal Army Medical Corps and 500 palms and potted plants bought from a Southampton florist. Attended by a rustling silk and gold-braided selection of her extensive royal family with their Germanic titles – Battenberg princes, a Schleswig-Holstein princess* – the Queen's visit took advantage of a new development, one which was soon to see more use than its constructors could ever have imagined: the hospital's own railway station. The line which had been built to serve Netley in the 1860s now branched off directly to the hospital itself, and like a delighted little old lady, Victoria pronounced it 'a remarkable improvement'.

The difference was that, from her seaside villa on the Isle of Wight, this little old lady had ruled over a third of the world. A year later, her body lay in state in Osborne's Dining Room, surrounded by four motionless Grenadier Guards in scarlet and swathed in clouds of white silk; after decades of dressing in black, Victoria forbade it for her own mourning, stipulating white and

---

* Vicky, her grand-daughter, who had also knitted a shawl for the benefit of the hospital's patients.

purple, the colours of bridal innocence and imperial triumph. As the sun set on the evening of 1 February 1901, the Queen was carried across the Solent for the last time. The Victorian era had ended, and its presiding spirit was gone. An Edwardian lull overtook England, but its brief gaiety was a mere afterglow. A sense of darkness and doubt would descend on the Empire, and without its steadfast patron, Netley's great hospital was set adrift in an uncertain century.

Enter His Gates with Thanksgiving

As I stood there, trying to trace the line of the ancient walls I thought: 'Shall I write about the Lion Heart who sailed from Southampton in 1189; or about the *Speedwell* and the *Mayflower* which set off to found Broadway a little later; or about that last most glorious of Southampton epics when the long troop-trains came in, one after the other, that August night in 1914, before most people knew of the thing that was to change our lives and our thoughts?'

H. V. MORTON, *In Search of England*

———

The hospital, and the railway that bore it, had brought order and industry to this quiet Hampshire shore. Anywhere else Netley would have been little more than a minor stop on the mainline of the great spider's web of rail, but since its arrival the hospital had turned a village halt into the third busiest station in the country, constantly thronged with casualties arriving from Southampton Docks, supplies from around the country, or staff such as Professor Longmore on his way from Sholing. The platform was often so busy that the local vicar claimed to have once seen no less than 500 men on it.

A photograph shows Netley's station staff assembled by a bench, in their tight buttoned tunics and smart caps, dedicated to their jobs, sternly overseen by the station-master, serving the passengers going to and from the hospital on its new branch line. Only a youthful figure lounging on the end of the bench strikes a different note: the bookstall manager, somewhere in his twenties, sits back on his hips, legs astride, hat pushed back, stiff collar straining around his neck, looking sullen and handsome in a vaguely foreign, faintly spivvish manner. Perhaps, besides his newspapers and sweets and the postcards displayed on the regulation W. H. Smith revolving stand, he sold 'exotic' photographs as a little under-the-counter sideline.

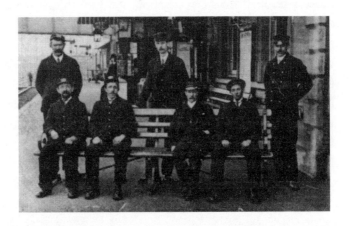

It's 1910: down the line that diverts deceptively into the trees, the great hospital is lulled by the Edwardian peace. Its corridors and wards are quiet after the clamour of the South African War, returning to the regular trickle of casualties and convalescents. But within a few years, the freedom of the dandy bookseller will be curtailed by the summons of military service, not in South Africa or India, but just across the Channel; an expedition from which he might return to Netley as a casualty in the first summer of a world war.

Back at home it would be business as usual under an August sun. On Southampton's much-admired High Street, with its Georgian bay windows and bicycles and trams riding under the

Bargate's great medieval arch, women in short skirts and men in boaters strolled the warm pavements, and the sea lapped at the old stone walls that still circled the town and even now seemed ready to defend island Britain. Secure in the victories of the past, in those photogravure scenes of heroism, they believed it would all be over by Christmas; that the volunteers they cheered to France in flag-waving send-offs from the quays of Southampton Docks would return in glory and in time for their Christmas dinners. They could not know, as those at Netley's hospital knew, what was really going on across the Channel.

The boats that bore the men away were coming back, but with cargoes of broken bodies. At Netley, the ambulance train with its beds like shelves in a cupboard would bring back the young bookseller's body, down the branch line, the familiar skyline rising out of the trees and sea mist, a city of the sick. The carriage would pull slowly into the hospital platform behind the chapel, and disgorge its load into the dark interior.

The new line which had so gladdened the old Queen now brought a war which A. J. P. Taylor described as 'an unexpected climax to the railway age'. Just as the railway had spread across the country, the creator of new suburbs and their commuters, so now it shunted young men into the heart of Europe's darkness, as though they had taken the morning train, not from New Malden to Waterloo, but from placid England to the blasted Western Front, and on the return journey delivered their wounded bodies to the hospital's back door.

Another photograph, taken five years later on just such a summer's day, shows a busy morning at the hospital station itself. The platform is crowded with waiting soldiers. In the foreground stand three railway workers with shovels at the ready; shirt-sleeves and high shadows indicate the heat of the day; their coats are thrown over the nearby wire fence.

But this summer is shrouded by war. Some of the soldiers are in regular uniform, upright and healthy, but others wear hospital undress, propped up on crutches, arms in slings or legs missing. Some have kitbags at their feet, returning to duty; some are in

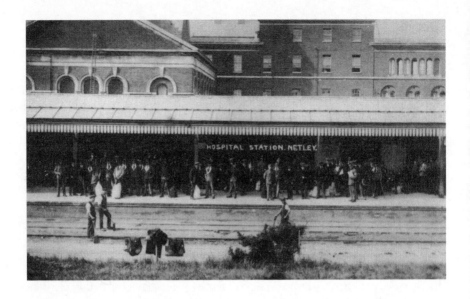

civvies, gratefully discharged; and some are mere blurs in the background, already ghosts, having moved as the camera's slow shutter opened. Visible behind the station canopy is the chapel's gable with an empty ladder propped up against it; beyond are tall walls, unadorned like their façade with dressed stone. This is the back of the hospital, the view most familiar to most of its inmates in their daily grind.

Each room could tell its own story, but from the outside, these windows betray only darkness as they stand open to let in the breeze, to air the stifled wards so disdained by Florence Nightingale. (She had died in 1910, before the beginning of a war which would have both appalled her and proved her reservations correct.) At one window is the tiny figure of one of her doughty nurses, resting her elbows on the sill, taking a moment away from the matron's stern gaze. Unobserved, she watches the photographer releasing his shutter on the far side of the embankment, watching us down the years, watching down the line to see what the next train will bring.

Through the sliding platform doors that admit the new arrivals – doors symbolic not of abandoned hope, but of suspended life – the diurnal industry of the hospital continues: unstoppable, continual, perpetual motion, running to order like an enormous machine. The hydraulic lifts moving up and down in their cages; the kitchens clattering with pots and pans; the children chanting times tables in the school. The horses stamping the ground in the stables; the carriages being polished. The baskets of 'foul linen' going into the laundry, the starched white sheets coming out. The x-ray equipment powered by a great turbine like one of Brunel's engines; the brass wheels turning in the generating station and the gasworks pumping gas. The spiralling snakes like embryos in their jars, the silent eyeless skulls in the museum. The traction wards with rows of shattered limbs suspended like lines of hammocks in the bowels of a drunken ship, holding arms and legs at weird right-angles to their owners' bodies; the doctors in their surgeries; the students at their laboratory benches. The operating theatres, with their blue and white enamel kidney dishes on tubular metal stands, and their tables with drains emptying into buckets below; the rubber tubes, the urine flasks, the metal syringes; the rolled-up bandages and the blue and brown glass bottles locked in rows of cupboards. The lime pits and incinerator; the sluices and latrines; the nursery and the mortuary. The countless rooms and occupations, the men and women scrubbing and washing, learning and dissecting, cooking and sleeping, eating and dying to the subconscious rhythm of military drill, compressed and quickened by the urgency of war.

Suddenly war was no longer remote battles of imperial troops in foreign lands. Now it was audibly, almost tangibly just across the sea. Troopships which had come to Netley from outposts of the Empire now had only to travel the short distance which pre-war steam packets would undertake twice a day, ferrying men back and forth on deadly military day-trips. The Channel might have insulated England from the theatre of war, but Netley, where men arrived with the mud of the trenches still on their khaki puttees, was as much a part of the war zone as any field dressing station.

On this secured site, the inhabitants were privy to the truths being denied to their civilian counterparts on the other side of

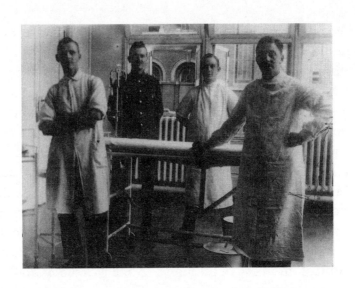

the hospital gates. Military police guarded German prisoners on surgical wards; the mutilated bodies and minds of allies and enemies shared darkened rooms, facing the reality of their changed world, a world closed to outsiders, for fear of undermining their morale. Denial and misinformation were becoming invaluable tools of war. For the first time, war exerted social control over the population, proscribing normal life by the despised Defence of the Realm Acts, known as Dora, applied to football matches and drug abuse, licensing laws and espionage, newspaper censorship and the keeping of pigeons alike. It was as if the entire country were under the same discipline that ruled the hospital, the same military rule book.

Armageddon might be in progress, but at Netley everything was determined by rigid routine, marching to a martial beat: polished, buffed, filled out in triplicate, signed and stamped and filed away. The regime altered only on one day of the week. On Sundays the inmates in their blue suits and red ties would be trooped, wheeled or pushed into the chapel under the high doorway which enjoined them, in bold gothic script written over its arch, to 'Enter His Gates with Thanksgiving'. Just as we schoolboys had filed into our chapel from our classroom corridors for Mass, so Netley's inmates shuffled in to fill the wooden pews and the galleries above, Catholics to one side, Protestants to the other; only the bed-ridden were excused.

Here the men assembled under plaques to doctors who had died in exotic wars that now seemed the stuff of an ancient civilisation: Surgeon Major Peter Shepherd killed by an assegai 'at the massacre of Isandula, [sic] Zululand'; Surgeon Joseph Heath 'killed in Upper Burma in 1886 whilst attempting to rescue an officer of the Hampshire Regiment ... shot ... by Burmese Dacoits who then savagely hacked off his head'. Under such vivid reminders of their carers' mortality, the soldiers sang a mournful hymn, were preached at about God and Country, Providence and Duty, then returned upstairs, and down corridors with row after row of uniform windows on one side and glass doors painted dark green on the other.

Their Victorian cloisters were 'excellently protected promenades' claimed optimistic press reports; yet the men that could walk them might as well have been monks, trapped in Netley's new 'horrible' site, where visitors were a rarity. The cell-like wards and tunnel-like passages seemed more than ever to be an earthly limbo: the innerspace of the hospital ceaselessly paced by staff going about their business by flickering daylight or gaslit night, while limbless soldiers on crutches reached one end of the building and had to turn and face the other, as if they hadn't left the corridors of the trains that brought them here.

At Netley the movement was never ending; a place designed for recuperation in wartime had ironically little time or space for rest. Its corridors became crowded alleys where the swelling population of the hospital spilled out, iron bedsteads crammed into every bay. In another irony, the very enormity of the war and the limitations of the hospital allowed a few patients a glimpse of the sea view denied to their mates in the sunless wards. As nurses bustled to and fro, those wives and girlfriends who had made the difficult wartime journey to Netley crouched by soldiers' beds which stood in the passageways like posh passengers in steamer chairs on the quarterdeck, the faded stripes of the canvas blinds pulled down against the glare of the sun.

Snapped by local photographers, postcard views of these makeshift wards were sent home by recuperating casualties to those loved ones who couldn't make it this far. In the sepia and silver nitrate images which had become the signature of Netley's hospital, each corridor stretched into infinity, past the faces of nurses and orderlies looking tentatively towards the camera, waiting to get on with their work. The lights covered with brown paper shades, the framed pictures, the wicker chairs and potted palms attempted to create something domestic out of the great passageways, although the result was more like one great railway waiting room, its passengers uniformly clad in blue.

The sheer scale and function of the hospital defied such attempts to cut it down to size. A junior VAD nurse who served at Netley during the First World War recalled life in this 'badly-designed and useless building':

> I clearly remember as I walked through the corridors of the ground floor daily, thinking how amazing it was that all the suffering men lying in their beds there did not die of double pneumonia and not of the wounds sustained in that terrible war . . . Netley Hospital was full in every floor and the corridors were lined on either side with beds and patients, leaving a narrow passageway between the beds. Behind all this glass so admired by some of the public the poor patient either froze in winter, or blistered in heat in the summer. Of those in the dark wards behind, theirs was an unhappy existence too. No view from the front and only the kitchen, coal heaps and general administrative collection at the back, not very health-giving to stricken soldiers. Excellent surgery and nursing by the doctors and Army sisters was unstintingly given to them all, in the most appalling working circumstances.

The reservations of Netley's nineteenth-century critics had been proved correct – even though they could not have imagined the contingency which would do so. In 1881, the Red Cross had sent its nurses to train for 'future emergencies' at Netley, but the pattern of Victorian wars for which they were prepared – fought out of England in the Khyber Pass or the Sudan, their victims decorously inhabiting Netley's wards, all neat in their moustaches and hospital undress – was overturned by the mayhem and mud of the Great War. Uncontained by its now bursting wards and untidy corridors, the hospital had already spilled out into the fields that surrounded it during the South African War when the Red Cross organised the construction of German 'Doecker' huts of canvas and felt, 'presented as a sort of advertisement of their firm in Berlin'.

Now the 'future emergencies' had come to pass, and soon after war was declared, the Red Cross offered the War Office a 500-bed 'hutted hospital'. The offer was accepted on condition that it was designed to be dismantled and shipped to France if necessary. The result was a camp of twenty-five prefabricated 'Fairley Fieldhouses', each accommodating twenty-five patients and funded by appeals – the greatest donations coming from Australia and New Zealand. Beds were sponsored by local organisations and individuals, their contributions to the war effort marked by thick brass plates above the metal-framed beds.

Towards the end of the year, another 'hutted hospital' was added, donated by the Welsh Ministry of Pensions. It held 200 beds, and cost £16,600: the *South Wales Argus* noted that 'The Welsh hospital has come from the generosity of the Welsh people ... it costs £250 to endow one bed and £2 to equip a bed.' It was becoming clear, as the war refused to end by Christmas and casualties escalated, that the temporary huts would not only become permanent, but would multiply over the months and years. In March a third hospital of ten huts was officially opened on St Patrick's Day and was known as the Irish Hospital after its donor, Edward Guinness, Viscount Iveagh, who had pledged £10,000 a year for its upkeep.

These new medical suburbs, named after the constituent nations of Great Britain and raised on sometimes competitive philanthropy, grew in direct proportion to the action on the Western Front as an echo of its expanding trenches and field stations. Soon what had been open land became an entire settlement in its own right: gated and fenced and patrolled, part military camp, part charitable donation; a hubub of humanity in varying states of health and disease. Spreading out over the windy plateau, this overgrown cottage hospital was hidden from the traffic passing through Southampton Water by the main building, as if to conceal from the troops the true extent of the war to which they were being sent, and its likely consequences for them. Only the revealing lens of the latest aerial photograph of the site could expose the massive scale of Netley during wartime.

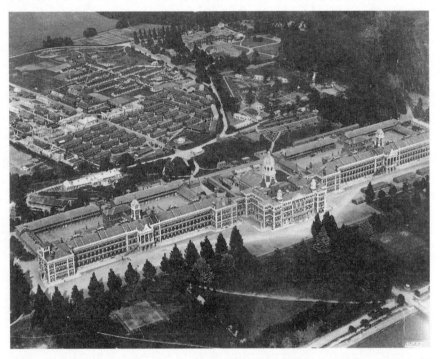

The hospital during the First World War. A walk around the site would find the hospital at its greatest extent, an inflated settlement of huts eddying in the main hospital's wake, from the A, B and C Blocks of the central building to the encampments of the Red Cross, Welsh and Irish hospitals. Later, as the overspill increased, an encampment of bell tents would appear on the fields behind them. At the top is the military asylum; in the triangle between, the isolation hospital and the stables.

Where the older hospital replicated itself in its eternal rows of windows, the new establishment was made of countless rows of huts, stretching back into the hinterland like an army town, coursed with lanes and paths. Expanding ever outwards just as the war itself spread across Europe's plains, this was utilitarian, pragmatic construction. Unlike the grand edifice of the older hospital – its façade now marred by wooden scaffolding-like temporary stairs which had been built out from the elegant porticoes, and dining huts for nurses constructed on the gravel driveway in front – the hutches of the hutted hospital aspired to no architectural distinction; it could spare no time for such niceties. This was a temporary, single-minded community, its business evident in the arterial thoroughfare funnelling the wounded up from the hospital station and dubbed 'Piccadilly' in the same ironic spirit that gave Spike Island its name. It was yet more ironic that a settlement partly funded by Australians should echo both those mythic camps on Sholing Common and their New World destination, 'the pad on which England drew its sketches for the immense Gulags of the twentieth century'; as though Botany Bay and Spike Island had come to Hampshire's coast, from one fatal shore to another.

Captain M. S. Esler was a doctor at the Norwich Hospital, Norfolk, when he volunteered for service with the RAMC in August 1914, and was sent to Netley. 'Many new huts were being built there to house the large number of wounded that poured into Southampton daily in the hospital ships', he wrote. 'As staff quarters had not been completed, we were housed temporarily in an hotel in Southampton where we had breakfast and were then conveyed by car to the ferry which crossed Southampton Waters [sic] and, by road again, on to Netley. I always remember the delightful fresh seaweed smell as we crossed the water.'

Lulled by its apparently idyllic setting, Esler's initial impressions of Netley were cheery. After a month, he and his colleagues moved on to the site, 'slept in a hut, and had our meals in the original hospital. Life was pleasant enough there, it was like being a house surgeon again. For recreation there was a private golf course and billiard rooms where we regaled ourselves after dinner in the evenings. I knew that I would be there only for a short time, as the younger men were waiting for a posting to more adventurous surroundings.' But in the coming weeks, Netley would give Captain Esler 'two warning notes on the future'.

The first came as he watched the troopships passing in and out of Southampton Docks: 'There were still plenty of young men who were ready to cheer and to sing "Tipperary" on their first trip out'; but the returning vessels were hospital ships, 'full of wounded and suffering humanity, and from these ships no sound emerged, the illusions of a rapid and glorious victory had ended in maimed bodies and in many maimed minds'. The second warning came 'when talking to an officer in the Scottish Highlanders who had had his knee blown off, and had received chest wounds, and suffered much on the Mons retreat'. Esler told the officer he was 'anxious to get out and see how things were at the front. He stared at me and said "Do you really mean that?" I told him that I did, and, to quote his exact words, he said, "I think you must be bloody well mad".'

Three months later, Captain Esler left Netley to serve on the Western Front and in Salonika, where, like so many others, he was quickly disabused of any optimistic ideas he had about war, not only through his work with the wounded and dying, but in his witness of a military court martial and execution of a deserter. For him the war was brought to an abrupt halt not by a bullet, but when he was captured in Champagne and taken as a prisoner of war to another bleak settlement of huts, the Denholme (Stralsund) camp in north Germany.

Meanwhile, back on the English south coast, war had turned the whole of Southampton into one gigantic military camp. Wyndham Lewis had envisioned England as an 'industrial island machine', a Vorticist image which seemed to have become reality in this southern port, this martial engine. Designated 'Military

Embarkation Port Number One' – as if to emphasise its conversion from civilian status to extended theatre of war – Southampton was the point of departure, supply and repair for the massive movement of men and materiel, its grey cranes, dazzle-painted ships and khaki platoons resembling the angular futurity of a William Roberts painting. Every twenty-four hours saw shipments of ammunition worth one million pounds; twenty-five to thirty transports a night would leave the docks, fed by the twenty-four-hour production line of the armaments factory which had been built on the Chamberlayne estate at Weston, where my great-grandfather was employed. With its own great brick bulk ranged along the waterside, it was the industrial equivalent of Netley's hospital, working day and night to feed the insatiable military machine.

Southampton Water was black with ships. This was military movement on an unprecedented scale. In the South African War the town had dealt with half a million men, 400 troopships and 27,000 horses, and welcomed back in return Lord Kitchener and the heroes of Ladysmith and Mafeking. Now, as the British Expeditionary Force – even the name seemed to recall colonial wars – shipped out, it returned chewed up by the mechanised process of modern warfare. From August 1914 to December 1918, twelve hundred ambulance trains arrived at Netley, almost daily, 'and if there had been an offensive in France, two or more in a day', recalled one Red Cross nurse. In the weeks after the battle of the Somme in 1916, 151 trains brought 30,000 from Southampton Docks, decanted down canvas-sided gangplanks and placed in stretchered rows on the platforms at the dockside terminus, there to wait for the ambulance trains, their bandaged bodies on public display while the business of the station went on around them.

One nurse serving on the Front wrote of the injuries she witnessed. Some had 'Blighty' injuries, lightly borne and enough to get them home, but 'there were other wounded men from whom no laughter came, nor any sound'.

They were carried on to the train on stretchers, laid down awhile on the wooden platforms, covered with blankets up to their chins, – unless they uncovered themselves with convulsive movements. I saw one young Londoner so smashed about the face that only his eyes were uncovered between layers of bandages, and they were glazed with the first film of death. Another had his jaw clean blown away, so the doctor told me . . . A splendid boy of the Black Watch was but a living trunk. Both his arms and legs were shattered. If even he lived after butcher's work of surgery he would be one of those who go about in boxes on wheels, from whom men turn their eyes away, sick with a sense of horror . . .

Outside a square brick building . . . the 'bad' cases were unloaded: men with chunks of steel in their lungs and bowels were vomiting great gobs of blood, men with arms and legs torn from their trunks, men without noses, and their brains throbbing through opened scalps, men without faces . . .

An ambulance train was 'one of the grimmest sights of the First World War', not least for those nurses who had to deal with its consignment. 'Its arrival was announced by a bugle, and all the hospital gates were closed', recalled a Red Cross nurse. 'No one could go in or out . . . until the coaches had been unloaded . . .' As the wounded were brought into the hospital, both trained military nurses – Nightingale's protégées – and 'amateur' VADs worked alongside each other to deal with soldiers who arrived labelled like luggage with their name, number, regiment, type of wound and whether or not they had received an anti-tetanus injection, 'but sometimes the label read GOK (God only knows)'. Young women who might never have left home now found themselves syphoning obscene-smelling pus from deep wounds, bandaging gangrenous feet from which toes would fall off like pegs, and carrying out baskets of severed limbs from operating theatres. 'Pain-killers were distributed sparingly, blood transfusions were in their infancy and there was a constant fear of haemorrhages after amputations'. One VAD recalled being sent round the wards on night duty with a torch 'looking under the bedclothes for the first eight or ten days after an operation to make sure nothing had gone wrong'.

With the majority of British wounded arriving via Southampton, many were destined for the building they passed on Southampton Water. For a casualty shipped over the Channel, having come through field hospitals and stations, arriving here must have seemed like nothing had changed. Looking forward to coming home, they found themselves shunted into yet another camp in this south coast cul-de-sac; one returning soldier wrote 'I cannot believe myself back in England in this unknown region.'

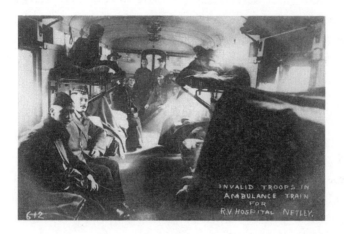

As the ambulance train slowed towards its final destination, it would be apparent that you were approaching the heart of a huge medical-military operation from the traffic coming in and out of the gateway and its sentries; the flat land still largely unsheltered by trees was filled with a teeming, ever-shifting population of doctors and patients. Then, as the train passed the hutted hospital and rounded the bend, the main hospital would reveal its bulk through a pine curtain. For some, the sight of its dead end brick walls produced a sinking weight in the pit of their

189

stomach. It must have been a trepidatious moment, inspiring a mixture of relief, awe and fear. For many, Netley's towers and domes signalled England; some seemed to hold out just long enough to see their homeland again. But for the Belgian, Canadian, Serbian, Russian or Indian soldiers brought here, they might as well have been on another planet as on this foreign shore.

In the hutted hospital, a phalanx of twenty-two Japanese nurses, faces knitted against the sun, sit serenely for a group photograph. Arranged diminutively in rows around their leader Dr Jiro Suzuki, this deputation had come from the land of the rising sun to offer their services for free. In other photographs, other, less exotic figures are scattered around the site: some hopeful, some taut with pain, some bored, looking out from the album compiled by Lady Emily Crooke-Lawless, wife of the camp commandant, Surgeon Lieutenant-Colonel Sir Warren Crooke-Lawless.

Camped on the plain like some colonial outpost, the huts stand in line, apparently little more than wooden tents, or, from the air, a particularly regimented model village. But on close examination, you can see more permanent-looking buildings with glass verandahs, pebble-dash walls and vaguely Arts and Crafts timbering; echoes of suburbia. One postcard displays the Maxine Elliot Operating Theatre, named after the famous stage star who 'equipped' it. This was a modern establishment, after all, sponsored by celebrities and purpose-built to accommodate twentieth-century warfare and its demands. Large huts contained electrical equipment – funded by a donation from the Maharaja of Gawalior – used to treat nerve-damaged legs, or special baths in which burns victims could be kept for up to five weeks, lying like Marat in the curative water. In others were treated the victims of chemical warfare: gas wards were also set up in the main hospital to deal with this terrifying new weapon.

The hutted hospital, for all its temporary nature, contained examples of the scientific developments which Thomas Longmore and Almroth Wright had worked towards; as one album assembled by a Red Cross nurse noted, in slangy rhyme:

V is for Vaccine just now all the fashion
For which Captain Steven has got quite a passion

and

Y stands for Yanks who to Netley have come,
& of up-to-date surgery they're now learning some

The same album displays a photograph of the arched gate to the 'Power House Camp', yet another addendum to the hutted hospital. Even when 'we seemed to have got to the end of the extension', noted one doctor, 'it was not, however, to be so, for the Senior Physician (Major Snowden) had always wished for an open-air hut for tubercle cases, and eventually the Committee decided to build one . . .'* In another row of balconied rooms facing the sea on the edge of the plateau, other convalescents could lie in the sun as they breathed in the ozone. The doctor concerned was relieved that with the building of the TB hut the hospital's expansion had finally come to a halt, 'for the very good reason that no more ground remains . . . Indeed, it is just as well no more space is available. Distance lends enchantment to the view, but when you have to cover the ground many times a day it gets tiresome . . .'

The hutted hospital was a sharp contrast to the building it overlooked. Its open structure was conceived with the ability to reassemble it on the battlefield in mind; unlike its brick counterpart, it was built for a modern war, and the result had the air of something between a French field station and a barracks on Salisbury Plain. Soldiers sat out on the stoeps, watching the new arrivals wheeled up 'Piccadilly' on bier-like hand carts. Filled with men and women and movement, the camp echoed to a Babel of tongues – another byproduct of modern war and its

---

* Arthur de Winton Snowden was Hon. Major RAMC in charge of the Medical Section of the Red Cross Hospital. A specialist in tuberculosis, he had served as a civil surgeon in the South African War for which he was awarded the Queen's Medal with four bars.

assimilation of colonial culture and imperial values. When Indian soldiers at Netley were deprived of their puggree headdresses, they 'were a little upset about the loss', noted the local paper, and 'not at all enthusiastic about the head wraps provided as a substitute'. Hearing of the situation, Queen Alexandra 'at once' sent 400 yards of lawn muslin, but, as the paper reported, the Indians did not use the material, but carefully packed it away 'for safekeeping'. With thousands of Hindus serving in the war, Netley also catered to their other religious requirements: a funeral pyre or *ghat* was built in the woods where their bodies could be cremated in the open air and the ashes scattered into the stream below, there to flow into Southampton Water and back, eventually, to meet with the waters of the River Ganges.

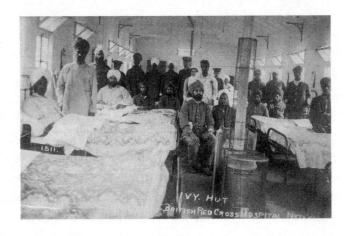

With no Queen Empress and her retinue of Indian attendants to alight from Osborne, other royal figures came to represent the Empire for which these men were fighting. On 30 July 1917 King George, Queen Mary, Princess Mary 'and their Suite', visited Netley. The King, bearded and taciturn in his uniform, walks solemnly through the camp, accompanied by Crooke-Lawless; Queen Mary, her toque rather like a turban itself, looks down on a man propped up on a wheeled stretcher, joined by two nurses, each crowned with starched white butterfly, and an officer in his khaki peaked cap. The object of their pity is hatless, his head covered, not by a turban, but by a bandage. His eyes appear half-shut; he does not even seem to register their presence as the visitors talk over him. In another scene in the main hospital's corridor, the Queen, her daughter beside her, halts over a soldier, a parable of patronage and philanthropy.

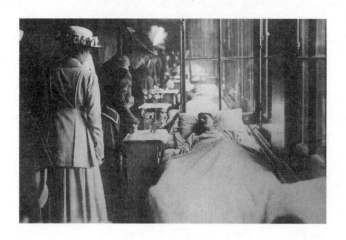

As with Victoria's visits, reports of such events strove to exemplify the spirit that had built the Empire; *The Times* was almost inspired to poetry: 'As you turn aslant towards the grey buildings and the Red Cross flag you become aware of the recumbent figures in blue suits lying in sunny spots quietly reading ... A gay infectious laugh is heard, and looking up an alley between the wards we see two men in blue approaching on two legs – not two legs each – and two crutches; and they have some merry jest between them! This happiness is the dominating spirit of the British Red Cross Hospital at Netley.' It was the same distillation of national war spirit displayed on generic coloured postcards, overprinted with Netley's name, which portrayed a remarkably healthy-looking and handsome invalid soldier in neat hospital undress, a pretty nurse hovering over his shoulder, and the caption below, 'Are we Downhearted? No! not at NETLEY.'

In hundreds of war hospitals – from Netley's huge sprawl to the few-roomed annexe that Mayfield House in Weston had become – these were the sentiments which carried people through;

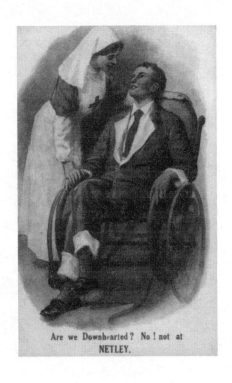

Are we Downhearted? No! not at
NETLEY.

the people at home, at least. Such happiness-in-adversity – the
bulldog spirit, the backbone of empire – may have presented itself
to a reporter on a day-trip from London, briefed by his editor and
steered about by officers determined like apparatchiks to show
him the best aspects of the place: its progressive treatments and
cheery wards of recuperating patients, the cinema where men
laughed at the antics of Charlie Chaplin, the Godwin Reading
Room where they could indulge their intellect. All this was
undoubtedly the good work of the Red Cross – unencumbered
by the military history of their counterparts in the older, darker,
decidedly old-fashioned building (which, as the nurse's albums
showed, already had cracked windows and an air of faint derelic-
tion about it). But for all his well-meaning enthusiasm, the man
from *The Times* could return to Netley station without the aid
of crutches, leaving behind the flat monotone of those utilitarian
grey garage-like sheds, broken only by the saturated crimson of
the Red Cross itself, a vivid symbol of care, the mortal imprimatur of war, a crusader's emblem; a multiple of suffering just as

194

those mass-produced cards were a multiple of patriotism. It was prescient of things to come, just as the huts' Berlin-built predecessors had been constructed of canvas and felt, and just as future huts would rise from European fields.

In those grey huts, and inside the brick behemoth that blocked their view of the sea, lay the deconstructed shapes of humanity, victims of the technological advance that had built the hospital, marked out by the blue of their 'pyjamas'. Where medieval victims of the plague had their doors painted with red crosses, wartime hospitals would paint park benches blue to warn the public that their occupants might have mere holes where their faces should be.

The blue of 'hospital undress' gave patients seats on buses and kept them out of public bars; it indicated a halfway existence, a limbo outfit that was neither military uniform nor civilian clothing; an inescapable branding that could also prevent desertion and curtail their freedom. In that it foreshadowed a later uniform, the broad stripes of another sort of institutional outfit worn two decades later. Less than twenty years after the British had pioneered the concept in South Africa, Netley itself – with its rows of huts, its railway terminus and its corralled, pyjama'd inmates being shunted to and from the Front – had begun to look uncomfortably like a concentration camp.

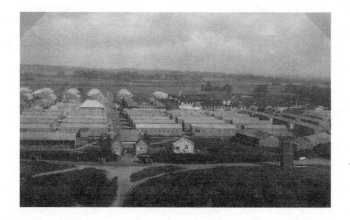

Remembrance Day

Footfalls echo in the memory
Down the passage which we did not take
Towards the door we never opened

T. S. ELIOT 'Burnt Norton'

M y mother was born in Southampton three years after the end of the First World War. On days out with her father, she would often visit Netley, and watched as the blue-clad patients taking the sea air, some laid prone in 'spinal carriages' like prams for grown men complete with fold-up leather hoods. For a little girl, these shuffling figures were a vivid contrast to her own adored and healthy father who had been lucky enough to survive the war unscathed.

My grandfather, Frederick, a bandsman corporal in the Hampshire Regiment, had spent the war in Meerut and Amballa, northern India (his territorial battalion had been sent to free regular soldiers for service on the Western Front) and Aden (where 'rounds were exchanged' with the Turkish enemy). Family photographs show the men on a training exercise before they left for India in January 1915. My grandfather, a lean young man looking older than his nineteen years, stands proudly to attention outside his bell tent. Elsewhere he and his mates are snapped in the middle of ablutions, one man with his feet in a bucket, others

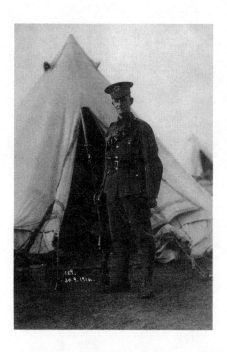

bare to the waist, their red-brown tans stopping abruptly at their necks where lard-white skin begins. Arm-in-arm, they are ready to do their bit, 'keeping the King Emperor's peace' in a foreign land.

Frederick's war belonged to the dusty campaigns of Egypt

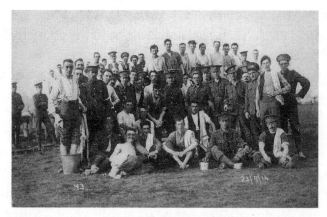

1/7th Battalion, Hampshire Regiment, September 1914 – Frederick seated, second on right

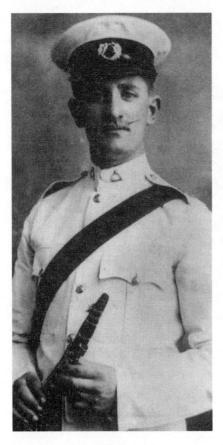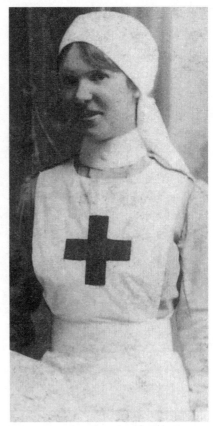

and South Africa, with their lancers and pith helmets and orderly formations, rather than the mustard gas, tanks and trenches of Europe. His war was invested with earlier, optimistic, imperial actions which we could win, and which underlined our benevolent dominion over other races (who would pay the levy for their loyalty by contributing one-third of the forces that fought in the Great War). My grandfather's twirled moustache, his smart uniform and his ivory and brass clarinet, his faith in his officers, all stood for another age. The ebony elephants and etched brass plates he brought back from India – suburban versions of the contents of Victoria's Durbar Hall – still stood on our shelves as I was growing up.

The couple had met when my grandmother, Florence – a

Christian name made popular by the heroine of the Crimea – was nursing the daughter of the Spanish ambassador in Bournemouth. Frederick was then a bandsman playing in the local park along with his father and uncles; Florence would sit in front of the bandstand, mischievously sucking a lemon to put her boyfriend off his clarinet. When war came, she followed in the footsteps of her namesake; in August 1916 she enlisted as a VAD and was sent to work at the 3rd West General Hospital in Cardiff. The family album shows her diminutive and sweet in her stiff high collar, her fair red hair tightly wrapped in a wimple-like scarf around her pale, small features, the picture of my sister, her white apron emblazoned with a red cross on its bib; even in black and white you can sense its redness. In another picture she poses with a wardful of soldier patients in their blue pyjama uniforms.

It is Christmas: the gas pipes and lamps are entwined with holly and ivy, and a large Union Jack has been pinned to the wall. Later, she would serve in military hospitals in Bath and

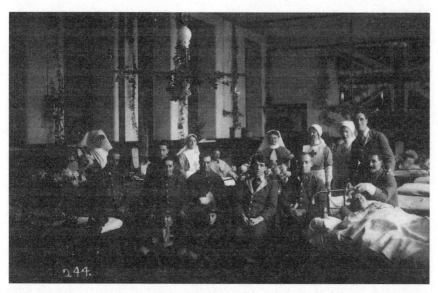

3rd West General Hospital, Cardiff, 1916 – Florence second nurse from the right

Birmingham, winning her scarlet 'efficiency stripes'. Pretty and lively, Nanny was a popular nurse: when she left, in March 1919, she gathered autographs of her soldier boys in an album, in which one wrote, 'To the only nurse who can take my eye out without it hurting.' Afterwards she kept a bottle of chloroform hidden in her bedroom drawer, which my mother, as a little girl, would go up and sniff. My grandfather had proposed marriage to her before he was posted abroad, before the War put a continent between them. Either doubting his affection, or hers, my grandmother broke off the engagement twice, sending her engagement ring all the way back to India, only for it to return as they made up. When peace was declared, Frederick returned to the building trade – helped by his army officer and friend, also a builder, even through the depression that quickly followed the brief post-war boom. Only then did they marry, my grandfather in his new suit, his wife in her veil and lace, standing in the porch of her parents' house, the thin smiles on their faces the smiles of survivors, of witnesses.

Frederick built their own house in Bitterne, where they would conduct their musical evenings, his wife on the violin, Fred on the clarinet, playing the plaintive songs of their time. For me, Netley became associated with the Great War through their music, through their memory at one remove. Peeling potatoes at the kitchen sink, my mother would sing the First World War songs which had been her lullabies: 'A Long Way to Tipperary', 'Pack Up Your Troubles', 'Roses of Picardy', 'Take Me Back to Dear Old Blighty'; wry, sentimental songs of loss and home, full of emotion (and, for me, anxiety) even generations after those who first sang them had died. In our house, as in thousands of others, stood brass-framed photographs of young men in khaki, distant participators in the War To End All Wars.

My father was born in 1915. He grew up in Bradford during the war, and his first memories were of wartime, overcast by the events around him, by the greater dramas that impacted on his small world, and on his family.

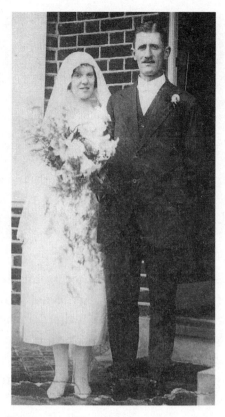

Florence and Frederick, Bitterne, 1920

Two of his uncles served on the Front; one was gassed and would never recover. There were few photographs of these vanished men in our house: only one was identifiable, standing next to my father's father at his wedding in 1914, photographed in a Shipley studio, an omnious year in which to marry. In the group of pre-war figures, laden with flowers that already look funereal, and centred around the substantial Victorian figure of my great-grandmother with her great grand face, stands Uncle Tom – neat moustache, sharply-dressed, head at an angle, but eyes fixed by the camera flash, as if suddenly aware of what the future held in store. He would die long after the war, which left him physically and mentally scarred, in the huge mental hospital of High Royds, near Shipley on the Yorkshire Moors. My father inherited

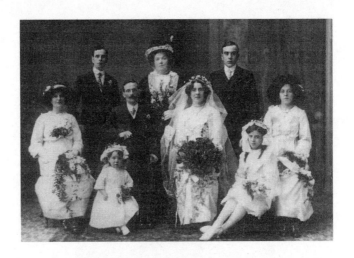

his gold signet ring, and passed it on to my brother, its entwined gothic initials saying as little of their owner's life as my father spoke of his past, rooted as it was in the dark romantic North, hundreds of miles away from Southampton's airier world.

His grandfather, my namesake and Tom's father, had lived in Whitby, working as a fisherman, then a coachman; he was originally from Ireland, from whence his family, and his wife's, had fled during the Great Famine. I imagined him as a young man, pushing out in his boat from Whitby Harbour, overlooked by its ruined abbey, site of Bram Stoker's *Dracula*, on one side, and on the other by its whalebone arch. The shops below it would be selling jet, the shiny fossilised mineral of Victorian mourning mined from the local cliffs and carved by workers – many with our family name – whose hands were turned black by their trade.

After my grandfather, Dennis, was born, the family moved again, down south to Bradford, where the mills offered work; there Dennis married in the year war began. As a tailor, his was a reserved occupation, and he too survived the war, only for his wife Josephine, my grandmother, to die suddenly when their eldest son was a teenager. One Saturday night, with Henry Hall on the wireless, she was dancing with my father, mother and son arm in arm, gently stepping around the room. Moments

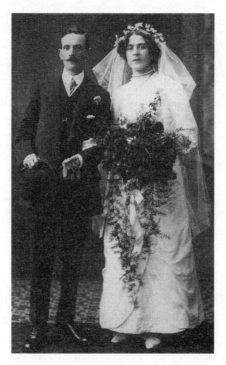

Dennis and Josephine, Bradford, 1914

later, after she had gone upstairs to bed, she collapsed with a heart attack, and was gone.

Three months later Dennis married his wife's best friend – someone had to look after the children – but members of the family refused to speak to him for months afterwards, their silence accusing him of disloyalty. His tailoring business burgeoned: he made suits for J. B. Priestley and a trench coat for Winston Churchill, and would make my father's wedding suit – photographs show its beautiful cut, as trim on my father as his father's suits were on him. Dennis always dressed elegantly, even in old age, in neatly-cut coat and waistcoat and fob-watch; he had a dandified wit to match, silver hair when I knew him, and bright, amused eyes.

But in the Depression, business slumped, and instead of pursuing his education, my father had to go out to work to help support his younger brothers and sisters. It was a harsh time.

He remembered a suicide found on waste ground near the factory in which he worked; there was a shed of some sort in which a man had slit his throat. In my mind – as I heard the story, as I remember it – I saw a bleak industrial landscape, the flat-capped crowd gathered silently round the victim, the policeman bringing a blanket to lay over his supine, drained body. Perhaps he had suffered from the same post-war despair which I imagined drove the inhabitant of a house at the top of our road in Sholing to slit his throat at the kitchen sink, standing with razor in hand (according to the local newspaper) as he bled, and discovered by his wife whose reported response in the 1921 newspaper – 'What have you done?' – sounded as though he'd broken a plate rather than cut his carotid artery.

Life was desperate for those who had survived Armageddon only to face deprivation. Their fate was easily forgotten, washed over with nostalgia and our soft southern ways. My father would recount his work with the Society of St Vincent de Paul, delivering food parcels to poverty-stricken families in the Thirties. 'You wouldn't believe there could be hunger like that in this country,' he would say, 'they would just grab the food out of your hands as soon as you came in the door.' For this we would feel grateful for the bread and jam on our plates in our comfortable suburban home.

Once a year we'd be roused before dawn, the windows still dark and the kitchen yellow with light as Mum filled the flasks. Outside in the wooden garage with its ladders suspended across the rafters, Dad, for once without a tie, packed our bags into the boot of the car, followed by us children, sleepy dust in our eyes, smuggling as many toys as we could into the Wolsey's deep leather seats. Then we'd set off through the empty streets, driving north, north for ever.

There was no motorway to speed us up the backbone of England, just A roads and B roads weaving through countryside. Through the dawn we'd recognise landmarks: the big house near Winchester, marked by its avenue of poplars, its distant windows hiding the ghost of an eighteenth-century royal mistress; the unbypassed Midland towns with clanking milk carts and news-agents just opening up; and the familiar sense of being drawn away from the south coast, irrevocably northwards. We'd stop on the way for our breakfast, the sun creeping up on our holi-day's horizon, drinking tea on the bonnet already hot from the journey, its engine ticking over in respite beneath. Then we'd drive on, the buildings around us exchanging their effete southern bricks for tough northern stone.

Compared to the seaside air and white stucco of Southampton, industrial Yorkshire was a black-brown place; the sooty stone houses, the wool mills and their chimneys made our home town look scrubbed and clean. Where Southampton was ordered and open, this place was grimy and knocked about, coursed with back alleys and brick terraces that seemed to reach over the moors. The legacy of industry was everywhere: in the very scale and monumentality of Bradford's public buildings, in Cartwright Hall with its Victorian beds of marigolds and salvias, a giant clock set surreally among them – I wondered how it could work in the rain – and huge petrified tree trunks, rusty brown like iron ore, oversized versions of the little chunk which stood on our rockery at home, a witness to passing dinosaurs.

On the hill stood Lister's mill, and all the other mills whose chimneys dominated the city's skyline. In a wooded valley was Sir Titus Salt's enlightened Saltaire, a workers' Utopia where every amenity was provided for employees so tyrannically treated elsewhere, Shelley's 'helots of luxury' weaving cloth for the Empire. Aunt Maureen said many of our Yorkshire relatives worked in the mills, including her mother, who had to have a certificate to allow her to be employed part-time while she was still at school. Nearby was the village of Haworth, its parsonage haunted by Bröntes in tiny-flowered dresses dying of consump-tion and destined for its graveyard of black-brown stones, while the shops sold souvenir rock shaped like walking sticks, as if they would help you climb the steep cobbled hill.

High on another hill in the Bradford suburb of Fagley, we'd

pull up outside our aunt and uncle's house, huge and solid in comparison to our southern semi, with its three floors, thick walls, and cellar full of home-made ginger beer. We were back in the world of my father's upbringing, and all our aunts and uncles: one aunt's endless hospitality, always in the kitchen, catering to her family's Yorkshire appetite; another aunt in her stone house on another hill between Bradford and Leeds; and Cyril, whose home was High Royds in Menston, the mental hospital on the edge of the moor in which my great uncle Tom had died. As a boy, a pan of scalding water had been upset on his head and he was 'never right' thereafter. But he seemed pretty normal to us, if a little taciturn and faintly shambling in his gait – the result of his medication rather than his condition, I'd only later realise. We would take him out for the afternoon to Ilkley Moor, walking to the strange flat stones of the Cow and Calf Rocks. Once we all got ice creams from a van parked on the moor: a drug-induced tremor shook Uncle Cyril's hand as he raised the cornet to his mouth and he missed, leaving a splodge of ice cream over his face; my mother went up and wiped it off. Then we'd drive back to the hospital and Dad would give Uncle Cyril the cigarettes he'd bought for him, and he would vanish back into the fluorescent-lit wards.

Late one summer night I came downstairs to watch the grainy footage of Neil Armstrong and Buzz Aldrin bumbling about on the moon, ghosts of the twenty-first century on a nuclear beach, delivered there by a craft cobbled together from scaffolding poles and bacofoil, awkward and ugly in comparison to the sleek, streamlined model from *2001* I'd make from a plastic kit. I watched this transcending moment of history through Victorian banisters in the house in Fagley Road, with its dark attic bed-rooms and a garden with roses made exquisite by Bradford soot, and the moon dust conflated with the soot in the air and the soot in the soil to produce miraculous pure white and crimson blooms, emblems of ancient wars which my parents too would plant in commemoration in our Southampton garden.

On our way to visit other uncles and aunts, we'd drive through

Cottingley, where fairies in Edwardian dresses convinced Conan Doyle of their existence, photographed at the bottom of a garden as if they'd become the fey spirits of the Flanders dead, its poppies psychically transformed. One year we stayed in our great aunt Lucy's terraced house, seemingly unchanged for a century. A little like a Cottingley fairy herself, Auntie Lucy was a fragile thing in a flowery pinny with the same sparkling eyes as our grandfather, her brother. A wistful, faintly sad sense of the past hung about her: it was her other brother Tom who'd been shell-shocked in the First World War. Later she'd married an Italian, and their seraphic daughter had died of meningitis at the age of two, an angel of mortality. Lucy taught my mother to crochet, and gave me an ancient copy of *The Pickwick Papers* with the original Cruikshank illustrations, its spine falling apart, and made tea in her tiny brown kitchen. We slept in the top of the house in iron beds with old quilts, the tiny dormer window looking out on a cobbled street, the light forcing its way in, fuzzy at the edges.

Aunt Lucy's was just like the house in which my father grew up, he said; it reminded me of what he'd told us about the harsh winters in Bradford, and how one morning Dad had woken up to find the snow drifted up to the height of his bedroom window, blocking the front door. The thick white snow must have appeared even whiter against the bricks and stone of a city where the streets seemed black. During the Depression my father had once seen a road in the town filled with a mass of rats coming towards him. He'd stood with his back pressed against the wall as the migrating rodents rushed downhill in full spate, a seething river of rats. It seemed these things happened in the North, where even the light was different. In another scene from a Bradford terrace, brown and black, bare tables and floors, Dad and his friends were playing cards one night. As they went to sit down, someone pulled the chair from behind another, a practical joke. The boy fell backwards to the ground, then asked who had turned the lights off; damaging his nervous system, the fall had sent him blind.

In such a world it seemed perfectly natural that the local shop where my father bought his sweets should be owned by Albert Pierrepoint, the public executioner. Some days it would be closed, and they'd know that the mild-mannered Mr Pierrepoint had taken the early morning train to London, carrying his black bag.

'Here at last was a town that had not fallen under the evil spell of our times', wrote J. B. Priestley, my grandfather's client, on his 1933 visit to Southampton. Following in the footsteps of Defoe, Cobbett and H. V. Morton, Priestley had embarked on an audit of England, touring a land suffering from the same malaise Cobbett had recorded a hundred years earlier. Yet Southampton in the Thirties was booming, saved from the worst effects of the Depression by its status as the country's premier passenger port. Once again it had reinvented itself, from spa town to commercial port and now the conduit of fashionable inter-war travel. From here embarked the Prince of Wales, in his check suits and floppy caps; Noël Coward, with bow-tie and slicked-back hair; Stephen Tennant, with his orchid buttonhole and his gilt-caged parrot; the glamour which would ensnare me.

Throughout the town, and even in its suburbs, ordinary-looking roads suddenly ended in the surreal sight of enormous ships towering over the houses; Priestley marvelled that you could 'catch the *Berengaria* or the *Empress of Britain* at the end of the High Street'. It was ironic that the privileged élite who arrived by the boat-train from Waterloo, drifting under the glass awning of the luxurious South Western Hotel and into the deluxe liners, were by one remove the saviours of Southampton's working class. And although Priestley – now one of England's wealthiest authors and having left Bradford for Highgate – discovered poverty in its back streets, he discerned that in Southampton, the romance of the sea undercut that sense of dispossession:

Once off that long High Street, I found myself in some very poor quarters. The only thing to be said in favour of these squalid little side-streets of Southampton is that they did not seem as devastatingly dismal as the slums of the big industrial towns. There was still a sea sparkle in these people's lives. They were noisy and cheerful, not crushed ... It might have been much worse. But it could be – and at first I thought it was – much better.

The transatlantic trade in film stars, businessmen and aristocrats had financed Southampton's new Civic Centre, a pale smooth-stone complex in neo-classical style topped with an obelisk-like tower and verdigris roofs. It stood optimistically – if not arrogantly, in this time of the Means Test and hunger marches – on the hill above the docks like a Roman fort, a gleaming new citadel of civic bureaucracy. Its clock, which I would hear striking the hours from my Sholing bedroom across the water, was Southampton's Big Ben, a monument, not to Victorian philanthropic imperialism, but to the new values which had overtaken it. It had the same kind of hauteur as Thomas Dugdale's 1936 painting of the Jarrow Marchers reaching London, an image which fascinated me. The arrival of the protestors in a dark city square is watched from a window by a languid socialite in a gold evening gown, kneeling on a sofa to get a better view. At her feet sits a dandified young man blowing smoke rings from his pursed lips; both figures could equally be leaving on a liner from Southampton's docks. The young man's attention is drawn by what is going on unseen in the room beyond; nonchalantly, he dangles his elegantly crossed leg, his back to the huddled masses outside in the gas-lit streets.

Back in depressed Bradford my father had been apprenticed to a printing firm, but when he reached twenty-one and was therefore entitled to the full wages of a grown man, he'd been sacked. A friend of his had gone south, not with the Jarrow Marchers, but in search of work, and on a trip back to Yorkshire he'd told Dad there were jobs down there. Just as his father had moved down from Whitby, so my father was drawn further south, down from the moors and the mills to the low-lying

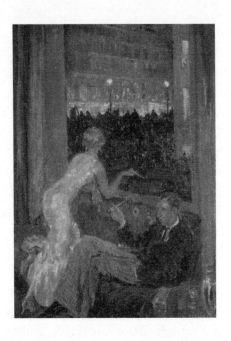

Hampshire coast, its sun and seaside promising a better future and cleaner air.

The prosperity of the 'Gateway to England' (and despite the bold promotion of its Civic Centre, it was still a town) had also financed the reshaping of Southampton as a huge crescent of muddy ground was reclaimed in front of the railway line. Here, in 1937, my twenty-one-year-old father stepped out of the modern streamlined station where the trains ran almost into the sea to be confronted by a huge power station belching black smoke, as though he hadn't left the industrial north at all.

And here, on this reborn land, lay his future. The Pirelli General Cable Works stretched greedily in red brick along the flat terrain, its jagged roof a new barrier between the medieval walls and the sea. A tall chimney, marked with the company's name down its length, echoed the neighbouring power station. I could never believe that a factory stood where there had once been open water; it was as though it was still floating, this great brick building which imprisoned my father, and at one point threatened to imprison me too, in its high gates guarded by self-important security men in their contrived uniforms.

By the asbestos-roofed cycle stands in the car park, I'd wait for a lift home from town, watching for my father to emerge from the unknowable innards of the factory. Somewhere inside he tested thick rubber-coated cables that wound round gigantic wooden drums ready to be laid on the ocean floor across the Atlantic, as if tethering England's island to its new colonial master. He would spend his working life in this institution, where the canteen was demarcated into white and blue collar sittings, and where your existence was punched away by a clock at the gate.

After forty-two years at Pirelli's, my father retired. The QAD – Quality Assurance Department – presented him with a green loose-leaf folder full of reminiscences, an 'Ode to Len,' illustrated by a set of Polaroids with witty comments written beneath them. 'I've shifted a few tons for you mate', says a fork-lift driver; 'Its my turn next Len', announces a nice-looking middle-aged woman; a bubbly blonde poses with a West Indian ('Here it is Len, in black and white'); and lastly, 'Happy Days': Dad with the rest of the department, he in white lab coat, a cut above the overalls, just as I was marked out by my brown and gold blazer, the uniform which meant I didn't have to wear his.

These memories stand away from me, folded up in a marquetry box with the embossed leather album and certificates of births, examinations, marriages and deaths beginning to fall apart at the creases. I never knew my mother's father; he died before I was born. There are only photographs now, and a wooden block stamped, like all his tools, with an iron brand, impressing his name deep into the grain. My grandmother, an elderly, elegantly-dressed lady in retirement in her New Forest bungalow, its ver-andah an echo of the Indian brasses and ebony elephants collected by her husband, never spoke of her experiences as a nurse in the war. My Bradford grandfather lived long enough to be a vague, slight shadow of my father, sweet and silver-whiskered with twinkling eyes, a man who loved books and history. Their memories, threaded between wars, seemed woven into Netley's hospital. Its very enormity, dwarfing ordinary lives like the wars that were beyond their control, made the past both palpable and distant; both nearer and further away, as though seen from the wrong end of a telescope.

As a young girl, my mother was taken by her father to the Remembrance Day services at Southampton's Cenotaph. There, across the road from the art nouveau memorial to *Titanic* off which echoed the sturdy hymns of loss sung to a brass band – 'Abide with me/ Fast falls the eventide' – the ceremony was almost drowned by cries of wailing wives and mothers. Like Muslim women mourning their dead or a Greek chorus masked by transfixed despair, the crowd of black-clad widows wept openly in an unEnglish lament. And as they cried, St John's Ambulance attendants carried overcome mourners away, still helpless in loss as the rest of the world was losing itself in a new age of jazz and suffrage and semi-detached suburbia.

One long generation later Netley's hospital would come to occupy my imagination in after-image; a cenotaph-like focus for my memories-at-one-remove. Just as my father had been born in wartime, his childhood overshadowed by its consequences, so we too lived under our own apocalyptic threat, governed by its own potent symbols: the white on black CND arrow and the haunting, recurrent motif of the mushroom cloud, the ticking of the doomsday clock. As schoolchildren we could hear the mournful wail of air-raid sirens being tested on police station roofs. Hindsight would indicate good reason for our apprehension: *Probable Nuclear Targets In The United Kingdom: Assumptions For Planning, 1967*, cited Southampton as one of twenty British cities expected to receive the blast of one and two megaton Soviet warheads. But I feared war because real war, as opposed to these jittery face-offs, didn't seem far away; it was part of my inheritance.

My parents had met in Southampton in 1938: the pretty girl from Bitterne who worked in a Portswood fancy goods store; the well-dressed young man from Bradford who'd come to make his life down south. On one of their days out, my mother snapped my father on Netley's shore. Looking dapper and handsome, he leans over a rail by the coast guard station, a four-funnelled liner steaming out of the docks behind him like something from another century, while out of sight of the camera, behind my mother's back, stands the hospital itself, unphotographed on this afternoon jaunt in 1939.

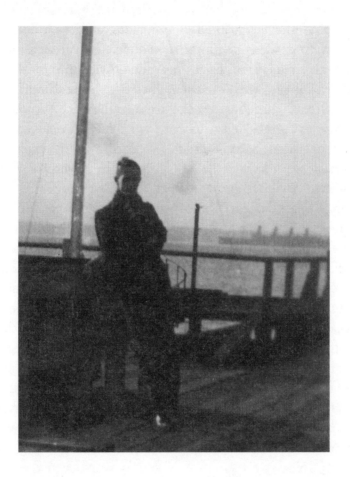

Like my father's father, my parents also married in wartime. Spending their honeymoon in a London hotel, seeing Ivor Novello in *The Dancing Years*, they dodged air raids on the way home, walking down the tracks from Waterloo, looking back to see the city's sky on fire. It must have seemed like the world had gone mad, although there was something exciting, too, in this sense of anarchy, a feeling of freedom from the authority which had governed their lives. Incendiaries as big as dinner plates would land in their Bitterne garden, and the household was drilled to put them out with stirrup pumps. Children playing in Mayfield Park ran for cover as the Luftwaffe burst out of peaceful skies, guns blazing; entire planes fell into suburban homes like plastic models whose strings had snapped. One evening my mother walked home from work and turned the corner to find their neighbour's house destroyed. My father, whose work for Pirelli's was a reserved occupation – like his father's in the last war – spent nights on Home Guard duty on an anti-aircraft gun outside the town, where he would watch, helplessly, as bombs fell on streets where his family lived. And my brother, then a baby, would look up and see the tracer bullets like incandescent rain and say, 'pretty lights, pretty lights', as if they were a firework display.

Twenty years later, when I was a boy, large parts of South-ampton were still bomb sites, and green-painted Anderson shel-ters were common in Sholing's back gardens, their corrugated iron turtle backs still braced to deflect that deadly rain. Ours contained relics of war, as though they'd been left there since the Forties (although we'd imported them from Osborne Road): a gas mask with its round, cracked glass insect eyes and the same stink of rubber lodged in my mind from the dental surgery, an association of blood and gas; a dented army helmet with its webbing straps to save the wearer's head from the impact of flying shrapnel; and my uncle's canvas kit bag in which he had packed his troubles, now stowed away among the garden spades and lumber, waiting for him to return.

My first memory of the hospital came through the windows of our big blue Wolsey. On Sunday afternoons, civilians were allowed to attend Mass in the Catholic chapel which had been established in a hut at the far end of the site of the hutted hospital, founded in 1920 by the same priest who'd donated Miss Enright's hut to our school. Passing the sentries at the hospital gates, we drove into the forbidden territory.

Sunk in the well of the Wolsey's cracked leather seats and carpeted floor, my chin resting on the walnut fascia, I looked out of the window as the car swung round away from the shore and up the hill to 'Piccadilly'. As we passed pine trees and toy-town-like road signs on narrow tarmac lanes leading to clusters of outbuildings, in my mind's eye I saw operations performed with toothed saws and gags, rubber tubing and oddly-shaped steel dishes; medical hardware that I conflated with iron lungs and polio victims, gothic x-rays and the army medical tents on display at the Aldershot Tattoo, with their khaki bandages and canvas stretchers.

At the age of eight, I don't know if I was aware of the great hospital itself – only its shadow, lingering after the event, like a figure glimpsed in the corner of the eye. Still less would I have known, as we parked the car at the end of the hospital grounds and filed into the chapel hut – like my classroom, only with soldiers in pews instead of children at their desks – that nearby stood another building, reserved for yet darker human stories.

D Block

Suffering is permanent, obscure and dark,
And shares the nature of infinity.

WILLIAM WORDSWORTH, *The Borderers*

'And this also,' said Marlow suddenly, 'has been one of
the dark places of the earth.'

JOSEPH CONRAD, *Heart of Darkness*

———

Lieutenant-Colonel Graham's article of 1897 makes just one
perfunctory and unilluminating reference to Netley's scion
in the woods, as if to shield his serving readership from its
fearful prospect: 'Accommodation is provided for cases of mental
disease in a Military Lunatic Asylum, which is isolated from the
other buildings.'

Back in the 1860s, part of the grand scheme for Netley had
included the first purpose-built military psychiatric unit. 'A short
distance behind the Hospital an asylum has recently been built',
noted a slightly more informative contemporary account. 'It is
intended to be used in the same way as the Hospital – to receive
patients sent from abroad, to test their curability, and if the cases
turn out satisfactorily, to serve as a place whence they may be
drafted off to their parishes or to other lunatic asylums.' If the

main building was to take care of sound bodies, then its sibling would see to sound minds – although the analytical culture of the main hospital would become positively obscure here, less sure of itself when dealing with such a difficult subject.

And like the main hospital, there was a certain degree of sensation about the building of the asylum, one which reached back to Britain's early history. When the foundations were being excavated, an early British earthenware crock was found, and in it nearly 2,000 Roman coins, dating from between AD 253 to 275. The *British Archaeological Association Journal* duly reported on this exciting discovery, noting that they joined thirteen similar coins found in Sholing, and speculating, 'A small creek runs in from the east of the Southampton Water alongside the high ground in which the urns were found, and there is a beach below where landing from a vessel could be effected. The spot may probably be considered an out-post, or look-out, from the Roman station of Clausentum . . .' The dark wooded valley and its stream which, like Spike Island's shore, once ran high from Southampton Water to the site of Netley's new asylum, held a memory of an older empire.

Until the building of the asylum, 'military lunacies' had been housed in a purpose-built extension, constructed in 1847 behind the massive stone walls of the Napoleonic Fort Pitt at Chatham, Kent. The Lunacy Act of 1845 had determined that by 'moral management' and supervised work, the mad could be brought back to sanity, thereby creating an imperative for new asylums. Thus the marvellously-named Commissioners in Lunacy – a group of silk-hatted gentlemen who sounded like an invention by Lewis Carroll – concluded Fort Pitt to be inappropriate accommodation. Their report prompted the decision to build Netley's asylum, which duly opened in July 1870 with the transfer of four inmates from Fort Pitt. This time there were no objections from Florence Nightingale or medical committees. The planners had learned their lessons, and the building was constructed along more enlightened standards employed in Britain's other new asylums.

217

Whereas the main hospital was constructed to treat the casualties of foreign service, the asylum's catchment area would – for the moment – be Britain itself. The new Lunacy Act had set a standard, and the military authorities were duty bound to extend the same benefits to their own mentally-ill soldiers. Taking its cue from its civilian counterparts, Netley's asylum was set apart, like them, from the rest of the community – for both the good of the community, and that of its inmates – in the furthest corner of the hospital site at the end of a tree-lined lane – literally round the bend. The soft red and yellow brick and low-angled blue slate roof of the new building were a contrast to the outlandish scale of its big brother; with its solid gables and arched windows, it seemed more homely, like an enlarged version of an archdeacon's country villa; or, as one writer described it, the Petit Trianon to the main hospital's Versailles.

But this was modern medical architecture, the 'pavilion' style championed by Miss Nightingale and her supporters: had Netley's main hospital been built ten years later, this is how it would have looked. It was as if the lunatics had benefited from the bureaucratic madness of its gigantean cousin. Yet it too deceived: the asylum's elegant proportions may have conjured up classical rationality, but for all its progressive faith in the effects of environment on its inhabitants, this was a fortified, walled institution, a place built to contain and restrain.

Inside the building, the superficial airiness was also deceptive. Windows which looked domestic from the outside were so constructed as to open only a few inches; what looked like ordinary offices were secure rooms with substantial locks. Passageways were divided by iron gates, and thick prison-like doors led into padded cells. The very wings of the building created a high-sided quad for the exercise of dangerous patients. And in the grounds specimen trees and lawns were laid out like a civic park, but they were encircled by high walls, beyond which the tree tops of the world outside were tantalisingly visible, over a parapet scaled only by squirrels and magpies.

*   *   *

218

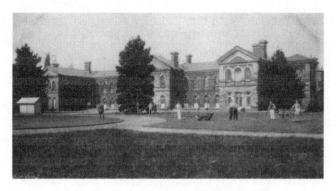

The Asylum, Netley Hospital

On 10 December 1870, the Commissioners in Lunacy drove up the lane from Netley station to make their first official visit to the asylum. They found forty-nine patients in residence – there had been a maximum of eighty-one – cared for by fourteen male orderlies and a cook. In the six months since its opening, records indicated four deaths from normal causes, and two attempted suicides. Of the 160 patients received, twenty were judged suicidal and seven more homicidal; solitary confinement had been ordered for five cases and there had been twelve escape attempts. Those high brick walls had been built for good reason, as an 1873 report from the local paper noted. Private James Hobbins, aged twenty-five, of the 1st Battalion, 21st regiment,

> was under the impression that he was being kept much longer at the hospital than necessary and exhibited a great desire to be allowed to leave, which, however, was thwarted by the opinion of the medical men. The unfortunate fellow appears to have ascribed this especially to Surgeon Sidney Keyworth Ray. As Mr. Ray was attending to the wants of another invalid Hobbins suddenly came behind him and cut his throat. It is hoped that he will survive his fearful injuries.

Few documents survive to give any idea of how the asylum operated during the nineteenth century, although 'Netley Form

21', issued from the Commandant's Office in the main hospital, tells what must have been a typical story. John Parratt had been a servant when he enlisted in the Royal Engineers, aged nineteen:

> Sir, Having received instructions from the Right Honourable Secretary of State for War to send the discharged soldier named in the margin to his place of settlement [Aldershot] . . . I have the honour to inform you that he will be sent to the Asylum under your supervision under the care of a [deleted and added '4'] guide[s] on the 2nd Nov. 1883.

The pre-set type of the form added applicable phrases to be struck out as required in a sort of psychiatric multiple-choice: 'This man is a lunatic but is reported to have sufficiently recovered to allow of his being removed'. Disconcertingly, someone has handwritten the word 'dangerous' before 'lunatic'.

Parratt was to be taken to Knowle, the 'County Lunatic Asylum' at Fareham, just east of Netley. In the accompanying medical certificate, Francis Welch, surgeon and pathologist at the Army Medical School, noted that Parratt's 'first attack' had occurred when he was twenty-seven, and that the 'Duration of Existing Attack' had begun on 5 August 1883:

> 1. Facts indicating dangeous insanity observed by myself (e); Essentially maniacal – irrational in speech, conduct and acts has numerous delusions and hallucinations' restless in body, gesticulates freely and addresses imaginary persons; no sleep with narcotics; very foul and blasphemous in language, noisy, disgusting, filthy, destructive. Requires the constant supervision of one or more attendants.

Like the main hospital, the asylum may have looked ordered, but what went on inside was not. The techniques it employed to deal with the strange maladies of the mind were at best experimental, at worst brutal, and its interior chaos, contained by its brick walls, was a challenge to the rationality of the Victorian

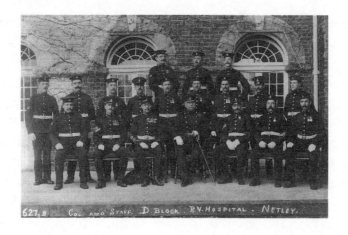

627.8 Co. and Staff. D Block . R.V. Hospital . Netley.

world, requiring the supervision of orderlies chosen for their physical strength rather than their nursing skills.

Yet psychiatric care was trying to keep up with its medical cousin, and new developments in the science of psychology slowly permeated its walls, leaving the prejudices of the past behind and finding new ways of dealing with lunacy. Although it was realised that victims of terminal syphilis – suffering 'General Paralysis of the Insane' – were pathological and incurable cases, other manifestations of nervous disorders were seen as treatable. By the turn of the century, the asylum was being held up as an exemplar of the modern, humane treatment of mentally-disturbed servicemen. '... The Military Lunatic Asylum [is] under the charge of Colonel Chester, whose kindly, sympathetic disposition eminently qualifies him for the post', announced a newspaper report in 1900.

> One fact in connection with the entire establishment should be brought home to every mind, and that is that no patient afflicted permanently with mental or other disablement is turned adrift. Unless such a man has a good home and friends to go to he is retained on the books of the Royal Victoria Hospital. Now depend upon it the country that adopts this thoughtful provision, that treats its invalid soldiers with such tender solicitude, will never want for an

221

Army, nor the Army for a reserve! Conscription is wholly unnecessary.

But just as the main hospital had proved insufficient for the physical – and conscripted – victims of modern warfare, so its mental wing would have to accommodate a new influx. In 1908, a neo-Georgian, pierlike extension was built, complete with large bay windows and a long communal ward. It too appeared light and airy, but jutting out into the asylum's grounds, it seemed to hold its inmates at arm's length. Military bureaucracy now referred to 'the Asylum' by its abbreviated designation: D Block. On this alphabetically-ordered site, the anonymity of the title discreetly disguised its function. And like its hard-pressed cousin across the fields, D Block was about to acquire an even more urgent role.

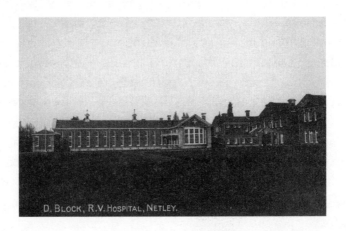

D. BLOCK, R.V. HOSPITAL, NETLEY.

With the general asylum population having trebled in the past fifty years, D Block was ministering to an increasing number of inmates. Blame fell on an industrialised society which some saw as weakening the British race and prompting this apparent epidemic of insanity. The right-wing polemicist, Arnold White, put the problems to his readers in 1911:

To-day we fly to Scotland in eight hours, whereas our fore-fathers required three days' coaching or a week in the saddle to reach Edinburgh. Fifty years of stimulating, tinned and frozen food, easy travel, and constant strain have made us an asthenic people. Our pulse is soft and compressible. The type of disease has changed. Mental instability is no longer rare – it infects large masses of the people. Nature having no favourites, we experienced in the Boer war the effect of the cerebral changes that have altered our racial character-istics. We all live constantly under overstrain, and what is called 'overstrain' among the well-to-do is insanity to crime among those less fortunately circumstanced.

In the yet more industrialised conflict which followed the South African war, the degeneration which White and his peers feared seemed to be proved. The rapidly evolving techno-bacillus of modern warfare had created a new disease, and D Block faced an epidemic. All over Britain disused spas, country houses and private mental institutions were commandeered to deal with the influx of traumatised men. Civilian psychologists from county asylums were given temporary commissions in the RAMC; female staff became probationers in nursing corps. By the end of the war, there were at least twenty such establishments in the country, whose inhabitants locals – and supporters of Arnold White – looked upon with suspicion as lunatics, cowards, or victims of venereal disease. In a hangover from the days of Bedlam, they were regarded as transgressors, confined for pun-ishment rather than cure.

The doctors and staff of Netley's asylum may have been shocked by the extraordinary nature of mental cases coming from the Front, but at least the authorities there seemed to have shown some sense of contingency with their recent extension – although they could have had no idea of the numbers the building would soon have to deal with. As the army's main clearing hospi-tal, D Block was the first place to which such casualties were brought, whether they stayed there or not, and it seems likely

– although I will probably never know for certain – that among the thousands of men who passed through its wards was my own great-uncle.

By the first winter of the war, the medical profession had begun to trace the cause and effect of the new disorder, forced by the sheer numbers to try and comprehend the nature of an affliction which seemed, as Arnold White had claimed of other mental crises, to be uniquely modern. 'From this time onwards interest in the nervous affection of battle became profound', noted *The Times* in 1916. 'Neurologists were attached to the military hospitals, and nerve cases were studied as closely and as carefully as were surgical and medical cases. It was realized that the coming of the high explosive shell ... had wrought a revolution in the types of war injuries and so in war medicine ...'

That year Dr Arthur Templer Davies addressed the Assurance Medical Society 'on the class of nerve cases which the War has brought into prominence'. He noted that a fellow doctor, George M. Beard – whose schemata rather recalled those of Almroth Wright and Arnold White – had 'assigned the chief and primary cause of neurasthenia to the complex agencies of modern life which he distinguished from the ancient by the five characteristics, viz., "steam power, the periodical press, the telegraph, the sciences and the mental activity of women".'

> If neurasthenia is due to the strain and stress of a civilisation different from those of other periods in the world's history, then we may regard the condition of War neurasthenia, if I may use the expression ... as due to the unparalleled conditions of modern War, to the duration of battles, the prolonged strain of responsibility, wakefulness, intensity of artillery bombardments and the devilish mechanical and scientific devices for slaughter.

Dr Davies went on to cite the variety of symptoms in a summary of contemporary medical opinion:

224

Dr T. R. Elliot ... describes as the effects of shell explosion a form of transient paraplegia, characterised by numbness, and complete paralysis of the legs immediately after the explosion ... *Dr Rolleston* ... says that the 'nervous strain of the War would naturally be expected to produce much insanity, mental disturbance and neurasthenia' ... *Major C. S. Myers* ... gives a long account of cases ... which caused total amnesia, rhythmic spasmodic movements, mutism and stupor which he treated by hypnotism...

Some believed it was the actual physical impact of bombardment which caused these symptoms; others saw deeper underlying causes. It was a highly complex and problematic issue for a science attempting to escape myth and superstition for rational progress, but which would realise that the emotional and the rational were not so easily separated. Netley had been witness to cultural swings from Cistercian and eighteenth-century rationalism to gothic romanticism and back to Victorian rationality. Now the new science of psychology encouraged D Block's doctors to attempt new therapies for what Charles Myers, a Cambridge colleague of W. H. Rivers and later 'Consultant Psychologist to the Army', had first described in *The Lancet* in February 1915 as 'shell-shock'. It was a term already being used in the trenches – although it would become clear to Myers and others that the bizarre symptoms produced by this phenomenon had less to do with exploding shells than with the intense and particular horror of modern war itself. Myers and his colleagues fought to have the condition recognised by the Army; it was only in 1916 that a more enlightened attitude to what had been seen as 'funk' or mere cowardice began to be adopted. In the investigation into this new neurosis of the twentieth century, both D Block and the main hospital would become laboratories. Here a new battle between the physical and the rational and the emotional and the romantic was fought over the fate of those quivering soldiers.

*   *   *

225

'On arrival from overseas at D Block, the patients are examined by the special medical officers attached to the hospital', reported *The Lancet* of 27 May 1916. 'All cases which are considered to be of a neurological character are removed for treatment to the Neurological Section in the Main Hospital Building...' This department had been set up in 1915; occupying several wards in the main block and consisting of about a hundred beds. It was an indication of how widespread the problem had become: other shell-shocked cases were apparently kept in bell tents beyond the hutted hospital, where one witness, a young boy visiting his father in the hospital, was told not to knock the guy-ropes as they walked past, for fear of disturbing the men.

'All patients suffering from the severer psychoses of a certifiable type are given two or three weeks' probationary treatment in D Block', noted the report, admitting that 'the number of cases which recover during their stay ... is negligible, but a certain number recover sufficiently ... to be no longer considered of a certifiable character...'

> The type of case observed and treated [in the Neurological Section]...are: Most forms of functional paralysis, especially paraplegia, disturbances of speech and articulation, amnesia, or loss of memory, the effects of terrifying dreams, mutism, deafness, deaf-mutism, amblyopia [partial blindness without any apparent damage to the eye], 'bent back', tremblings and motor agitations, tic-like movements, sleeplessness, nervous debility, indecision, loss of self-confidence, and the milder forms of neurasthenia, simple mental confusion, the anxiety psycho-neurosis, and simple mental depression.
>
> The treatment adopted consists chiefly of rest and feeding; massage and electrical applications in suitable cases; baths when these seem indicated; and psychotherapy in the form of simple suggestion and occasional hypnosis.

The Lancet reported an optimistic cure rate of 'forty per cent of cases returned to light duty, twenty per cent invalided, and twenty per cent transferred for further treatment to the special institutions'. The medical establishment, struggling to cope with the extraordinary demands of this war, sought to reassure itself, as much as anyone, that it was doing its best to treat its victims. The following year, 1917, Netley's surgeon-general agreed to allow Dr Arthur Hurst and Dr J. Symns to make a 'kinematography record' demonstrating the efficacy of the treatments at the hospital. A representative cross-section of symptoms were selected to appear in front of the Pathé brothers' cameras. The result was a remarkable and unique record of the hospital in operation.

The film's initial sequences were shot outside the main building, where the light was bright enough to register on the primitive stock. It is strange to see the vast splendour of the place suddenly brought to life. Sixty years after it opened, Netley's hospital appears as a virtual Victorian scene on film, fantastically anachronistic. The flickering, grainy black and white celluloid flares intermittently, luminous with ancient sunlight as though the viewer were rushing through successive days and nights in some weird time-travel, watching ghostly images of tremulous young soldiers in their baggy pyjama uniforms parade across the terraces. In between these scenes texts appear like the captions in a silent movie, compressing into case histories in one or two sentences. It is as though the hospital were being brought out of a nineteenth-century past via the twentieth-century medium. Netley had become one big medical bioscope, a filmed cabinet of curiosities.

The racked bodies replay the impact of war in a perpetually recurring mimesis, a syndrome the psychiatrists would positively induce as 'abreaction': the reliving of trauma in order to exorcise it, a particularly tortuous piece of psychoanalytic homoeopathy. These men seem condemned to recycle their pain, over and over again, for the benefit of this 'kinematograph record' made on a winter's morning at Netley. Private Reed, aged thirty-two, has an 'hysterical gait', the equally querulous lettering informs us; he repeatedly raises his hand to touch his nose. Blurred on film by the speed of his paroxysms, it is hard to focus on the

227

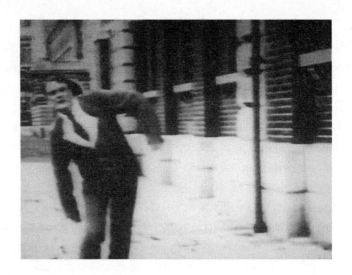

movement of his disconnected limbs. In yet more baroque chor-eography, Corporal Anderson, twenty-seven, has developed an 'hysterical "dancing" gait', twisting and turning to inaudible music from an invisible gramophone, while Private Williams's malfunction is likened to that of walking on 'slippery ice'. One soldier's attempt to control his shuddering body is termed 'battling with the wind' by the analysts; another is reduced to perpetually stepping up and down non-existent stairs in a Sisy-phean tape loop of torment. Products of the Western Front's mechanised madness, these are uniquely disturbing scenes, all the more fearsome for their setting in front of Netley's civilised, imperial façade.

Some of these men had been brutalised by a system which had yet to recognise their diagnoses. Charles Myers had noted that patients arriving from France reported that they had been badly treated there; some claimed to have been tortured with electric shocks.* At Netley the regime of D Block removed their

---

* In 1916 Dr Lewis Yealland, himself an avid proponent of 'electrical therapy', noted of one patient that 'he had been strapped in a chair for twenty minutes at a time while strong electricity was applied to his neck and throat; lighted cigarettes had been applied to the tip of his tongue and "hot plates" had been

ties and bootlaces like prisoners locked up overnight in a police cell, ostensibly to prevent suicide bids; like the weekly Sunday route marches on which they were sent, as if on public display, it was another mark of shame, a lingering suspicion of cowardice.

The film resonates uncomfortably with these suspicions, on the viewer's part as much as the participants'; it is the thin dividing line between care and abuse. These sufferers from a troublesome new disorder, potential 'lead swingers', were put under peculiar examination. On Netley's terraces they are made to display their dysfunction for the camera, as if it was there to prove the truth of their disability, this new symptom of war. Incapable of deceit, the unlying camera challenged their dysfunction just as it was rumoured that the execution of every deserting soldier was filmed as a record of military justice. As the century was already discovering, film was a potent force in the right or wrong hands.

One patient, Private Meek, is shown in a wheelchair, held by

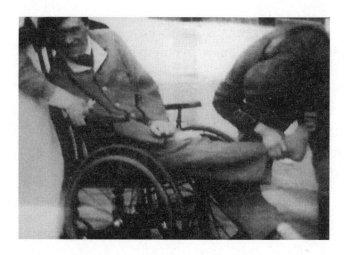

placed at the back of his mouth. Hypnotism had also been tried.' In Germany, the electrical treatments of Dr Kaufmann's *überrumpellungsmethode* ('surprise-method' shock therapy) at Mannheim had been so severe that at least twenty of his patients died and others committed suicide.

229

a nurse while an officer doctor – perhaps Hurst himself – attempts to straighten the grinning man's contorted limbs. When fighting at the battle of the Marne, Meek – a basket-maker before the war – had been confronted by a German soldier who fired his rifle at him, but missed. 'P.M. promptly struck him in the abdomen with his bayonet and killed him', noted his doctor. 'He felt rather proud of this incident and laughed over it with his two chums. Soon afterwards these two chums were killed, and P.M. began to see them come to his bedside at night and would hear them talk to him . . .'

Brought to Netley, Meek was at first treated by William McDougall, another Cambridge colleague of Rivers's, who used hypnosis 'as a method of exploration', to rid the traumatised man of another ghost – that of the German soldier he had killed:

During the night the figure appears suddenly in the ward, points his rifle at P.M., says 'Now I've got you, you can't get away', and fires point blank at him. P.M. hears the crack of the rifle, and sees the ghost sink to the ground. He takes this to be a real ghost come to take his revenge and every night he is terrified anew by this visitor.

Meek seemed to have regressed to his childhood – clutching teddy bears and 'small dolls' in his bent fingers. He would remain like that for a year, unable to remember the events that had brought him to this pass. In June 1918 he is walking, but with a bizarre gait, still waiting to be cured, although under Hurst's therapies his submerged memories were returning.

For the shell-shocked, memory had become part of the pain of war; but for the civilian world – the world outside Netley – the truth of the war was still unknowable, unremembered; although it was beginning to become apparent. A year before the film was made, the battle of the Somme, which produced huge new numbers of mental casualties, was also filmed, and the results shown in cinemas to give the population some sense of the reality of the war. The shock of seeing these moving pictures of Hell caused one woman in a London cinema to stand up and shout, 'My God, they're dead!' How much more disturbed would she have been had she seen this filmic proof of demented men – brothers, sons, fathers, lovers – quivering uncontrollably like cornered animals in a Hampshire hospital.

On film, out of the trenches and on the pavements of Netley, their ataxic gaits and shaking bodies still seem to reel from the explosions of No-Man's-Land. Their very bones seem bent and twisted – yet the cause of their crippled state is not physical (although the worst affected are emaciated from their inability to eat properly). They are boys who should have been playing football or drinking down the pub. Instead they are subjected to the camera's remorseless, hand-cranked record of their shattered nervous systems. Captured on film, they are too removed from the world to regard the act as glamorous, yet as they march towards the lens, each attempts a polite, pathetic grimace for the camera, their jerky walks and tics resembling nothing so much as those of silent comedians. All the while, behind them looms the hospital, elusive, never quite revealing its enormous bulk.

The next sequences are interiors, filmed in the hospital's wards. Private Preston, aged nineteen, dives under his iron bedstead every time he hears the word 'bombs' – an 'abreaction' which

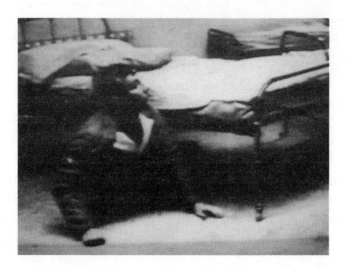

prompts the viewer to wonder at the necessity of using it. On another bed, a man's head is manipulated, rolled about in the doctor's hands until the image blurs into something resembling a painting by Francis Bacon, a mutated image of dumb pain. A third soldier, suffering from 'hyperthyroidism' induced by 'hysteria', stares at the camera, his protruding eyes a disquieting scene from a medieval nightmare.

Most dreadful of all is the last 'before' sequence, shot in a bare, empty ward. A full-length nude figure stands alone by a bed; the picture is exquisitely composed, a portrait in scratched chiaroscuro, a Renaissance Christ reborn in war. But instead of a beautiful Italian youth, we see the twisted body of an emaciated English officer, clad only in a handkerchief-shaped piece of material pulled round his hips and knotted at the base of his spine.

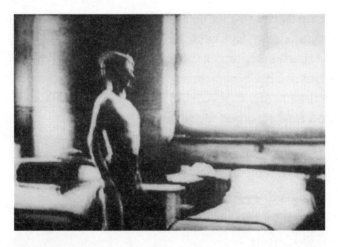

Slowly, stiffly, the man begins to move, walking across the ward floor, his limbs bent at right-angles to his bony ribcage; his frail body seems filleted by the dissection of the camera. There is something about his bearing, a residual normality beneath the terrible contortions. His angular gait and the stark slow/fastness of the image take on the air of a German expressionist film. As the man reaches the end of the ward, he stops by a row of metal-framed beds. The light is bursting through the window, the *lux nova* of a new, blasted century. Now the image evokes a starved prisoner of war in a labour camp. Standing as near to attention as his pathetically crooked, bone-thin body will allow, he fixes his stare straight ahead, awaiting release. This new world will have it all on film, from here to Belsen, Hiroshima and Kosovo.

Yet these scenes are classic before and after sequences, presented to a papal board of canonisation to prove the miracles of medicine; proof of the ability to repair what had previously been irreparable, or ignored, or dealt with by firing squad. The film's very existence says that science has moved on since Bedlam (although its portrayal of the hospital's inhabitants seems uncomfortably close to exhibition). In the sequences that follow, the contemporary audience – other men of science, dispassionately observing this new dysfunction and its remedy – were shown the same men after hypnotherapy and what is ominously described in the captions as 'persuasion' and 're-education' – a Cultural Revolution for their time.

Reporting on their experiments in *The Lancet* in August 1918, Dr Hurst and Dr Symns wrote, 'From the earliest days of the war we realized that recent cases could generally be cured quickly and completely by a variety of methods, including simple persuasion and re-education, suggestion with the aid of electricity in the waking state and suggestion under hypnosis or light anaesthesia ... We are now disappointed if complete recovery does not occur within 24 hours of commencing treatment, even in cases which have been in other hospitals for over a year.' A later report usefully summed up these techniques:

Persuasion
Here the medical officer ... persuades the patient to make the effort necessary to overcome the disability. In order to do this, he uses his authority as an officer, he brings into play all the moral suasion he can, appealing to the patient's social self-esteem to make him co-operate and put forth a real effort of will. If moral suasion fails, then recourse may be had to

more forcible methods, and according to certain witnesses even threats were justified in certain cases (Major Pritchard Taylor, Dr Dunn, Dr Elliot, and Lieut. Colonel Rogers)

Explanation
In this method the causes of the origin and persistence of the symptoms are explained to the patient in reference to his own individual case, he is reassured as to the fact that he is not suffering from some terrible and lasting nervous or mental disorder, and he is shown what direction he must turn to get rid of his troubles. This process, the inoculation of Autognosis, was of universal application and was much recommended by many witnesses of high authorative standing (Dr Head, Dr Rivers, Dr Myers, Dr Brown)

Suggestion
. . . the use of hypnotics to overcome insomnias, of electrical stimulation to restore function . . .

Analysis
By the method of Free Association or Reaction Time experiment, the unconscious factors behind the conscious symptoms are brought to light, the patient's mind is analysed, and by finally affecting a synthesis in which cause and effect are placed in juxtaposition in the consciousness of the patient, the symptoms are said to disappear. A full analysis in the Freudian sense (Psycho-analysis) was recommended by very few witnesses, while several witnesses spoke against its employment (Dr Mapother regarded it as unnecessary and impracticable, Dr Bernard Hart as hardly practicable at all, Dr Hurst as dangerous in setting up sexual ideas, etc.)

Re-education
Having cleared away the symptoms, it was found necessary to submit the patient to a course of graduated experiences which should prepare him for taking on his duty again . . .

Occupation
... The patient should be kept occupied consistently and not allowed to slip back into unprofitable habits ...

The atmosphere of cure.
All witnesses agree as to the supreme importance of the maintenance of the general atmosphere of cure in the hospitals where these patients are being treated; no influence is more potent for beneficial suggestion than this ... There should be no maudlin sentimentality about the hospital for functional nervous or mental disorder, there must be an air of practical cheerfulness supported by all the staff who must co-operate to produce a solid barrier against the development of any unwholesome attitudes of discontent or morbid doubting ... Sympathy which is misplaced is most harmful, and the deleterious effect of indiscrimate sympathy from the general public cannot be too strongly deprecated (Miss Cockerell). Hence cases of this type should never be treated in the unofficial VAD hospitals (Dr Mapother and Dr Hurst).

Doctors such as Charles Myers believed they had to be cruel to be kind to treat war's new disorders; later, an eminent psychiatrist would comment that a 'wave of sentimentality' made the 'sane treatment of shell-shock' impossible. The 'talking cure' and the long-term analytic methods of Freud (who called military psychiatrists 'the machine gun behind the front line ... driving back those who had fled') were frowned upon; Myers concluded – perhaps rightly – that it was best to treat victims as close to the front as possible, then send them back into action.

Doubtless Miss Cockerell would have disapproved of my grandfather and his daughter as they watched the pyjama-clad inmates of Netley from the seashore. Whichever aspects of the psychotherapeutic menu were chosen for their treatment, the *War Neuroses* film demonstrates – in the bland, simplified manner of its medium, its propaganda for military psychiatry – that just hours and sometime minutes later patients would emerge, as if from the wings, miraculously cured. They appear whole, functioning human beings once more, beneficiaries of medical advance, ready to return to normality – or the Front. They take their historical place in Netley's drama. It is as though they have been brought back to life, resurrected and redeemed by their living martyrdom, these crucified heirs of the Crimea having suffered for our sins.

In its final sequence, the film's dramatic resolution – its happy ending – shows convalescents decamped to Seale Hayne, a requisitioned agricultural college in the West Country, far from the mire into which Flemish fields had been ploughed. Private Meek, now apparently completely cured, is seen supervising patients weaving baskets, his pre-war trade. Yet these 'cures' were not all they seemed to be. The soldiers who had submitted 'to the all-powerful will of . . . Dr Hurst' may have been freed of their symptoms, but they were not necessarily 'good soldiers or more stable human beings': cynics suggested 'that many of Hurst's patients began to decline as soon as they left his charismatic presence and had usually developed new symptoms by the time the train away from Seale Hayne had reached Salisbury'.

The last scene of the *War Neuroses* film shows Hurst's cured men staging 'The Battle of Seale Hayne', a dramatic reconstruction of trench conditions in an idyllic English valley, complete with drifting smoke and 'wounded' being carried off on stretchers. It was *re-education* in action, a sort of mass 'abreaction'. It is also a bizarre piece of play-acting, an amateur version of the professional filmed re-enactments of Western Front battles which it was decided were less disturbing for popular consumption than the real thing. But for Netley's Pathé newsreel from the home front, for all its air of propaganda and instruction, there would be no public exhibition: such images were hardly suitable for the cinema-goers of Southampton's High Street. The power of film was all too evident, and to witness these disturbed minds and bodies might have had audiences doubting not only the cures themselves, but the war that had made them necessary.

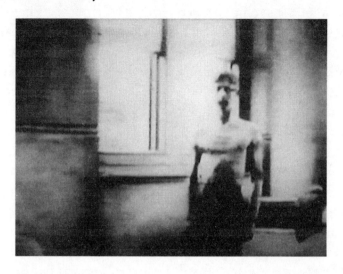

War could produce symptoms of mass hysteria even among the civilian population; the shell-shocked casualties were frontline sufferers of the altered states produced by the meeting of techno-logical and historical eras, grinding together like tectonic plates. To some psychologists, as to Arnold White, D Block's quivering soldiers were evidence of a modern, repressed civilisation; the mass unconscious manifested as the product of industrialisation. Such ideas bridged ancient notions of metaphysics and the modern sciences of the mind. They connected the nineteenth-century fascination with the science of psychology and the residual belief in magic and the supernatural that underlay Doctor Mesmer's experiments into hypnotism at the beginning of the century. It was no coincidence that medieval psychiatrists were known as 'persuaders', or that their eighteenth- and nineteenth-century counterparts were called 'alienists'. Even in 1918, psychology remained a strange practice, caught between science and myth.

Back in 1887, Madame Blavatsky had written, in a self-congratulatory article in *Lucifer* magazine, of how hypnosis had been 'denied and laughed at ... accused for the last century as being principally based on superstition and fraud ...' Now it had become a psychic science to deal with this disease of the psyche; a sympathetic magic created out of 'animal magnetism' and 'mesmerism'. Netley had embraced new techniques – Almroth Wright's inoculations, Röntgen's x-rays – but only war, and this new, unknown epidemic of nervous disorder had the power to both dignify and prove the efficacy of these new techniques. Even then, hypnotherapy seemed to some little more than a slightly less eccentric branch of spiritualism, that great mystical solace of the war bereaved. The suspicions still held, just as many (especially those who had not been to the Front) were suspicious of the very diagnosis of 'shell-shock'. There was something unmanly, if cowardly, about such 'funk'.

Yet like everything about this war, the new malady deceived. Its sufferers were not refined aesthetes living at their nerves' edge, decadently sipping from tincture of laudanum, but ordinary men, farm-labourers or manservants. One contemporary medical report observed, 'it is not generally the slight, nervous men who suffer worst from shell-shock. It is often the stolid fellow, one of those we described as being utterly without nerves, who goes down badly. Something snaps in him. He has no resilience in his nervous system. He has never trained himself in nerve-control, being so stolid and self-reliant ... But there is no law. Imagination – apprehension – are the devil, too, and they go with "nerves".' As much as any Romantic poet prone to reverie, they too were cursed with imagination. This was the dark reality to Netley's gothic fantasy, to its walled-up nuns and ghostly monks: the locked wards and contorted bodies of D Block.

Siegfried Sassoon, sent to the shell-shock hospital at Craig-lockhart, saw in this 'their evil hour ... now, in the sweating suffocation of nightmare, in paralysis of limbs, in the stammering of dislocated speech. Worst of all, in the disintegration of those qualities through which they had been so gallant and selfless and uncomplaining – this, in the finer types of man, was the unspeakable tragedy of shell-shock.' Here, as everywhere else, class mattered; even mania had its social division. One anonymous soldier complained to the press in 1916 that while shell-shocked casualties from the ranks were placed 'in a block in a county asylum, and under the same management as the rest of the ... certified lunatics', their superiors received 'all sorts of interesting methods'.

Officers were seen to suffer differently; their symptoms were more subtle, repressed, and for them a suitably refined diagnosis was produced: war neurosis, a martial elaboration of the Edwardian condition of 'neurasthenia'. This may have reflected their role on the Front, their life-and-death responsibility to their men, whom they would be the first to lead over the top, but it also distanced them from the degenerates who were seen as victims of poor heredity: of the 28,533 cases of shell-shock who were sent back to England during the war, the vast majority – 26,938 – came from the ranks (although as historian Ben Shephard points out, one in six of the shell-shocked were officers, compared to a ratio of one officer to thirty men at the Front). An estimated 80,000 British troops suffered shell-shock, of whom more than half were treated in the field, if at all. Of the 28,000 brought back – at least half of whom passed through Netley – 16,138* arrived in the second half of 1916 alone, victims of the explosive onslaught of the Somme and its shells and gigantic mines.

Reverting to images of racial degeneration, the supporters of new theories of eugenics reasoned that the rank and file were genetically prone to such instability. Arnold White condemned the culture of lunatic asylums which had grown up since the 1847 Lunacy Act: 'Hanwell [the mental hospital in London] is stud farm for deaf mutes, epileptics, lunatics, dipsomaniacs, kleptomaniacs, and sexual perverts', he claimed; they were what he called 'concentration breeding-camps of the insane'. White even discussed proposals made elsewhere for the setting up of

---

* A figure which, due to the Army's reluctance to diagnose shell-shock, Shephard recommends should be multiplied by at least three.

'county council lethal chambers' to deal with the problem, and endorsed sterilisation for the mentally ill.*

White's claim that the racial purity of the nation was under threat was a theme which would pervade psychiatric culture, especially in military medicine. Its supporters would cite evidence gathered by the Royal Army Medical Corps of such cases as that of the 1/5th Royal Warwick Regiment, whose commander complained of a 'large % utterly useless men' in his battalion. 'Have brought it to notice several times – cannot get rid of them', he noted in the brusque manner of an officer. It was

> not a question of Medical Examination. On 16/7/16 when Battn. attacked and held trenches at least 40 men were incapable – would not use rifles, bayonets or even move . . . This class of man is petrified with fear when he meets a German in flesh . . . I cannot be responsible for holding trenches while this stamp of man is in the Battn. There are about 100 such men and I would rather be without them.

Another commander, who transferred the offenders to a Labour battalion ('but not out of the danger area'), agreed they were wasters with a 'miserable physique', 'lack of intelligence' and a 'vacant, hang-dog look'. A further memo pointed out that 'these men are degenerates – a source of danger to their comrades, their battalion and the Brigade and this will be not be lessened by distribution to Warwickshire Bns. They should be replaced

---

* In the spring of 1918 Arnold White was called by the extreme right-wing MP Noel Pemberton Billing as a witness in the libel suit brought against Billing by Maud Allan, the Salome Dancer. Billing had alleged that Allan was involved in the 'cult of Wilde' – 47,000 members of the British Establishment supposedly addicted to perverted practices and subject to blackmail by the German Secret Service. In the sensational five-day trial at the Old Bailey, the 'Black Book' which was claimed to list their names was never produced. Nonetheless, Billing won his case.

by drafts. This will not be a dangerous precedent as the stigma (the transfer) will be a deterrent.'

The fine line between the physically unacceptable and the mentally unfit was not a matter for such men of action, but for men of medicine. However for civilian doctors recruited into the military to deal with these 'degenerates', the essential paradox of their work – curing men to fight again – was countermanded by their patriotic duty, in pursuit of which they employed the various psychotherapies – physical cures, if necessary – which were available to them. Not only were men forced to relive the experience which had traumatised them in the first place, the ultimate, subtle cruelty was that their recovery was effected with one pre-eminent purpose: to send them back to the Front. These ironies did not escape psychologists such as W. H. Rivers, who had no idea how long their beneficial work would last – perhaps for the duration of the war, only for the men to return to civilian life haunted, as his Craiglockhart patient Sassoon would be, by visions of dismembered corpses in Piccadilly Circus.

As with later psychiatric techniques, the strange new therapies employed at Netley were used because they seemed to work, without their practitioners actually knowing how. The thousands of traumatised patients being mesmerised and *re-educated* into 'normality' as they passed through D Block's wards also seemed to be manifestations of a world as querulous and troubled as these shaking soldier victims it had produced. At this meeting of epochs, the shifting shapes of Netley's pathological films appeared as living ghosts produced in the nether region in between; as much ectoplasmic extrusions as the blobs of psychic cottonwool that represented their dead comrades in spiritualist seances. On dark afternoons in provincial town halls, the desperate living sought to contact their beloved dead. Back at Netley, the living dead were summoned by the whirring camera of the film crew and the calm adjudicators of their sanity.

Throughout its history, the Royal Victoria Military Hospital, its great complex concealed around this blind corner of the English coast, was nonetheless impossible to ignore. Its existence, its teeming humanity and its economic power exerted itself through the county and beyond. For those who lived near it, the proximity of this sprawling locus of employment and healing, of disease and madness, of life and death, brought home, sometimes uncomfortably, the reality of war.

Even now a certain sensitivity about the place remains, a mixture of macabre fascination and a vague sense of guilt – for complicity in war and its institutions, or for being a beneficiary of its sacrifice. This schism between participants and onlookers was at its most acute in the years of the Great War when that sacrifice was at its height. Then loss and guilt turned to pagan belief; the spiritualism and table-tapping which tried to reclaim dead souls and overcome their traumatic bereavement. Netley's psychic power was never greater than in those years when the world itself seemed to have been turned upside down.

Like those suburban seances, like the temporary street shrines of flowers in cities and towns across Britain,* and like their civic cenotaphs and village memorials in the years afterwards, the hospital became charged with the desperate emotions of the war; with the emotions of its inhabitants, and those outside who could only imagine what scenes it and its inhabitants had witnessed. The enclosed nature and sheer size of the building fed the imagination of the outside world with notions of what might be taking place within its walls, on this *terra incognita*. Romantic imagination had imbued Netley's abbey ruins with a gothic charge; now its hospital seemed to produce the same effect, as if it were feeding in turn on that imagination. By its very scale and place in the national consciousness, Netley's medical citadel straddled the imaginative gap

---

* Spontaneous street shrines of flowers appeared on walls in Ealing, Hackney and Camberwell during the war, popular expressions of grief culminating in the enormous shrine made in Hyde Park in 1918 which had been 'quickly smothered by 10,000 wreaths of flowers', just as generations later another wayside shrine would spread outside the gates of Kensington Palace.

between reality and fantasy. The fact that the general public were mostly forbidden from seeing behind its towers, turrets and dark windows prompted all manner of speculation.

In 1917, a worker at Thornycroft's shipyard in Woolston returned from his dinner at 1.00 pm, summoned by the same works' siren which half a century later would be my cue to return to school for the afternoon. He found that a meeting had been convened by his workmates. 'The men had heard that down at Netley Hospital the German prisoners of war were being nursed inside whilst our own men were outside under canvas.' Others reported that 'German officer casualties were in beds while British troops were on the floor'.

In a war-heightened atmosphere of spy scares and tales of Russian troops with snow on their boots landing in secret at Dover, German factories making soap out of their war dead and poisoned sweets being dropped by the enemy to kill children in Hull, all manner of improbable stories circulated through the country, and this one was more credible than most. The truth was that the Germans had to be kept in wards on the secure centre floor of the hospital, with armed guards posted on floors above and below. (Other accounts maintained that Germans were also given grey uniforms with red discs on the front and back, supposedly targets at which to aim if they attempted to escape. At least two men did escape, climbing on to the buffers of a train at Southampton and making it to Waterloo station before being caught.)

The apparent inequality of treatment between British troops and prisoners of war at Netley aroused the ire of the ship-workers of Woolston (among them the now fervently patriotic parishioners of St Patrick's and Spike Island). They rolled up their sleeves, slung their jackets over their shoulders and set off. 'All the men from Thornycrofts marched along the shore lifting the gates off at the entrance to the rolling mills [in which my great-grandfather was at work, making shell cases] ... and ... at the seaweed hut end', recalled Fred Sutton. When they reached the hospital, the military police tried to stop them, but they lifted these gates off too. The protest simmered close to a public riot, demanding justice for Englishmen and 'stayed on the sports ground until our own men were re-instated, finally leaving about 6.00 pm'. One account maintains that the Commandant of the hutted hospital, Sir Warren Crooke-Lawless, to whom the men had sent a deputation, promised that the Germans would be moved; the following day a special train arrived to take the unfortunate men away. Another claims the Germans were moved to the camp of bell tents on the edge of the site – ironically, next to the railway where, presumably, two of their number made their getaway.

Such escapes – and the fear of possible sabotage by enemy spies – led to a twenty-four-hour armed guard being placed on the line from Southampton to Netley at the viaduct over Miller's Pond in Sholing. For these settlements, so intimately connected with the hospital down the line that wound through the woods and fields, the building became the focus for such fears, its evocative power circulating contemporary versions of the haunted cloisters of Netley Abbey. One such was the mystery of Otto Scholz, a German subaltern in the 3rd Uhlans who spent two years in the hospital, having originally been admitted suffering from 'light wounds' only to end up in the asylum, dying there, as his death certificate recorded, of 'Mania (acute)' and 'Exhaustion' on 14 December 1916. Scholz was buried, according to one interviewee, 'in mysterious [but unspecified] circumstances' in the hospital cemetery two days later.

A local solicitor, Simon Daniels, investigated rumours that Scholz had been a German spy who had been interrogated and kept in a padded cell for the sake of security. When he was told that the 'exhaustion' which his death certificate gave as cause of death was a term for loss of blood, he speculated that Scholz was 'a victim of experimentation, a test of trial and error which had gone wrong', the result of early blood transfusions carried out on human guinea pigs.

With the stakes so high, it is not impossible that radical experiments might have been conducted at this relatively remote and secure site; certainly the enemy's use of chemical warfare had led to the establishment, in 1916, of Porton Down in nearby Wiltshire, where tests were carried out on 'volunteered' servicemen, and the rumours surrounding such places inevitably encouraged notions of secret war work elsewhere. Netley, with its sprawling, secure site, its isolation hospital and other buildings dotted about in the scrubby woods behind the already ominous and apparently endless main hospital, was an obvious place for such intrigue; here there were enough dark rooms and little huts for all kinds of experiments to be carried out. 'It is a fact that ... researchers told how eye-witnesses from Netley let slip a reference or two to experimentation and then hastily shut up', noted Daniels. One former nurse recalled the 'scrap shop', an isolated building where animals were taken 'to test them on different things in the pathological room'.

Daniels could find no concrete evidence of what really happened to Otto Scholz. Those he interviewed who had worked at the hospital seemed concerned not to discuss the subject, although one, Sid Mills, talked of the rumour that Scholz was a spy who had been buried in suspicious circumstances. And despite his assiduous detective work, Daniels did not apparently consider the possibility that Scholz's death certificate cited 'exhaustion'/loss of blood because the German officer, suffering from 'acute mania' at D Block, may have committed suicide – reason enough for the cloud hanging over his internment, more especially so if he had been questioned as a possible spy.

Whatever the truth of Otto Scholz's fate, its mysteries reinforced the hospital's associative power, its impenetrable tree-surrounded site able to contain any number of gothic narratives. A sense of secrecy and psychic charge grew out of the hospital's institutional nature, more especially now when the nation's very existence was threatened. Like the abbey, its medieval neighbour, the hospital created its own ghosts, harbingers of mortality which the extremes of wartime brought into ectoplasmic manifestation.

Netley's legendary 'Grey Lady' was said to be the ghost of a heartbroken nurse who, in the earliest years of the hospital, had thrown herself from one of the towers because she realised she'd killed a soldier patient with an accidental overdose. Another version claimed that, against hospital rules, she had fallen in unrequited love with a patient already in love with one of her colleagues; the spurned woman poisoned the man then committed suicide by swallowing her own fatal dose. A modern version of the abbey's incarcerated nun, her unquiet spirit now wandered the corridors, a drifting monochrome figure in nineteenth-century dress whose appearance, like Queen Victoria's shawl, signified imminent death.

Like Arthur Machen's Angels of Mons (so widely believed that it was said German dead had been found with arrows in their breasts) or the soldiers who claimed to have identified men marching with them as comrades killed in previous battles and who in one case carried them out of danger, so Netley provided a spirit nurse as an immortal carer, a beneficent version of the ghostly German who haunted Private Meek's dreams. This phantom may have augured the end, but it could also be seen as a guardian angel easing the dying into the next world, an intimation of immortality. Like some race memory of the Lady with the Lamp – only bringing death instead of life – Netley's ghostly nurse was conjured up by the collective imagination of its inmates, as though the bricks themselves, charged with emotion, had produced a watchful phantom.

There were many who bore witness to Netley's Grey Lady, such as the Catholic chaplain who, on his first visit to the chapel, asked the matron who the lady was who had followed her inside. A switchboard operator also heard the rustle of her silk dress and smelt her perfume in the hospital: 'At the same time, a night nurse saw the same spectre pass along a corridor next to the telephone room in which I was on duty. True to form, one of her patients died the next morning.' For years to come the Grey Lady would continue to haunt the corridors of Netley, projected along them like a romantic, deathly film on a decaying loop, a constantly replaying reminder of the building's mortal state.

* * *

As Netley created its own legends, like a shadow that precedes its form, so its looming presence haunted me, just as the pale invalids my mother had seen in the grounds as a young girl had stayed with her, and just as I attended school in a hut from the hospital's fields. Years later I would discover a cache of diaries kept by Esme Wynne, Noël Coward's teenage confidante, written during the war when they were touring the country in *Charley's Aunt*. Their first date was the Grand Theatre in Southampton, and it was strange to read, in her minuscule handwriting in equally tiny leatherbound diaries, Esme's adolescent account of the visit made by the cast to the hospital:

> Friday 11 February 1916 ... In the afternoon we were motored to Netley – we had to cross the floating bridge – to entertain the wounded soldiers at the hospital. I recited in 'Ela' dress and did a trio with Noël and Kitty called Nonsense Rhymes then we did the second act of *Charley's Aunt* – it was all a great success – then we had tea in Major Stevenson's room overlooking the waters and long stretches of lawn and dark pine trees the sky was grey and pink with a big splodge of gold showing between the pines ...

The two theatrical teenagers must have presented a sharp contrast to the young men they entertained, a reminder of ordinary, everyday life for the hutted hospital, which strove to present a happier alternative to the haunted corridors and wards of its brick counterpart. The wartime hospital magazine, an inhouse publication of skittish cartoons and optimistic reports on institutional life, records that performers were regularly brought in to entertain the troops – men who ironically referred to their battles in the theatre of war as 'shows', the deadly, choreographed *son-et-lumière* spectaculars of the Somme and Verdun – 'The cot cases were entertained in the Recreation Room from 3 to 4 pm on the dates specified ...'

The camp magazine was evidence of Netley's cultural life; an assertion of civilised normality, of what Britain was fighting for. In other editions, the editor – the euphoniously-named Caesar Caine who gave his address as the Author's Club, SW – discoursed for the benefit of his readers on the ancient history of Netley (accompanied by a cartoon of Stone Age lovers and a snake-necked dinosaur by Southampton Water), and on such local antiquarian subjects as the 'Fisherman's Spring', a gothic porch-like structure on the shore, constructed in the last century by a local benefactor to cap the fresh water that ran out of the gravel and into the sea as though it were some ancient holy well.

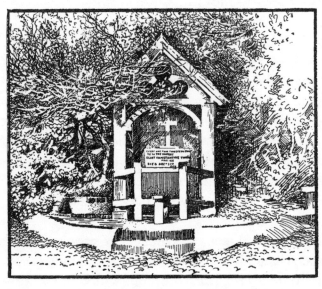

'We would suggest that those who used to benefit by the sweet spring water should help in these days to keep it in order, till the good times come again.'

A threatened time had recourse to history and philosophy and even myth; they provided necessary solace and a reassurance of national identity, as well as exploring new beliefs, new faiths to replace the old ones which had brought this situation about. In his running commentary, 'Impressions in a Great War Hospital', Caine contributed one instalment headed 'Intellectuality': 'Often I have been surprised and sometimes carried off my feet as it were, by finding plain Tommies who had read, to much advantage, Tyndal and Huxley. Others have studied Spiritualism and are familiar with the works of F. W. H. Myers and Sir Oliver Lodge. Others again, have been attracted to Christian Science, and practise its tenets in connection with their healing'.

Esme Wynne's romantic gold and pink diary description of the hospital was counterpointed by another wartime view, from the other side of its pine-fringed shore. In 1915 Vera Brittain left England for Malta as a VAD nurse. She too wrote in her journal of the setting sun over Hampshire. The omnipresence of war did not preclude the observation of beauty; indeed, the sense of mortality enhanced it:

> We sailed down the Solent just as the sun was setting; on either side of us the colours of the mainland were vividly beautiful. The sinking sun made a shimmering golden track on the water which seemed to link us in our tender to the England we were leaving behind, and in the evening light the aeroplanes and seaplanes which now and again flew round us looked like fairy things.

Brittain was on her way to *Britannic*, moored off Cowes, which 'appeared in the distance like a huge white mammoth lying on its side'. The sight filled her with 'sick dread'. Even in the beauty of this landscape – overlooked as it was by Netley's looming bulk – there was a sense of the war's perpetual process in which the individual was a helpless pawn. The following year Siegfried Sassoon would observe a similar scene, returning to the Front after home leave. '. . . My mind was unperturbed when we steamed out of Southampton Water', he wrote. 'I watched the woods on the Isle of Wight, hazily receding in the heat. And when the Isle of Wight was out of sight – well, there was nothing to be done about it.' The year was 1916, and Sassoon was on his way to the Somme. Like many others, he doubted that he would return.

*   *   *

The following summer, 1917, Wilfred Owen was brought up Southampton Water from Etretat in France. 'The Voyage was in a luxurious West Indian Liner', he told his mother. 'I had a cabin to myself, and fared sumptuously at Table'. It was a strange homecoming, moving slowly along this busy marine conduit yet insulated both from the real world and from the war which he had temporarily left behind. On arrival at Southampton Docks, Owen was abruptly pitched out of his deluxe surroundings and into the organised mayhem of military disembarkation; the lull of his Channel crossing was broken by the quayside chaos of shouting men and clanking cranes, and the contrary decisions of army bureaucracy. 'There was no choice of Hospitals when we were detailed off from Southampton, tho' I tried to get the Birmingham Train, which those officers who lived hereabouts had to take!' Instead, Owen was put on a train bound for Netley.

He arrived at the hutted Welsh Hospital on 16 June. His medical board, which he attended early on the morning of the 25th, briefly recorded the events which had brought him to the hospital, and the source of Owen's shell-shock, which was diagnosed as 'neurasthenia (143)':

... In March 1917 he fell down a well at Bouchoir, and was momentarily stunned. He was under Medical treatment for 3 weeks, and then resumed duty. About the middle of April he was blown up by a shell explosion while he was asleep. On May 1st he was observed to be shaky and tremulous, and his conduct and manner were peculiar, and his memory was confused. The RMC sent him to No. 41 Sty.H. Gailly where he was under observation and treatment by Capt. Brown RAMC, Neurological Specialist for a month. On 7/6/17 he was transferred to No. 1 G.H. Etretat, and on 16/6/17 to the Welsh Hospital Netley.

Like Sassoon, Owen had been serving on the Somme – 'at the edge of the world' – since the beginning of the year, living in waterlogged dugouts and resenting 'the illusory War Films'

250

which mediated the conflict for an ignorant public back home. On the night of 13 March he was trying to help 'a man in a dangerous state of exhaustion' when, like Alice, he fell into 'a kind of well', fifteen foot deep. There he lay for some time, concussed, before being taken to the 13th Casualty Clearing Station at Gailly, where he amused himself 'drawing plans for Country Houses and Bungalows, especially Bungalows. I worked my wits all day on one, and, within the prescribed limits, it is about perfect, for the intended occupant – solitary me.'

Owen's fantasy of a poetic retreat (like the Dorset cottage built by another literary soldier-outsider, T. E. Lawrence) was promptly demolished by his return to action. He rejoined his company at Saint-Quentin – 'a city dominated by the majestic, battered bulk of its gothic church' – from there to advance on Savy Wood. In their withdrawal behind the Hindenburg Line the Germans had laid an already devastated country to waste, removing all civilians from towns and villages, blowing up roads and poisoning wells. What had been countryside was now pock-marked with shellholes like acne, its woods and copses stripped to skeletons. A wad of aerial photographs kept by one RAMC officer show another view from a balloon; a deconstructed chaos compared to the ordered military might of Netley's hospital as seen from above Southampton Water.

It was the antithesis of the improved landscapes of the rational past. In this dimensionless perspective, the land had become a dispassionate pattern of destruction, a new manmade vista in which rows of houses were reduced to shells, like some future dream of Sholing's suburbia devasted by nuclear war. In such a wasteland, Owen's daydream of idyllic bungalows was blown apart by nightmare reality, and the very earth seemed ready to swallow him up. For nearly two weeks his company

lay in holes, where at any moment a shell might put us out. I think the worst incident was one wet night when we lay up against a railway embankment. A big shell lit on the top of the bank, just 2 yards from my head. Before I awoke, I

251

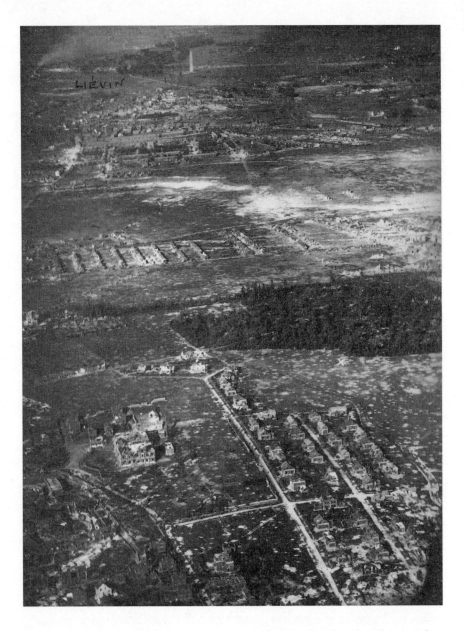

was blown in the air right away from the bank. I passed most of the following days in a railway Cutting, in a hole just big enough to lie in, and covered with corrugated iron. My brother officer of B Coy, 2/Lt Gaukroger lay opposite in a similar hole. But he was covered with earth, and no relief will ever relieve him . . .

It was more than a week before Owen's superior, Lieutenant-Colonel Luxmoore, observed his officer's strange behaviour.

'I shall have to stay here for a week or so', Owen wrote to his mother, Susan, from Netley on Sunday morning, 17 June. 'Visitors are allowed in the afternoons, but you will of course wait till I get my 3 Weeks at home.'

We are on Southampton Water, pleasantly placed, but not so lovely a coast as Etretat. The Town is not far off, and we are allowed to go in ... Nothing to write about now. I am in too <u>receptive</u> a mood to speak at all about the other side the seamy side of the *Manche*. I just wander about absorbing Hampshire.

In an antediluvian world, Gerald Manley Hopkins too had wandered through this countryside. The following day, back in the week's routine after Sunday's *longueurs*, Owen wrote again.

Dearest of Mothers,

I had your letter this morning – a great delight. This place is very boring, and I cannot believe myself back on England in this unknown region. I have just written to Leslie [Gunston, his cousin] asking him to come and convince me.

It is pleasant to be among the Welsh – doctors, sisters, orderlies. And nurses.

They kept me in bed all yesterday, but I got up for an hour & went out today, only to be recaught and put back in bed for the inspection of a specialist ... When I get away I shall try to journey through London. There are new clothes I want ... Here also we fare much better than anywhere in France. I sleep well and show every sign of health, except in the manipulation of this pencil.

Your own W.E.O.x

253

Having been treated with hypnosis by William Brown – 'a kind of wizard who mesmerises when he likes' – Owen had arrived at Netley stammering, in a nervous state, and with the possible shame of cowardice about him. He spent a week there, free, as an officer, to come and go from the hospital – at least, nominally. After a few days wandering the grounds, taking in the scale of Netley ('the "Welsh" is a hutment behind this Bunga-low', he wrote drily on the back of a postcard of the hospital to his mother), Owen was longing for company. He was duly visited by his cousin, Leslie Gunston, who, having been excused active service because of a heart murmur, was serving in a YMCA hut at a camp on Hazeley Down, near Winchester. Later that year Owen would return Gunston's visit, afterwards leaving him with 'the key to many of my poems, which you will guard from rust of soilure', and his poem 'Asleep', 'which came from Winchester Downs, as I crossed the long backs of the downs after leaving you. It is written <u>as from</u> the trenches. I could almost see the dead lying about in the hollows of the downs.' Plans were also made for Owen's mother and younger brother to come to Netley, but when Owen's medical board met on 25 June, it concluded, 'There is little abnormality to be observed but he seems to be of a highly strung temperament. He has slept well while here. He leaves Hospital to-day transferred to Craig Lockart War Hospital [sic], Edinburgh for special observation and treatment.'

Owen took the 11am train from Southampton to Waterloo, and stopped briefly in London to buy his new clothes and visit the Royal Academy Summer Exhibition. Afterwards he took tea at the Shamrock Tea Rooms, 'perhaps the most eminently respectable exclusive and secluded in Town', he told his mother. 'There was the usual deaf old lady and her Companion holding forth upon the new curate. I happen to know that a few storeys higher in the same building is an Opium Den. I have not investigated. But I know. That's London.' Five months later Owen met Sassoon at Craiglockhart ('this excellent concen-tration camp' as its own house magazine called it), and under

254

the older poet's influence began to produce the poetry which would achieve his immortality. Netley too had its part to play in that transition, its wooden huts a clearing station for Owen's fate.

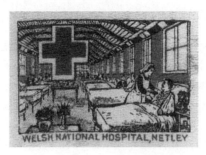

WELSH NATIONAL HOSPITAL, NETLEY

Here were treated the gassed soldiers of Owen's 'Dulce Et Decorum Est', their '... blood/ Come gargling from the forth-corrupted lungs/ Obscene as cancer, bitter as the cud.' Here, the broken minds of 'Mental Cases', 'Who are these? Why sit they here in twilight?/ Wherefore rock they, purgatorial shadows,/ Drooping tongues from jaws that slob their relish,/ Baring teeth that leer like skulls' teeth wicked?' And here the kilt-wearing god of 'Disabled', now no longer borne shoulder-high after foot-ball, but abandoned in a hospital ward: 'How cold and late it is! Why don't they come/ And put him into bed? Why don't they come?'

Owen left England the following August, in the last summer of war. On the day that he sailed for France, Owen went swim-ming on Folkestone beach, where he met 'a Harrow boy, of superb intellect & refinement; intellect because he hates war more than Germans; refinement because of the way he spoke of my Going, and of the Sun, and of the Sea there; and the way he spoke of Everything'. Four months later, as the bells announcing the Armistice rang, Susan Owen received the telegram announ-cing her son's death.

In 1922 the War Office 'Committee of Enquiry into Shell-Shock' reported its findings to Parliament. In the post-war elegiac mood – symbolised by the now annual rituals at cenotaphs and memorials in every town and village, and by the publication of verse such as Owen's and Sassoon's – even officialdom, perhaps suffering collective guilt, seemed to have become sentimental. The report's introduction quoted from Lady Percy's speech to Hotspur in *Henry IV, Part 1*: 'Why hast thou lost the fresh blood in thy cheeks . . . O what portents are these?'

Lloyd George may have announced that 'the world is suffering from shell-shock', but there was still scepticism about the nature of the illness that had brought so many thousands of men to D Block. Concerned that diagnoses of shell-shock might actually encourage its proliferation, the committee tried to rationalise its cause and effect. One witness cited a checklist, '*Behaviour Characteristics*', as used in the training of recruits by the US Navy during the war:

1. Resentfulness to discipline or inability to be disciplined.
2. Unusual stupidity or awkwardness in drills or exercises.
3. Inability to transmit orders correctly.
4. Personal uncleanliness.
5. Criminal tendencies.
6. Abnormal sex practices and tendencies, including masturbation.
7. Filthy language and defacement of property.
8. Distinct femine [sic] types.
9. Bed-wetters.
10. Subjects of continual ridicule or teasing.
11. Queer or peculiar behaviour.
12. All recruits who show persistently, the following characteristics: Tearfulness, irritability, seclusiveness, sulkiness, depression, shyness, timidity, anti-social attitude, overboisterousness, suspicion, dullness, sleeplessness, sleepwalking.
13. Chronic homesickness.

Some might have remarked that had this list of exclusions been adhered to, there would have been no British Army, certainly not in its conscripted form. Sir James Galloway somewhat sensibly informed the committee: 'I have been reading of the exceedingly elaborate methods put into operation by our colleagues in the United States ... From experience of what did happen to the American troops, I do not think it did much good. I do not think their casualties so far as "Shell-shock" was concerned were much minimised by this elaborate examination.' (Some blamed the Americans themselves for introducing British troops to subversive habits: in 1916, a concerned *Lancet* had commented on the case of two persons imprisoned in Folkestone for supplying cocaine to privates in a Canadian regiment, 'in the course of the hearing of which it was stated by an officer of the Royal Army Medical Corps that there were forty men in a barracks hospital suffering from the cocaine habit...'. The magazine also noted 'a traffic in morphine' with the 'palatable little gelatine discs' which were easily obtained by both officers and men.)

Among the other witnesses called to the 1922 enquiry – along with such eminent names as W. H. Rivers and the neurologist Henry Head (another friend of Sassoon's who in 1908 had allowed Rivers to sever the nerves in his arm in an experiment on the physiological basis of sensation, and who in the 1920s developed a therapy for 'converting' homosexuals) – was Dr C. Stanford Read, commander of D Block and now 'Neurological and Mental Specialist, Ministry of Pensions':

Dr Read defined 'shell-shock' as 'a mental abnormality brought about by emotional shock, of which a shell explosion is only a frequent type. Mental disassociation is the main mechanism involved, and the symptoms may be manifold, and either mental or physical or a combination of the two. A previous mental conflict usually can be traced which mainly involves the impulses towards self-preservation and duty.' 'When the Armistice came,' said

257

the witness, 'the neurosis stopped, and psychoses went on, showing that they were different conflicts.' Those service patients, who were still in asylums and whose histories Dr Read had been able to follow, were nearly all suffering from dementia praecox. The witness thought that they would probably have broken down with any comparatively small strain under any circumstances. The great stress of war produced psychosis, or expedited its development.

Like the lower classes of the previous century who were pathologised in Netley's laboratories, these mentally-disturbed men continued to be seen as predisposed – by social conditions or genetic circumstance – to their maladies. Thus the Army was not responsible, and thus officialdom drew a line under the traumatic memory of the war. Britain, its army and its empire, could return to normality once more. To the likes of Arnold White, the 'Condy's Fluid' of war had disinfected the country of that very decadence and degeneracy which had threatened the pre-war state. Madness had made the Empire sane.

The emptying wards of D Block were proof of the efficacy of the new therapies and the temporary nature of shell-shock. But Netley continued to repair the damage done by the War To End All Wars, and its hutted hospital took on a sense of semi-permanence, the air of a colony of sickness and healing. Ornamental shrubs and gardens had been planted in between the rows of huts, their plots demarcated by rustic fencing in imitation of the new English suburbs; a mimesis of normality caught somewhere between Owen's imaginary bungalow and the bombed and shelled towns of France and Belgium.

It was a medical version of the estates being built by Herbert Collins on the other side of Southampton in Highfield; neo-Georgian utopias to fulfil the Prime Minister's promise of homes for heroes. A contemporary photograph shows Lloyd George visiting Netley, making a joke as his driver climbs into his car, watched by patients and a welcoming party of the commandant and his officers. The informality is in marked contrast to Victoria's measured visits of the previous century.

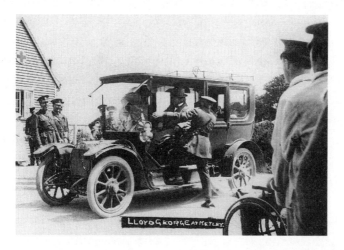

A new society was emerging, with new calls for reform and equality; war veterans marched past the Whitehall Cenotaph with pawn tickets pinned to their chest instead of medals. But Netley's ailing population was unlikely to rebel against the process which had put them there. For them, war had bequeathed less rather than more freedom. While their healthy compatriots would spend their summers in holiday camps organised for a populace accustomed to a new sense of social control, they were confined to permanent, medical equivalents of holiday chalets.

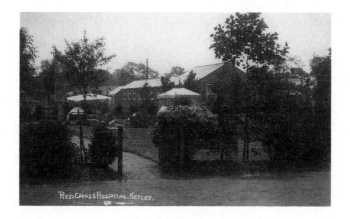

Sere, sunk in their beds, they faced the unknown clean and tidy for the camera. Photographs show boys barely out of school uniform bearing up bravely, propped up on one elbow while proudly disregarding their shattered legs below. Others portray men holding up embroidered panels, sewn to raise funds and pass the hours. There were tailor's shops and basket-weaving classes; some made poker-work boxes and dolls houses out of wood; some made models of tanks; all sold for the Red Cross, for the support of their fellow men. Yet for all the homespun activity, for all the roses, the sad roses of Picardy, around the trellises, and for all the postcards with their cheery captions, the sewn-short sleeves and trousers of these men and boys betray what their faces try not to show: that their legs will never feel warm again after swimming in a chilly sea, nor the sun tan forearms brown as they roll up their sleeves. For all their brave expressions, they are ultimately pathetic, these faces made pallid by the intensity of their experience, as if the life has been drained out of them by so much emotion and pain.

In a group photographed in August of 1919, a summer picnic of disabled men and their nurses sit out on the lawn, the main hospital high behind them. Their crutches lie in the grass. Beside one soldier sits a little girl in white; another little boy sits slumped in the end of the basket stretcher in which lies his wounded father or brother, his legs covered by a flowered quilt, the pain

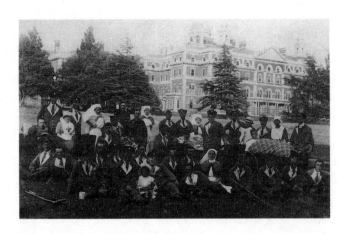

on his face reflected in the child's discomfort. Such posed groups do not include the disfigured and mutilated victims of shrapnel or burns; still less would anyone want to photograph the shell-shocked, chronically-psychotic or syphilitically-deranged of D Block, safely locked away out of sight in their padded cells.

Up in 'Piccadilly', Red Cross nurses pose in starched white skirts that billow in the breeze, their bosoms covered to their necks in cotton aprons; they look just as my grandmother did in her new posting at Birmingham, her fiancé still out in India. Inside their mess hut, on their afternoon off, blonde girls with fresh faces and blue eyes sit reading the papers and smoking surreptitious cigarettes on chintz-covered sofas, while in another wooden hut men dressed in black and white pierrot costumes, their necks surrounded by ruffs and heads encased in two-tone skull caps, rehearse some 'Co-Optimists' numbers. They look as incongruous as the other fancy-dressed soldiers in costumes made out of giant polka-dot material, with spiky wigs and cardboard bow-ties, oddly abashed by their silliness, in contrast to the military discipline under which they labour. Or the trio in comic colonial uniforms, painted and made-up, one effete-looking man standing akimbo in jodhpurs, the make-up a little too neatly applied to his face, as if the coming years might see him make a living in a bar in Weimar Berlin.

For all their attempts to forget, the figures in these scenes reflect the afterglow of the war – the bodies which Sassoon 'saw' in the streets of London; Vera Brittain's fear that her face 'was changing' as she lived with the 'dark hallucinations' left by her experiences. In the freneticism of the coming decade, lives flared into indulgence and escape, if they could; a world in which the brittle wit and hedonism effected by the characters in Noël Coward's plays seemed merely a delayed symptom of shell-shock, as much an expression of discontent as those Jarrow marchers in Dugdale's painting. Meanwhile the long corridors at Netley fell quiet, waiting for the next patient.

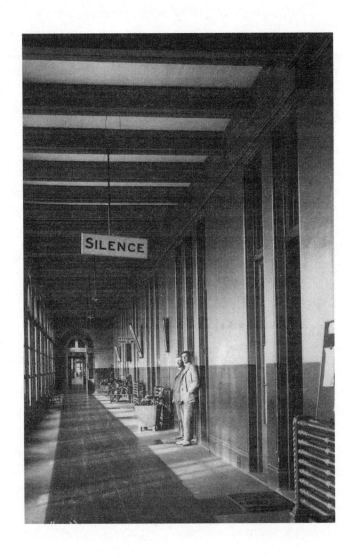

Towards a Better Britain

Before a building can take visible shape, it ought first to
have been created as a thought; imagination must precede
action; without ordered imagination action is likely to be
wasteful and productive of chaos.

W. H. AUSELL, RIBA

'I will not again curse the ground for any man's sake;
for the imagination of man's heart is evil from youth . . .'

Genesis 8:6

———

Along the south coast of England appeared modernist white
blocks with Crittall windows as suburbia joined the dots
along the shore. Symbols of a new optimism – as though they'd
been manufactured from the chalk cliffs – their clean lines and
European design expressed a new sense of freedom. Compared
to these forward-looking new buildings, the ponderous architecture of Netley's seaside hospital seemed ever more outmoded in
the inter-war years. Behind it the huts of the Red Cross hospital
were slowly dismantled, some destined for the new suburbs as
bungalows or changing rooms on recreation grounds, while the
Catholic chaplain donated the matron's quarters to the head-
mistress at St Patrick's in Woolston, who employed a gang of

local men, laid off in the 1921 coal strike, to reassemble its corrugated iron in the playground where, forty years later, it would become my classroom.

The main hospital's once pristine bricks were now beginning to show their age; the precision-cut stone, so elegantly dressed by Victorian masons, was blunted by the years, an acute contrast to the ever-sharp, angular architecture of the modern era. The young pines, once whippy and lithe, had grown old and gnarled around the building, darkening the site with their nineteenth-century planting. Without a war to service, and with the empire it served rapidly diminishing, the hospital seemed forlorn and empty, beginning to lose its grip on the national consciousness. Now, more than ever, it was out of step with the times.

But the hospital did have one particular function in those apparently unclouded, optimistic years. One wing was given over to the care of sufferers from tuberculosis, a disease which remained a potent killer, responsible for 50,000 deaths a year. Röntgen's rays might reveal lungs pitted with tubercles, but with the discoveries of Almroth Wright's assistant Alexander Fleming yet to hold out any hope, little could be done to treat the sufferers beyond exposing them to fresh air – as they were in Dr Snowden's huts at Netley. Like the influenza epidemic of 1918–19 and the 'sleepy sickness', *encephalitis lethargica*, which left its victims as living statues, TB in the Twenties and Thirties was a modern disease of dense populations and no respecter of class, although its romantic overtones remained for Siegfried Sassoon's lover, the tubercular young aristocrat Stephen Tennant, attended in his Wiltshire mansion by the same Dr Snowden and advised, via Sassoon, on his own neurosis by Henry Head. Meanwhile in Southampton my mother watched from her bedroom window as their neighbour's son sat in a wooden summerhouse, a pale boy dying of tuberculosis in a suburban garden, and at Netley, other young men lay coughing into their handkerchieves, staining the linen crimson.

These dark rooms, the antechambers to the Jazz Age's bright freneticism, conjured up Netley's gothic inheritance in the dim-lit wards and the decaying half-life of their doomed inhabitants.

One summer night in 1936, 'warm and as usual quiet', the orderly in charge of the TB ward heard a patient coughing 'very harshly',

> so I went into the ward where the coughing was coming from, and I found a patient sitting up in bed . . . he said that he had been dreaming, of being choked . . . At 2 am I made out a temperature chart and just having given the man his medicine I wrote this in the treatment book, and then, I felt as if I had left this world, although the pen was still in my hand, I could see the entry, and yet I wasn't part of it, I was at the door of the duty room looking at the Sister who passed by without speaking. I was trying to speak, but no sound came from me, it seemed that my body was fixed and rigid, my mind was alert but nothing came from my voice.

Somewhere in the room he saw a dark shape, moving slowly; then it was gone.

> The 'Grey Lady' had passed into nothing, and I jerked into life, wondering what had happened. I looked at the clock. It was 2.2 am. For two minutes I had been in the presence of the unknown. What did it mean – a death? . . . The patient was due for a discharge to a civil hospital at 8 am that morning; he didn't make it, for he died at 6.20 am. I had my thoughts that morning as I laid him out, something must have happened years ago but the official side kept a tight and 'stiff upper lip' on such things.

The hospital seemed to retain the mortality of war; indeed, some of its staff appeared to cultivate such morbidity. One patient recalled a visit from the padre, who stopped near his bed and asked, 'How long do you think a dead body remains whole in a coffin?' That afternoon a number of Belgian war dead had been repatriated from the hospital cemetery, and 'those in oak coffins remained in good condition, but in coffins made of elm, the bodies went to dust'. 'The padre's question did not do my temperature chart any good', remarked the hapless patient, 'but in those days Netley Hospital had rather an eerie, depressing atmosphere . . .'

Yet for those whose existence was not proscribed by illness, life between the wars at Netley was actually rather enjoyable. The park-like setting, the balmy sea air in summer, and the sense of solitude which to someone confined to a hospital bed was a reminder of his own isolation was, to the healthy and carefree, an almost idyllic state. In a world once again freed for leisure and travel, with Southampton Water now thronged with paddle steamers rather than hospital ships, the pines and tamarisks along the shore seemed to evoke the newly-fashionable resorts of Europe, now no longer a place of destruction but of recreation, a Mediterranean destination for the celebrated writers, business moguls and aristocrats who set off from Southampton's docks or travelled across the Atlantic in its luxurious liners.

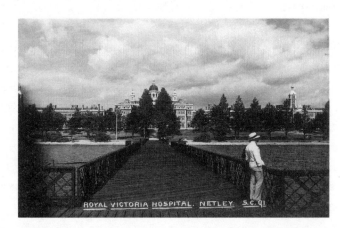

Such an image of inter-war glamour, transferred to Netley, was a sunlit contrast to the gloominess of the hospital's interior. One dedicated nursing officer, Colonel Kneebone, of QAR-ANC (Queen Alexandra's Royal Army Nursing Corps), was posted to Netley in 1933 and found it a peaceful place between the 'trooping seasons'. 'The Commanding Officer had a very nice speed boat', she recalled, 'he was a dear, very benign, and he used to take us out on it along Southampton Water, and we were able to swim at the end of the Pier, because in those days, the water was fairly clean.' Her sister, also a nurse, remembered the troopships returning from foreign service would lay off Netley before going into port, and the nurses would wave at the soldiers on board. They'd throw their tropical helmets into the sea, leaving the shore 'littered with soggy topees' when they were washed up days later. At night the nightingales would sing so sweetly in the coppice by the TB ward that the BBC came to record them, and from the windows the nurses watched as ships strung with lights passed up and down the water, 'a fairylike sight' to Sister Kneebone, although she too experienced strange incidents.

We were all told the story of the Grey Lady, and I believe one night I saw her very much in the distance, because it could be very spooky along those tremendously long corridors. One night my Orderly, I was going round about two o'clock in the morning, to my amazement I found him wide awake . . . He said: 'But you have only just been round', and I said, 'Oh, no I haven't.' I think he was very frightened, he said: 'It must have been the Grey Lady.' Well he was so frightened he kept awake for the rest of the night . . .

With her commanding officer's speed boat, nightingales singing in the woods and the frisson of a Victorian ghost, Kneebone painted a romantic scene. Her brave soldier patients were rallied by their camaraderie, determined not to be conquered by the 'depressing' building around them. On Sundays, after compulsory Church parade – which she considered 'broke the monotony of the day, because Netley being so far away, we had no visitors for patients' – the men 'amused themselves with singsongs from ward to ward . . . they would start spontaneously with all the hymns. It was quite a common thing to come on Night Duty on Sunday evening, you opened the door and there was this lovely sound of men singing – it was so spontaneous, and I think it was one of the best therapies they had, because they got it out of their system . . .' In this cross between a seaside resort, a sanatorium and an army barracks, life seemed caught in the lingering strains of old hymns, as though every day was Sunday. Through the long summer of peace, Netley idled by the sea, until its services would be needed once more.

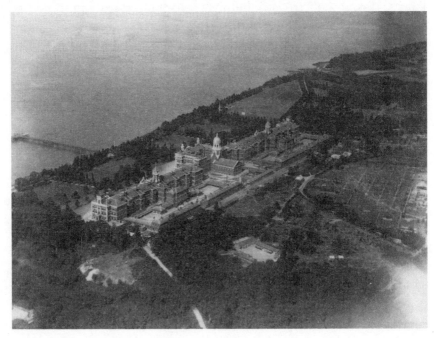

A rare view of the rear of the hospital, late 1920s. The hutted hospital has been cleared; in the foreground are the hospital stables and isolation ward

Then hell fell out of the sky. From 1940 to 1944, intensive German bombing raids on Southampton killed or seriously injured nearly 2,000 people, and destroyed or seriously damaged 10,000 properties.

Viking and Norman raiders had come by barge and galley up Southampton Water; now the estuary provided a flight path for Heinkels and Dorniers, and its hospital dome a landmark for their lumbering drone, their foreign shapes dark against the sky as they brought the European war into the heart of southern England. Invasion seemed imminent, and set along the shore gun emplacements and pillboxes – concrete versions of Henry VIII's forts – awaited the enemy's next move. When it came, its *blitz-krieg* ferocity was unparalleled.

It seemed the end of the world had come. Within the space of ten days Southampton was raided seven times, and on 24 September enemy bombers turned their attention to the banks of the Itchen, sweeping low over the riverside. Woolston, with its shipbuilding and aircraft works, was heavily hit, and St Patrick's Church set ablaze with incendiary bombs. Once again Netley escaped unharmed, perhaps protected by its hospital status, but three miles away, Southampton's centre 'had largely crumbled into unrecognisable wreckage'; its once gracious High Street now resembled a bombed Belgian town from 1918. It was as if the horror of that war had returned, this time to England's shores.

With the destruction of the town's commercial spine, the very fabric of life appeared to break down. As the bombs began to fall on the suburbs too, inhabitants left each night to sleep in the safety of the open countryside. In 1940, a Mass Observation commentator recorded that morale was low: 'The strongest feeling in Southampton today is that it is finished. Many will not say this openly, but it is a deep-seated feeling that has grown in the past fortnight. Yet many householders continue to come in every day, and quite a number of women spend the day in their homes and the night in outlying billets – even as far as Salisbury.' Contrary to expectation, the civilian population proved remarkably resilient to a war which had come directly into their own homes, defining their day-to-day existence.* As a vitally important strategic port, sentries were placed on roads

---

* Before the war 'the aerial holocaust, it was assumed, would not only kill civilians; it would also send them mad'; an estimated three to four million psychiatric casualties were expected, and 'large psychiatric hospitals were established on the edges of major conurbations' to deal with them. Yet the expected 'trembling hordes' did not materialise. In fact, 'clinics emptied [and] cases of neurosis and attempted suicide declined dramatically . . .'

in and out of Southampton and permission was required to enter the town; like Netley, it was a settlement under military manners.

The town also had a new official designation – Area C – and Military Movement Control set up its headquarters in the dockside South Western Hotel. The glamorous interior with its murals of the *Mayflower* and mirrored ballroom became a centre of war operations, resounding to the march of military boots rather than patent pumps. The town's parks, with their band-stands and flower-beds, were turned into army camps, and lorries and tanks rumbled down the High Street. Churchill arrived to instil courage in the battered town, watched by my mother from the doorway of Rose & Co. as he passed in his car, smiling and giving the workers the Victory sign. In turn, they placed their trust in him.

Faced with imminent invasion, Southampton turned itself into one offensive, defensive entity. In the docks, smoke bombs were let off during air raids, billowing plumes drifting over the site like an artificial cloud to obscure it from the enemy's sight. My mother left the fancy goods of Rose & Co. to work at a lathe making machine gun parts, while my father manned the Home Guard ack-ack emplacements outside the town. Down at Netley, their counterparts launched missiles at enemy aircraft from an experimental rocket station in Westwood, and the beach was strung with medieval-looking defences of concrete and barbed wire where children had paddled. Barrage balloons were tethered above Sholing Common, and on the low cliffs at Netley the pillboxes were ready to repel the invasion everyone knew could come at any time. The hospital's pier was severed to prevent its use by invading Nazis and, sensitised to a new war situation, Netley continued to breed rumours: when in 1942 a long, closed-off train arrived at the hospital station, it was said to hold either Russians, Germans, or coffins from the London blitz. In fact, it contained cavalry horses, sent for their own equine recuperation on the hospital's lush pastures.

Then, as the tide of war turned, and as the graphic smoke

trails of aerial combat cleared from the skies, other, friendly invaders arrived up Southampton Water.

In November 1943 Helen Luker, a nurse in the Queen Alexandra's Imperial Military Service, was sent to Netley. 'What have I done to deserve this?' she wrote one evening in her little red leather pocket diary. 'The cold is bitter, and how to make myself get up early for 7 am breakfast, I didn't know. Mess about all morning in the ward – it is a shambles – never have I seen such messes, even in Egypt!' Luker, a sweet-looking, bespectacled young woman from Petersfield, kept her journal assiduously in neat handwriting, adding bus and train tickets as mementoes, and writing brief reports on the war's progress after her daily accounts of life in the hospital – an intimate, inconsequential record of the monotony of existence in this rambling shell.

Since Dunkirk the hospital had been full to capacity, dealing with thousands of sick and wounded from Europe in wards still furnished with Victorian beds and tables and looking distinctly shabby and outdated. In that harsh mid-war winter of 1943, Netley's nineteenth-century rooms were so 'punishingly cold' that the falling temperature actually woke Nurse Luker, her sleep already disturbed by a 'fog horn going all night, 270 times per hour'. Rising at 6.30 am for morning service in the chapel, she would put on all her jumpers and an overcoat, yet still be 'simply freezing'. The days stretched in front of her like the great long corridors. At times she was hopelessly idle, painting pots and jars 'for want of something better to do!'; then, suddenly, she was attending to tens of burns patients in chilly operating theatres. Precious half-days were spent in Southampton, going to the cinema or meeting friends in tea shops in Shirley.

On New Year's Day 1944, Nurse Luker took a snapshot from her bedroom, Room 28, a garret on the top floor. Through the arched window she saw dark conifers against the lawns, the same trees which three decades before Esme Wynne had noted in her own pocket diary. Nine days later, Luker left the hospital, 'not

271

sorry to see the back of Netley'. As she and her colleagues moved out, the US Army moved in.

On 15 January 1944, five days after Helen Luker's glad departure, the Americans rolled up the country lanes to establish the 28th US General Hospital at Netley. The BBC was back with its big black microphone ready to broadcast, not peaceable nightingales singing in the woods, but the speeches of Lieutenant-General Sir Alexander Hood as he presented the hospital's keys to Brigadier General P. Hawley of the United States Army on the steps of the main entrance.

Suddenly the place was filled with sexy Americans, with their sweatshirts, crewcuts and baseball matches on the football ground; Netley's new occupants looked more like lovers than victims. Two million of their countrymen passed through Southampton, and at the factory where my mother worked, some of the younger girls 'went silly' over the Yanks, with their neat uniforms and movie star accents, and they misbehaved in dance halls and back alleys. Meanwhile, American tanks and trucks were parked on suburban streets, and the whole of Weston Shore became one giant US army camp shut off from public access. Across the water at Hythe, enormous Mulberry harbours were being constructed, their concrete pontoons defying the water. It seemed the south coast itself was about to invade France.

The Americans found 325 British patients still in the main hospital, 'mostly suffering from respiratory and minor medical problems', as one US psychiatric nurse, Roberta Henry, recalled. Coming from a land of refrigerators, chrome and gasoline, the Americans were appalled at the state of the hospital and its archaic facilities. The hospital's new tenants were so impatient with the sprawling, old-fashioned behemoth that it was said they drove down its corridors in their jeeps – a gesture of cultural appropriation as surreal as the sight of their state-of-the-art equipment installed in crumbling Victorian wards. Here boys from Brooklyn or Nebraska were x-rayed and operated on in surroundings which to their doctors seemed little more than Dickensian. If the nurses of the hutted hospital had joked about giving 'the Yanks' a lesson in modern medical techniques in the last war, the lessons were vividly reversed now.

With the facilities of the main hospital outdated and rundown, the American army were given the use of a new single-storey concrete complex which had been built at the end of 'Piccadilly', on the northernmost edge of the hospital's grounds. Like the Red Cross's 'fieldhouses' it too was a semi-prefabricated construction, hurriedly assembled in 1940 to a standard design, providing new operating theatres, wards, barracks, officers' quarters and ten outlying bomb shelters for its inhabitants. Known as a 'spider' hospital because of the way its network of slab-roofed huts spread outwards like an arachnid's legs, the extended initials it actually formed were more reminiscent of prison compounds – the H Blocks of Northern Ireland a generation later. But in 1944 this new settlement on the south Hampshire plains was adopted as American territory, flying the stars and stripes as the US Army 110th Station Hospital and all but surrounded by a wooden palisade. Typically, the new hospital proved too small to contain its influx, and most of its staff had to sleep under canvas. They would treat more than 37,000 patients, including German prisoners of war, all ferried across from France to Southampton, by rail to Netley and then up Piccadilly into this field full of flat concrete blocks.

In February, a second wave of Americans arrived at Netley; the US Navy had come to occupy the main hospital which their Army colleagues had found wanting. They were equally unimpressed: Navy Nurse Sara E. Marcum Kelley declared, 'When we reported to the hospital we were impressed with the beautiful setting. Outside the hospital looked great but [we] were horrified how antiquated it was inside, especially the plumbing . . .' This being the highwater mark of civilisation for an American, Nurse Kelley was horrified to watch as 'water ran from the bath tub and sink into a groove in the floor next to the wall, then went halfway around the room before finally down the pipe'.

Preparing for the invasion of Europe on D-Day 1944, the

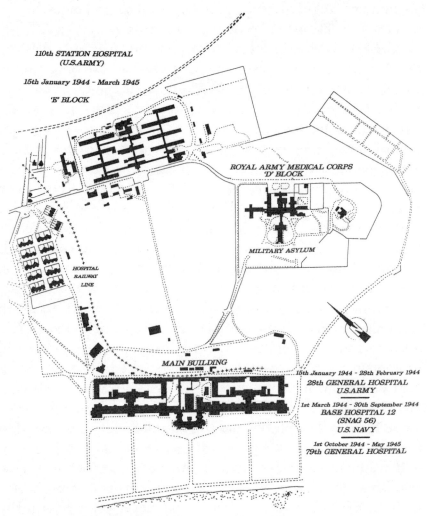

110th STATION HOSPITAL
(U.S.ARMY)

15th January 1944 - March 1945

'E' BLOCK

ROYAL ARMY MEDICAL CORPS
'D' BLOCK

MILITARY ASYLUM

HOSPITAL
RAILWAY
LINE

MAIN BUILDING

15th January 1944 - 28th February 1944
28th GENERAL HOSPITAL
U.S.ARMY

1st March 1944 - 30th September 1944
BASE HOSPITAL 12
(SNAG 56)
U.S. NAVY

1st October 1944 - May 1945
79th GENERAL HOSPITAL

LOCATION OF MEDICAL UNITS AT NETLEY 1944 - 1945

Americans at Netley had learned from the last war and made provision for their mental casualties. With the walled asylum of D Block still in British hands, they set up a psychiatric unit on the second floor of the main hospital; here new therapies were applied to the reinvented, US version of shell-shock. 'Treatment for combat fatigue consisted of deep sleep, good nourishment and psychiatry', reported Roberta Henry. 'Sodium pentothal (also known as the truth serum) was administered and closely monitored to maintain complete sleep and relaxation. The patient was only allowed to be awake for brief periods of nourishment. After a few days they were gradually brought out of the deep slumber and interviewed by the Psychiatrist. This was known as Narcoanalysis.'

It was also modern psychotherapy: pioneering, conquering, rational, exorcising the old demons with drugs and benign interrogation. The therapies used by the Americans at Netley were the product of a forward-looking country which regarded it as their duty to dispel the evils of the past, a feat accomplished with certain faith in their techniques for dealing with deep human trauma. Their modern world, all chrome and gasoline and straight-talking, had no patience with failure. (It was also one sensitised to the science of psychology in a manner which would set the tone for generations to come – the historian Ben Shephard has spoken of the 'pampered' GI victims of combat fatigue as precursors of the modern 'culture' of post-traumatic stress disorder.)

'Most patients talked freely of their experiences and fears and relived many of the demons that were troubling them', wrote Nurse Henry. 'I recall one patient, a US soldier, who couldn't respond, a blank look on his face as if he couldn't hear. An examination revealed no physical hearing problem. While in Narcoanalysis, he recalled that a mortar shell had blown up in the fox hole, killing all of his buddies. The experience was so traumatic that he was in shock. His recovery was remarkable and he returned to duty.' Yet for all these scientific advances, the paradox remained the same: healing to send men back to the war which had brought them there.

In the wake of D-Day, Southampton's invasion of Americans was replaced by an influx of wounded: 68,000 of them, including 10,000 wounded Germans. Prisoners of war – haggard, unshaven men beaten down by battle – were kept in secure compounds and transit camps in the docks and surrounding countryside. Pitted with bomb sites and wrapped in barbed wire, the area looked more like a piece of war-torn Europe than part of the English south coast. It seemed as exhausted as the old world it represented, as though the tide had gone out, and wasn't coming back.

Virtually an American colony for the latter half of the war, the hospital was officially handed back to the British on 14 July 1945. But the great assembly of Allied military power that had gathered in and around Southampton Water had heralded a new empire, a modern world anticipated even as the war was being fought.

'The new aesthetic. We need not lose many words over it. You know it, even if you are not always conscious of it.' So announced the Royal Institute of British Architects in the illustrated brochure, *Towards a Better Britain*, produced in 1943 as a statement of faith in a democratic future freed from fascism. Its preface, written by Churchill, speculated that reconstruction was 'one of our essential jobs after the war: not only because so much has been knocked down by Hitler, but also because we, over a century or so have allowed a fantastic muddle, a mountain of dirt and debris, to accumulate'. In the last war the Vorticists had envisioned an 'industrial island machine'; the new Britain would in turn be marked by democratic monuments. In an uplifting, regenerating embrace of constructivist collectivism, bricks and mortar were to be replaced by steel and glass:

> This **giant object** is the wheel of an aeroplane, but it is also a piece of abstract art like Paul Nash's menhirs, or of sculpture, comparable with Moholy Nagy and Henry Moore. Again, how the **funnel of a liner** combines the qualities of machine precision with those of an entrancing abstract art, delicate and full of spatial eloquence. And what do these shimmering flasks mean with their exquisite spiral steel trimming? They are **gas containers** in America, a monument as telling of the ambitions of our age as were the aqueducts of Rome.

276

In 1951, London's South Bank sprouted futuristic structures, a centennial reprise of the Great Exhibition to embody this soaring new spirit, a tonic for the nation. That same year, on the New Forest shore opposite Netley, the spikes and cylinders of Fawley's new oil refinery rose like multiples of the Skylon and the Dome of Discovery. For the nineteenth-century visitor to Netley, one of the most impressive aspects about the hospital had been its 'comprehensive view ... the blue-grey masses of the New Forest, bordered by the bright green waters of the tidal way, in which several vessels were lying at anchor'. Now that far horizon had a new skyline of spires and towers, industrial versions of the abbey's gothic arches and the hospital's Italianate campanile.

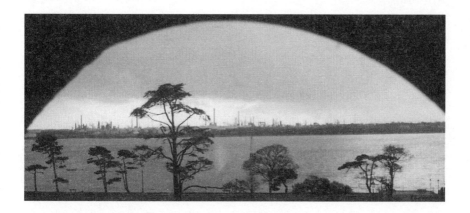

Built in the grounds of Cadland House, a Capability Brown-designed estate, the new factory had grown out of the Atlantic Gulf West Indies Refinery constructed in 1921 (even in 1917, Siegfried Sassoon had been told that the war was being fought for 'Mesopotamian Oil Wells'). With the end of the Second World War and the increase in oil consumption, Fawley expanded to become Europe's second largest refinery, taking up nearly two miles of Hampshire shoreline and erasing Cadland's eighteenth-century estate in the process. A view little changed since Cobbett's first glimpse from Weston was now broken by the dull jagged metal of silos and flares; instead of picturesque vessels at anchor, lumbering tankers moored off the shore to suckle the plant with black liquid, while burning above them was the refinery's eternal flame, as though in commemoration of some unknown warrior of the future.

The mid-twentieth-century sky, suspended with the by-products of refineries around the world, was filled with Ruskin's storm-clouds and plague-winds. Vivid orange-red sunsets hung over Fawley as though its flares were licking them into incandescence, and at night, as I slept in my bed, the electric lights gleamed on the refinery's towers, turning them into a futuristic city across the water, the tanks and silos silhouetted against the inky blackness. This was the future Netley and Britain faced: new forms of energy, new cloud shapes forming in the dark sky and contaminating the ground. In later assessments of the environmental impact of the refinery, Esso's researchers would date their core samples from the saltmarshes by the radioactive traces left by the Pacific hydrogen bomb tests of 1953.

In 1956 a special correspondent for *The Times* was sent to report on the changes going on in this part of southern England.

The first view of England which the ocean traveller gets at Southampton to-day is very different from the one he had in 1939. This is not just because the town was severely bombed and now, half-reconstructed, mixes modernity with ruins. It is also because economic logic is carrying out a revolution in the Southampton area which Whitehall and the local authorities are having to face.

Entitled 'Gateway to Britain' – an echo of the ageing road signs which informed visitors that they were approaching the 'Gateway to the Empire' – the survey marvelled at Fawley's 'incessant burning of waste gases which ... look like blazing wind-socks attached to their chimneys', but discovered that 'an unattractive product' was its smell, 'which the refinery superintendent freely admits is "pretty vile". The New Forest has been largely spared by westerly winds, and most complaints have come from ... across the water. Esso have already spent £3m trying to control it; and, for the day to day battle, they employ men whose sole function is to go about in search of smells.' Almost exactly a hundred years ago the objections to the hospital had focused on the notion of a poisonous atmosphere; now the same concerns returned to these shores. As a new miasma threatened Netley, its memory seemed cast into shade by Fawley and its refinery towers. In the bright white light of the modern age, Netley's Victorian vision was rapidly fading, receding into the shadows of history.

Riven with doubt since its creation, the hospital's fate now looked distinctly uncertain. The site was visibly decaying. Its truncated pier had rotted away and the remains demolished in 1955; over its stump stood Scots pines, wind-whipped as young saplings, now twisted into melancholic shapes, bent back from the shore as if frozen in the breeze.

Unable to comprehend the future, Netley took refuge in its past. After the war it continued to function as a reception point for the sick and wounded arriving from overseas, from actions in deliquescing colonies and the post-imperial struggle for resources that marked years not of peace but of continual war. Decreasing in usefulness in disproportion to its size, as a general and convalescent hospital for the army, Netley was less popular than ever with those who worked there. 'It was frequently one's first posting within the Army', recalled one nurse, 'and long remembered as the worst.' It was also a holiday venue for red-coated Chelsea Pensioners, with whom my two older brothers were photographed as boys on Lepe Beach in 1951, just as Fawley's towers were rising along that same shore. Eyes squinted against the summer sun, their fair heads rather solemnly bow at the shiny black feet of the bemedalled, scarlet-tunicked and equally solemn-faced old men who had been bussed to the seaside for the day from Netley's nineteenth-century military hospital, where their archaic uniforms were suited to the scene like toy soldiers on a wooden fort.

The building was certainly more appealing as a reminder of past glories than it was for the put-upon staff who worked there and in its still-functioning asylum. One upstairs ward of the main hospital was used to discharge patients from D Block; from here, one guardsman watched an inmate take a running jump through the window and land gruesomely on a pillarbox below in a repeat trajectory of Netley's suicidal Grey Lady. Another witness was convinced you could still see the bloodstains on the stone where she fell, and that D Block's suicides were driven to perpetuate the process on the same spot.

By the mid-Fifties – as CND protesters were writing 'Go Home Yanks' on walls in London – the great bulk of the old-fashioned hospital so despised by the US Army had fallen into disuse. Its railway had ground to a halt: the ambulance carriages languished in sidings, fireweed and sorrel grew between the sleepers, and the steep embankments spilled over with brambles and gorse. There was no longer an army of staff to care for the huge building. The floors of wards and corridors once buffed daily to a military polish had lost their sheen; the cracks started to show and the paint began to peel.

Photographed again from the air – even now, only an aerial view could convey its scale – it was clear how far suburbia had begun to encroach upon the site. The housing estates and the light engineering works were steadily marching up to the hospital perimeter, and in the aeronautical factory next door stood car parks full of employees' cars, taking up more room just as the countryside was being tarmacked to carry them there. In the middle of this expanding post-war development, Netley's Victorian folly held out against the twentieth century, protected by its sentinel trees.

In 1956 the general duties of the hospital were moved to the American hospital, and its convalescent wing transferred to Chester; the main building had finally given up its medical usefulness. That year Cold War refugees from Hungary were housed in its drafty wards, and it was subsequently announced in the local press that 'male patients – of about military age – at Southampton

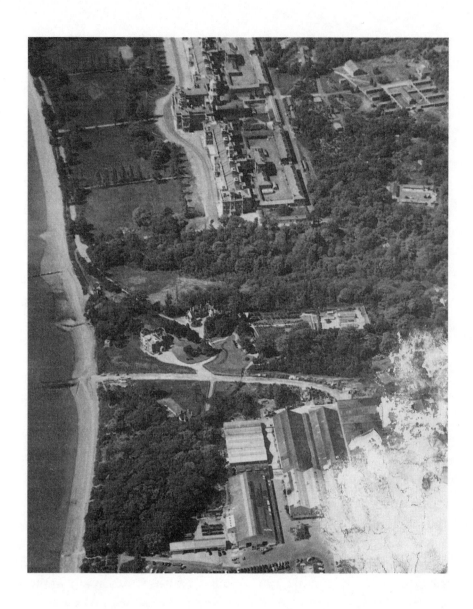

hospitals will be "posted" to the Royal Military Hospital at Netley to finish their convalescence'. But by then the great white elephant had become dilapidated, its bricks decaying in their mortar, slowly crumbling into the clay from which they came. In the dark unlit interior, laboratory benches lay unused, operating theatres gathered dust, and the 'Radiant Heat Department' stood as cold and empty as the slab in the hospital's post-mortem room.

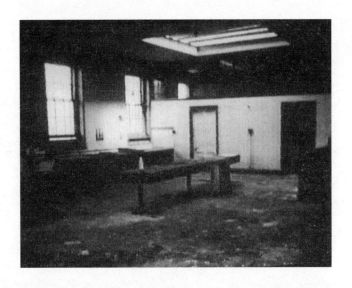

In the same year General Sir George Erskine of Southern Command (even now Britain was divided into military zones) declared in bluff army jargon that the building was a 'shocker', requiring £50,000 a year just to keep the exterior watertight and painted. Architectural sentimentality had no place in service life; Erskine declared that Netley should be sold and pulled down, finding no better use for it than 'to make "hard core" for roads'.

With no one to defend the unloved building, its fate was sealed by the General's words. The hospital stood empty, prey to interlopers and trespassers. One night my teenage brothers broke in and climbed the chapel tower via an iron ladder fixed to the inside wall, a vertiginous feat which they celebrated by ringing the great bell at the top and sparking off new ghost stories in the process. By January 1963 Netley's future was again under scrutiny: it does not seem coincidental that six months later a 'mysterious fire' substantially damaged the central block, fierce enough to be seen from miles around, throwing the chapel dome into relief against the night sky as though the blitz had returned for its unclaimed victim. The heat was fierce enough to buckle iron girders, yet it was claimed that the fire had been started by children – the Army Special Investigation Bureau were reported to be questioning three boys, aged nine, seven and five years old. But the local paper also received an anonymous letter, signed by 'Y', claiming that the fire had been started deliberately.

Some speculated that the Army had good reason to precipitate the demise of this architectural albatross; others that potential developers wanted to free up its land for building. More darkly, however, it was said that the fire had destroyed the hospital's records with whatever secrets they might have held – maybe the truth behind Otto Scholz's mysterious death, the conspiracy myths of Netley which the still-classified files at the Public Record Office encourage. Perhaps the fire was a convenient way of getting rid of incriminating paperwork; worse has happened in the corridors of Britain's bureaucracies. It is undoubtedly strange – some might say unbelievable – how little survived to document a hundred years of Britain's biggest military hospital. In the 1950s, even Netley's Commandant had professed ignorance of the whereabouts of its records. Perhaps they had been taken away over the years by doctors and surgeons, squirrelled away among private papers that even now could be mouldering in some attic. But the probable truth is that no one cared enough to keep them. Visitors to the derelict building remember seeing files filled with documents in abandoned offices, their ink as faded as the lives whose stories they told.

An army which no longer policed the world had no need of a huge hospital to service its casualties. Like a dingy shopful of camouflage nets and billy-cans, Netley had become army surplus. After a brief spell when it was suggested, somewhat bizarrely, that the place could be turned into a holiday camp, a deal was done with the contractors, and the order was given to demolish the building.

As the hospital was about to be pulled down, it was realised that there existed no film of this historic and soon to be demolished structure, and so a BBC crew were hurriedly dispatched to Netley. Their footage is the only remaining film of the entire building, a last audit of its immensity.

Fifty years after the shell-shocked were made to perform on

the hospital's terraces, the unedited, monochrome film hardly seems a technological advance. In its grey silence, you almost expect captions to flash up, but its only text is the numbered leader that counts down to its start, as if marking off the time left for the building. Two generations after those shaking, fugitive figures shuffled across these stone flags, it is almost shocking to see the hospital brought back to life, a great grey ghost, its breathtaking size undermined by the knowledge that it no longer exists in real time.

The establishing shot is filmed from a boat on Southampton Water. Slowly, as though viewed from a stately barge on a royal progress, as though some last monarch were making a final visit, the hospital hoves into view, the trees revealing the majestic building, austere and serene, as empty now as it once was full. Its sublime bulk fills the screen; like that nineteenth-century visitor arriving at the newly-built hospital, the camera cannot take it all in. At the rear of the building, following the ghosts of its inmates, the camera moves along the disused railway line like an ambulance train drawing on to the platform where it shoots straight up into a stretcher's eye view, the glass canopy and metal-shaded lights above as it wheels into the dark interior; a transition from light to darkness, beckoning into the emptiness.

Inside, doors hang uselessly from their hinges, paint peels from the ceiling like bark from a silver birch, and puddles of water stagnate on the floor, reflecting cracked sash windows. For the sake of scale, a man is made to walk down a corridor and up a pair of sweeping staircases that divide into nothingness; there is no dramatic sound of echoing footsteps. The lone figure looks oddly familiar; someone says he looks like me. Then, abruptly, the film ends, as if someone or something had interrupted this snatched and somehow illicit exposition of the hospital's secrets. The crew retreat; with its demolition about to begin, perhaps they were wary of the entire massive structure collapsing over their heads.

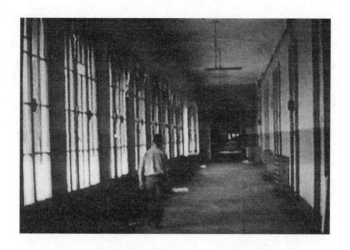

Bending her flaxen-haired head, a girl creeps into a barrel-vaulted tunnel, deep into the earth, moving from the light, the trees, the grass outside and into the darkness.

Curtains billow in the sea breeze that blows in through half-open windows. She runs, pursued or pursuing, down corridors and stairs that bend back on each other, past walls shedding ancient skins of paint, gripping serpentine banisters on iron railings, her close-miked, muffled voiceover imbued with unidentifiable sexuality as she recites Victorian prose. A stone has been thrown through a window: the light spills out, or in, through the star-burst crack. The hallway below is empty, and, still running as if pursued by some invisible spirit, Alice reaches the ground floor and a great arched doorway, a dead stop.

Beyond these double-height doors, in some unknown space on the other side, the trial of the theft of the Queen of Heart's tarts might be in progress; or Oscar Wilde could be asking if he might not be allowed to speak; or Noel Pemberton Billing could be brandishing his fantastic Black Book of corrupt persecution. But the girl is standing in the entrance hall of the Royal Victoria Military Hospital where, in that last year of its existence, one final crew had arrived to film Jonathan Miller's *Alice*. Using only the interior of the building, the place was transformed into an enormous and decrepit set, like an early studio long abandoned.

In a final starring role, Netley's quarter-mile corridors melded into the trippy, 1960s gothic version of Lewis Carroll's weird Victorian fantasy, invented a century before on a river in Oxford just as the great hospital on Southampton Water was being completed.

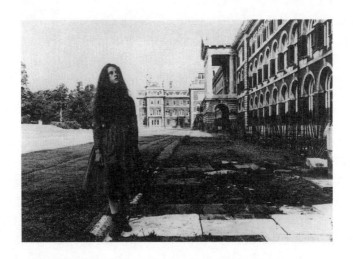

In Miller's film, the characters appear in Victorian dress, each as mad as the other, as though Alice had entered the cells of D Block itself. Looking through a tiny door, she sees, not the jerking puppets of its shell-shocked soldiers, but sombre nineteenth-century figures in black taffeta and silk, processing across a cedar-lined path. It looks like the same view Nurse Luker snapped from her wintry cell. For a brief eternity, the hospital's empty rooms live again, recostumed in their own gothic spirit. It seems fitting that the hospital's final act was to slide into a fantasy, as though, like Alice's adventures, the whole thing had been a dream.

But this was no romantic reverie, and unlike Thomas Dummer who had transplanted the abbey's north transept to his country park, no twentieth-century goth considered this semi-ruin sublime enough to transpose bits of it to their stately pile. Nor was there a heritage lobby vocal enough to halt the irrevocable and demand its preservation for future generations. Where the abbey had been able to escape the predations of time, the hospital was less lucky. There was little use for sentiment in the white hot technology of the 1960s. Along the shore, next to the abbey, Weston's tower blocks rose up over the trees, the kind of concentration of humanity which the English Array – obscure rural fascists with 'a name of Gothic derivation' – would describe as 'Birth Control Barracks'. Concrete monuments to a world ridding itself of its memories, they would 'form effective landmarks from the water' declared David Lloyd optimistically in *The Buildings of Hampshire*. That year, 1966, in the same book, his editor Nikolaus Pevsner called Netley's hospital 'a monster of a building', although he conceded that its own skyline was 'distinctly romantic, with the rhythm of towers, turrets, cupolas, and central dome, rising above the trees which hide the main bulk of the building'.

It was a vista which was about to vanish.

To mark the beginning of the end, an 'Open Day' was announced, and the press and television crews were invited to witness the fall of the first chimney. With a rope attached to its waist, it splattered to the ground, buckling like a soldier sniped on a parapet, a mournful demise concealed from the outside world by the park's sheltering pines. As the bricks tumbled to the earth which had produced them, the visitors watched from the barrack's first floor galleries, recording the moment of destruction. A final aerial view of the hospital would show the centrepiece of the vast structure stoved in, as if a giant crowbar had violently rent it asunder. And if Wagner had been recalled to provide the soundtrack to the hospital's demolition, then his *Götterdammerung* might have played out its gothic ruination, the ultimate test of the survival of the fittest.

In the weeks to come the dinosaurian machines advanced on the hospital, eating into its walls, tearing it apart with their metal jaws, doing what nineteenth-century reformers and the Luftwaffe had failed to do. Section by section, floor by floor, ward by ward, in the same methodical manner in which they had been

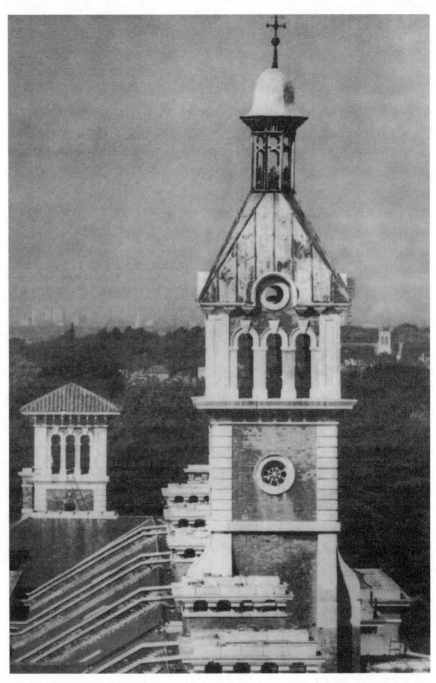

a monster of a building . . . distinctly romantic, with the rhythm of towers, turrets, cupolas, and central dome,

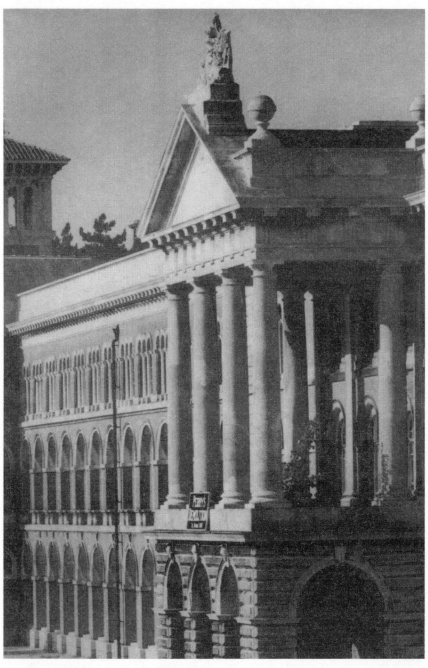

rising above the trees which hide the main bulk of the building

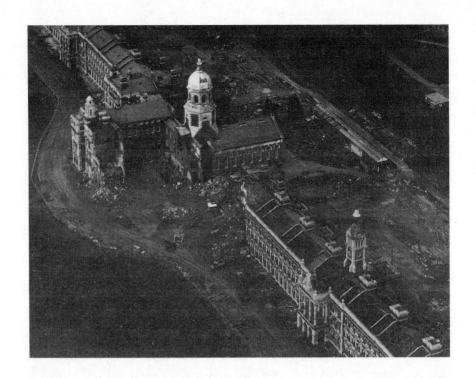

constructed, its hundreds of rooms were destroyed: the railway station and the grand entrance hall; the long corridors and the dark barracks behind; the great towers and the granite facings of the façade. The grand vista of this improved landscape was reduced to a bomb site. It was a humbling end for Netley's planners; a strange, destructive revenge for its critics. The hospital's unfitness for purpose was, finally, the cause of its demise. Over in D Block, preserved by its continuing function and insulated by its own walls and trees, the asylum's commanding officer remarked ruefully of the main hospital that 'had Florence Nightingale's plans been adopted it may have been in use even to this day'.

It was another irony that, just as the sons of Netley Abbey's builders had been the instruments of its dissolution, so it was the hospital's own workers who enthusiastically took part in its destruction. A naval psychiatric officer working in D Block recalled that 'the demolition contractor . . . advertised for casual labour. As a result, most of that labour consisted of off-duty staff.' For these moonlighting destroyers, demolition was better paid than wrestling with the inmates of padded cells. 'At the rate of pay of 6/- per hour', he and his friends were making £20 a week. 'It was a gold mine', he recalled.

It was also terribly hard work. The technique was to start at the top – one had to have a head for heights – and remove individual slates for salvage. These were of excellent quality and sold for 1/3d each. There were many thousands. After a section of roof was completely stripped, we moved to the room below. The windows were stripped out and the cast iron sash weights rescued for salvage. All the floorboards were removed and the cast iron fireplaces and all the decorative wooden mouldings were salvaged for sale. After the floor boards, we would drop the ceiling, that is with a sledge hammer a few hefty blows would be delivered through the floor joists to the ceiling below, which would collapse leaving us standing on the joists, which we then removed one by one, working towards the door. Everything of value was salvaged for sale, this included cast iron decorative hoppers on gutter downspouts, all cast iron most bricks. All the lead, which was apparently more valuable than modern lead in that it had a high silver content. I must say I enjoyed the experience as it is the only time that I was ever paid for destroying government property.

Month after month this process continued, until the human locusts reduced the once proud building in which they worked to a quarter of a million cubic yards of rubble. Historic Portland stone, 'reported to be of a perfect texture which cannot be quarried these days', was conserved, but the rest was loaded on to lorries which rumbled through Southampton like the trains and carriages that had brought the wounded to the hospital wards. On the far side of the city the debris was tipped into the foundations of the Totton flyover; at the same time, the demolition contractors issued a press release proudly stating that metal from the hospital was to be recycled for use in the motor industry: 'Thus next year's new car may contain traces of Netley Hospital. And next year's new road may have some of Netley Hospital in its foundation.' The building's deconstruction was complete: a passive victim to voracious combustion, literally consumed by the despoiler of the age.

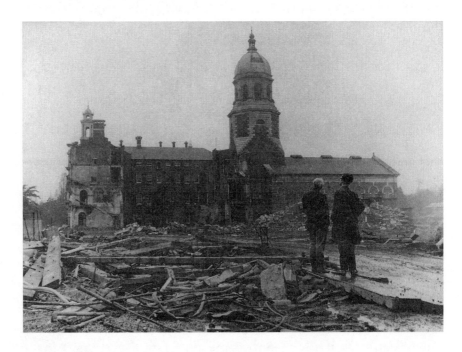

And among the ruins came other scavengers, as though they had lain in wait for the great beast to be mortally wounded. A chaise longue was carried off from the matron's sitting room, said to have been used for Queen Victoria's visits; a pair of ten foot Georgian cannon were uprooted like iron molars from the hospital entrance where they had stood as bollards; and in the settling dust were found invitations to nineteenth-century balls. Like the body of a medieval bishop divided for burial at separate sites, bits of the hospital were dispersed throughout the area. Six years later a walker discovered that Milford's sea wall, some twenty miles further down the coast, had been constructed using dressed stone blocks from the hospital.

As the rest of the building fell apart, only its centre withheld: its sacred heart, the Royal Chapel. The elegant green dome – landmark to a century of inmates and sailors, troopships and bomber pilots, immigrants and movie stars – stood defiant before the advancing machines, facing the final assault, awaiting the *coup de grâce* of the wrecking ball as it too was scheduled on the demolition timesheet. There remained only the question of the crucifix which surmounted the dome. It would be sacrilegious for it to fall into brick dust at the blow of a ball and chain, so it was decided that it would be removed by an RAF helicopter. For a few minutes, the Christian symbol of the Victorian edifice would hang in mid-air like a giant censer, dispensing the last traces of its memory.

But at the last minute there came a reprieve. Just as objections had been raised to the hospital's inexorable construction, so someone somewhere introduced an element of doubt into the progress of its destruction. Perhaps the vision of its dangling crucifix appeared to a latterday Walter Taylor as a warning; or perhaps it was mere sentimentality which prevailed. For whatever reason, the decision was made to save the chapel, although even then the architects declared that the tower must go, lest it mar the building's sense of proportion. But the tower stayed. Its survival seemed a minor victory, yet it was actually a monument to the entire site's failure, a giant memorial to imperial hubris.

As the diggers came to a halt before the chapel's sacred interior, they also reached the foundation stone, set into the bare brick earth a hundred years ago. Acknowledging public interest, the army agreed a date for the disinterring of the steel box known to be buried under the stone. In the act of its destruction, as its innards were exposed to the light of common day, it seemed that the hospital's secrets were about to be revealed. With the sudden flurry of media coverage and letters in the press, it was as if, as with the obituary of an obscure figure, the public only now realised the extraordinary nature of the place that the newspapers had so triumphed all those years ago. The hospital's history had come full circle, as though some preordained cycle was complete: just as that first ceremony had installed Netley's hospital in the national consciousness, so now it was being removed. The great lump of granite, tapped down by a royal trowel, was about to be raised up in a twentieth-century defoundation.

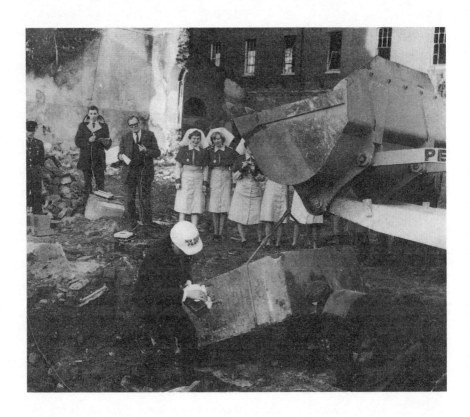

The press were summoned to witness the unsealing of the box on 7 December 1966 ('Uniform or Lounge Suit' stipulated the invitation), in a ceremony attended by a guard and the Lord Lieutenant of the county in lieu of royalty. None of the television viewers sitting at home listening to the reporter's commentary could know that the stone had already been lifted and the contents of its time capsule opened the night before to enable army officials to ascertain that there was actually anything in it. What they discovered was the dull bronze of a VC and a set of the hospital plans placed inside the oblong box by The Queen-

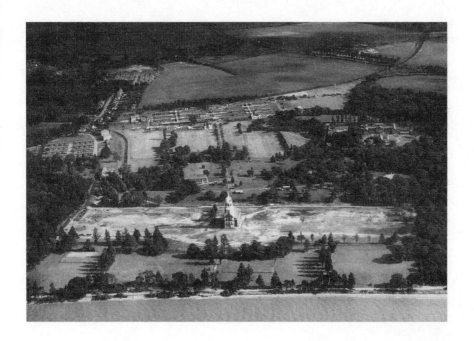

Empress Victoria – as its intricately-engraved lettering declared – as a relic of her reign and a reminder to future generations of the hospital's great mission. In that decorated tin were contained the hopes and aspirations of her age.

With the removal of this reliquary, the site was deconsecrated. What was left became a dissolved, modern version of a gothic ruin, imbued with the same powers of evocation as Netley's abbey. The hospital was dead, an empty space on the Ordnance Survey chart; but its memory remained.

PART

III

His Dark Estate

My Days & Nights are so much alike, so equally insen-
sible of any Moving Power but Fancy, that I have sometimes spoke of things in our family as Truth and real
accidents, which I only Dreamt of; & again when some
things that actually happen'd came into my head, have
thought (till I enquired) that I had only dream'd of them.

ALEXANDER POPE

The sixth of the sixth, sixty-six. We dutifully wrote down
the date in our exercise books, instructed by our teacher
that it would be eleven years before we could do the same again.
To us, eleven years seemed an impossible amount of time, greater
than the life we'd already lived. The idea of the future, just like
the past, seemed fantastic.

As I sat in our green-painted school hut, the sun shining
through the windows and the door tantalisingly open to the
summer heat, my older brother was watching out of his classroom window at St Mary's as the lorries carrying the hospital's
remains trundled incessantly down Lance's Hill. Although I was
perfectly old enough to remember it, the demolition didn't register in my world. Waiting for the home-time bell, looking forward
to playing in my Red Indian wigwam on the lawn, I had no idea

that the hut in which I sat had once stood in Netley's fields, nor would I have cared. The past I remembered was full of myths, of dinosaurs and lake monsters, of Aztec warriors and ancient Romans, and it came, not from the lessons I learnt in our school hut, but from Woolston Library.

Dad would take us there on Thursday evenings, an exciting expedition; the only other time we went out at night was on our annual visit down town to see the lights and receive our presents on the knees of a cottonwool-bearded Father Christmas at Edwin Jones's department store. The library had grey lino floors and a wide staircase segregating the junior section from the adult; the buff card tickets in wooden drawers as neat as a bus conductor's machine were overseen by bespectacled, matronly librarians in an atmosphere as hushed and polished as the church we attended over the road. Its contents were semi-sacred objects, date-stamped and warning of punitive fines and the dire consequences for any borrower who failed to report any infectious diseases in the household. They were the source of my fantasy world – a world which darkened with my brother's sudden loss and the events surrounding it in the year I left St Patrick's. Unlike the hospital's demolition, these were incidents I thought I remembered, even the ones to which I was not a witness, as if their vividness had deceived my memory into thinking I was there.

Around that time there had been odd, unsolicited callers, both at our house and at the friend's house where my brother had been working on the day he died. The man was Indian and ostensibly a salesman, but like some fakir whom my grandfather might have encountered in wartime Calcutta, he gestured to my mother with his hand the descending heights of her children, my brothers and sisters, and seemed to indicate a gap in between. A week before the accident, his clairvoyant compatriot (or was it the same man?) had looked across the farmyard to where Andrew and his mate had their heads in the bonnet of a car and told his friend's mother that he felt sorry for the boy's family.

It was as though the ghosts we had left behind at Akaba had followed us across town. From the school bus I'd look at the

300

Spiritualist Church at the top of Lance's Hill which advertised its services like any ordinary place of worship, and wonder what rites went on in its strange little hut. Under the suburban ordinariness, secret sects still operated, like the Masonic Hall that stood behind our church, with its roundel depicting an eagle and the word 'Clausentum' evoking the mighty power of Imperial Rome (as opposed to the Popish power of modern Rome across the street). Closed off from the curiosity of passersby, it had just one great circular window set high in the wall, its glass blanked out in white like a Communion wafer in a giant monstrance. I imagined the Holy Ghost in that milky white glass, the mysterious unknown third of the Trinity, a sanctified phantom.

One afternoon I came home to find my parents seated round a table, their fingers on an upturned glass. Messages to his wife located my brother's lost keys, even an asphalt lump on the roadside which seemed to have caused his accident. Later my mother heard someone come up the drive and call out in my brother's voice, and one night they woke up to find the house pervaded with the smell of the hospital ward in which he died. My elder sister, whom my brother loved – in his wedding photographs, as he puts his hand on my shoulder, he looks down at her, and she up at him, the connexion visible over the years – thought she saw Andrew come to her bed, as though to kiss her as she slept. And I too lay awake on my top bunk, and watched as a fuzzy after-image of my dead brother took shape in the doorway. I still don't know if I really saw that; but one autumn evening I did see tiny black crosses on every door leading off the upstairs landing. I could touch them, but not rub them out. No one downstairs seemed particularly interested; I don't think they even bothered to go up and look.

One year – as monumental a marker as the day I took First Holy Communion in my white shirt, red tie and grey shorts, my sins absolved from behind a metal grille in my first confession – I got my tickets to the adults' 'Downstairs' library. Leaving the Chronicles of Narnia and *The Eagle of the Ninth* behind on the upstairs shelf, I'd bring home books about Borley Rectory, 'the most haunted house in England', fascinated by their grainy plates of a Suffolk parsonage surrounded by tall trees, and a bosky 'Nun's Walk' where a weeping sister appeared like Netley's Grey Lady to witnesses in the garden's gothic summerhouse. But my favourite story – because it seemed so convincing – was *The Ghosts of Versailles*. In 1901, two British women, Misses Moberly and Jourdain, Principal and Vice-Principal, respectively, of St Hugh's Hall, Oxford, claimed, on a visit to Versailles, to have witnessed eighteenth-century apparations at the Petit Trianon. Here, on Marie-Antoinette's ornamental farm with its cottages and pavilions they had seen the Queen, together with servants and gardeners, with whom they spoke.

On their return to England, in the unforeign security of Oxford, they compared notes and attempted to come to terms with what they had experienced. As Miss Moberly wrote in their original account, *An Adventure*, even the very landscape they had walked seemed to have changed: 'Everything suddenly looked unnatural, therefore unpleasant; even the trees behind the building seemed to have become flat and lifeless, *like a wood worked in tapestry*.' They had moved through these scenes, believing them to be real, yet acknowledging their uncanniness. One man they encountered 'slowly turned his face, which was marked by smallpox: his complexion was very dark', recorded Miss Jourdain. 'The expression was very evil and yet unseeing, and though I did not feel he was looking particularly at us, I felt a repugnance to going past him.'

It was as though they had walked into a film set (which was exactly the explanation given by some of their critics), or a re-enactment of the dramatic adventures of the Comte de Cartrie. But the stern spinsters diligently researched their experience, establishing its historical accuracy; to them, it seemed they had entered the *memory* of Marie-Antoinette, in which more was happening than they could actually see; the rustling of silk skirts and the sound of running figures invisible about them, voices in their ears. This apparent transportation of events – of memory – from the late eighteenth century to the beginning of the twentieth, and its notion of entire scenes rematerialising like pastoral water-colours out of a psychic cathode ray tube, fired my imagination. Perhaps Netley and D Block, with their own lost memories, would inhabit my mind as a mad – or madder – version of Versailles and the Trianon, with its Grey Lady as Marie-Antoinette.

An Adventure was first published in 1911, but became increasingly popular in the psychically-sensitised period during and after the war, when many were eager to prove life after death, and when Oliver Lodge's experiments into psychical research caught the attention of Almroth Wright and even the soldiers of the hutted hospital. Moberly and Jourdain's account was taken quite seriously: one writer claimed that the two ladies had in fact been witness to one of the Marquis de Sade's experiments in time, and even the sceptical A.J.P. Taylor admitted that it was 'the best authenticated ghost story in the world'.

I believed it, implicitly, just as I believed a plesiosaur could exist in Loch Ness, as though it were a ghost of the prehistoric past. I would examine the detailed reconstructions of Jurassic and Triassic scenes in my library books, with their landscapes of lush tree ferns and spiky cycads, and brooding volcanoes visible on the horizon. I'd memorise every scale, fin and bony bump of their antediluvian population, cataloguing the complicated names in my head. Yet these illustrations which I took to be scientific fact were as much fantastic reconstructions specific to their time as were Crystal Palace's concrete monsters or the swan-necked swamp-dwellers of the officers' mess at Netley; they were sections from one huge panorama, *The Age of Reptiles*, painted at Yale's Peabody Museum from 1940 to 1945, recreating prehistory when civilisation itself seemed threatened with extinction.*

---

* 'A dinotopic refuge from World War II', as W. J. T. Mitchell writes of Rudolph Zallinger's 100 foot mural, with 'the 170-million-year evolution of ancient life as a single, unified landscape ... a symmetrical tableau of stately reptilian demigods in a peaceable arcadian kingdom'.

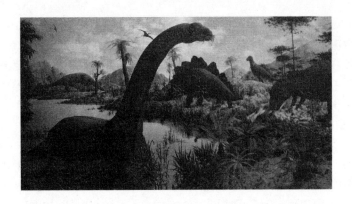

This was how we saw the past: one long wallchart like the one I'd bought on a visit to Osborne House on another sunny day, the car radio playing 'If You Go To San Francisco' as we pulled up on the gravel under the cedar trees. The great white villa of Victoria's suburban Versailles seemed sombre as we walked through its gated rooms and past the Queen's bed overhung with her dead Consort's portrait and fob watch, and the surreal replicas of children's hands and feet under their glass domes. In the grounds were a Swiss chalet and a miniature fort, another Trianon. Down on the shore was the Queen's bathing machine, where Victoria waded into the sea in her voluminous bathing suit which I imagined to be as black as the rest of her post-Albert wardrobe. At the end of our tour, in the gift shop, I bought a poster preserved in a plastic tube which made it seem serious and documentary. It displayed the reigns of British kings and queens in Corinthian columns, a scientifically proven past plotted on a mathematical graph; a sample of unchanging history like a medical specimen in its tube.

But there were new challenges to that past, and they came from across the sea and up Southampton Water. I shared my realm of ghosts and dinosaurs with sci-fi superheroes, future myths to those eighteenth-century apparitions and reptilian ancestors; boys with x-ray eyes and angel's wings, visibly different, in the way I was different, too. Dad disapproved of such American imports, so I hid my Marvel comics under my bed, guiltily bringing them out at night to read, eating a clementine, sealing the pulpy coloured strips and pneumatic spacemen with the pungent orange oil in my memory.

But my father's concern was a rearguard action and even my encyclopaedias saw the world from the other side of the Atlantic, with their coloured illustrations of miraculous ice-cream makers and Yellowstone geysers and their potted biographies of historic figures – the blank after Churchill's date of birth neatly filled in by my father after we watched the statesman's coffin carried by barge down the wintry Thames. The black-and-whiteness of England stood in contrast to America's Technicolor, and the crewcut boys we saw in Disney films were comic book heroes in embryo, supermen heirs to those dinosaurian demi-gods.

Yet for all the brash, petroleum immediacy and magnetic glamour of that transatlantic drift, the ghosts of the old world still haunted our Hampshire shores, in the Seaweed Hut and the crumbling abbey and the absent hospital surrounded by pines. I was still convinced – sixty years after the Oxford spinsters had made their sightings – that I too could experience the past; that it might be possible to reinhabit its surroundings, and see Gray's spirits at noonday.

As I was reading in my Sholing bedroom, bedclothes pulled over my shoulder against the night, a mile or so down the road D Block was still functioning, its wards full of the mental casualties of war or military life. Now the British Army Psychiatric Unit, 'You'll be sent to Netley' was a familiar joke – or threat – in the services.

In 1937 Roger Hall was at the Royal Military College, Sandhurst, training to become an army officer. He was nineteen and at the end of his intermediate term when, on home leave, he met his seventeen-year-old cousin, Anne, who had come to stay. He had not seen her since they were children; now, quite unexpectedly, he fell in love with her. 'I used to lie on the grass and look into her eyes, not speaking. It seemed that a bond existed between us that made speech unnecessary.'

From this romantic idyll Hall was rudely awakened by his

return to Sandhurst. Whereas before he had tolerated, even enjoyed the institutional discipline, the lectures, the drilling, the endless parades, he now felt discomfited. A future without Anne was intolerable – yet he convinced himself it was impossible, that his parents would object, citing 'ancestral archives [which] might produce evidence of some abnormality or minor defect that, between us, we might help to perpetuate'. Overshadowed by some unspecified genetic threat – as though the ghosts of a *fin-de-siècle* degeneration had returned to haunt him – his concern turned to obsession. 'My imagination started to override my reason and I began to know the meaning of madness. Not the insanity of love, but the madness of doubt and the unreason of imagination and its mastery over the conscious mind.' For Hall, his literally romantic imagination had tipped his mind from rationality into madness.

The young cadet 'contemplated entering another life, a life in which no way could be worse. The thought of suicide was in no way repellent to me . . . From initial exaltation I went downhill, quickly, suddenly and seemingly irrevocably. One bad habit followed another . . . There were only doubts, fears, evil thoughts and forebodings. I was moving rapidly into a world of total unreality . . .' He was no longer able to face the duties of the day: 'If this were hell I no longer felt wonder or surprise that people, in order to avoid it, killed themselves. I was going mad.' Hall confined himself to his bedroom, brooding, writing no letters, chain-smoking. When he saw Anne again that Christmas, 'I was not in the same realm.' She was offended that he had not written: 'Perhaps she thought me unfaithful. What could I tell her?'

In February 1938 Hall was gazetted as a second lieutenant. He was waiting to join his regiment, but 'one day I could go on no longer and so I left'. Still in uniform, he bunked his lecture and set off across the heath. 'I became tired and I stopped and sat down and smoked a cigarette . . . There were pine trees and I was secluded among them. I was late now and would be missed . . .' He slept there, returning at nightfall to hide in the shadows beneath the barrack block and the 'wooden huts that were our sleeping quarters'. From the bushes, he watched as his fellow officers dressed themselves for dinner.

'I must wait. I must wait a long while before I can go in. I must wait until they are all asleep and then enter by the window . . . I was hungry but I would starve myself to death. That seemed easy. I walked back to the heath and it was cold. The stars were brilliant and the night dark.' Hall returned to the camp after midnight, took off his boots and crept into bed, setting his alarm for 5 am. Waking fully dressed, he left again by the window, 'softly, silently, stealthily and quickly. I had the sharpness of the devil. I was the devil, the devil was in me, in complete possession.' He returned to his heathland nest, and waited for the inevitable alarm to be raised. Slowly they came, men in overalls, 'as if beating for pheasants'. Still in uniform himself, he jumped up and told one of his pursuers that the man had 'gone down there'. He ran, now camouflaged in his khaki, determined not to be caught; at one point he picked up a piece of broken glass from the undergrowth: 'I would cut my throat rather than face the music.'

Darkness fell again; he crossed a road, and a sports field, and hid in its pavilion. The camp hospital lay on the other side of the field. He began to walk towards it. The next thing he remembered was being given hot milk in bed in one of the wards. A few days later, Hall was taken in custody to Netley.

Extracts from Netley Form 6, Medical Instructions for Guides in carrying out Station Order No. . . . regarding the man marginally named.

3. In the event of his becoming insubordinate, giving trouble, especially whilst waiting for trains, you will ask the assistance of the Civil Police and with them take means to have him removed to a place away from the crowd (to a Police Station or otherwise) until such time as the train starts.
4. You will be very careful of him at Railway Stations,

307

keeping him from the sides of the platforms and passing trains. In the carriages he must be kept from the doors and windows.

'I was placed in "D" Block, the mental block, the psychological block for observation. The heavy self-locking door clanged behind me. I was a patient in a lunatic asylum.'

Hall was told to undress and get into bed, 'an iron-framed army bed in a small room at the end of a second floor corridor'. His cell consisted of a chest of drawers, a barred window that opened nine inches at the top and bottom, and a light built into the ceiling. Everything was secured to the floor or the wall. On a chair just inside the door sat an RAMC private 'with eyes all round his head. I was never addressed as "Sir". I had forfeited that privilege in the mud on the heath.' It was not the only human privilege he lost. Soon D Block had imposed its terrible geography on his disturbed mind.

'Outside were high brick walls with glass on top. There were other blocks, one-storeyed blocks with windows barred on the outside. There was some grass with bushes and trees on the edges of it. Behind the trees, little trees mostly, there were more high brick walls. There was a cemetery in a corner of the enclosure. "The evil that men do lives after them." Everything seemed to fit into place exactly. If I died now I would be buried there and my grave would live after me as a reminder of why and how I had died; in a lunatic asylum.'

Hall was examined by the Medical Officer, and was kept in his room for six weeks, 'fit only to wear pyjamas and to smoke cigarettes in bed under surveillance.' Allowed no matches, he had to chain-smoke; forbidden knife or fork, he ate his meals with a spoon. All the while, he was conscious of eyes watching him through the door, through the glass spy-holes. Sometimes he would throw a fit and chuck his food about. His reward for such behaviour was to be dragged from his room and thrown into a padded cell. If he showed no remorse for his actions, the orderlies would set on him 'like thugs and beat me up, making sure my most vulnerable parts received the preponderance of their attention'. In 1938 a man who affected madness to evade his military duties deserved no human respect. 'Sometimes this would go on for minutes and sometimes for half an hour. Always at the end I lay prostrate on the floor. I was, in this state, considered no longer a potential menace. They were quite right to do it, I thought. I deserved it. I was filth.'

In the master-slave community of the asylum, the internal workings of D Block had become a world within itself, self-dependent as the hospital was self-reliant, operating beyond the normal bounds of human rationality. Who was mad and who was sane? And in his maddened state, who would believe Hall's account? Self-abased, reduced to the status of an animal, he could only wait, in the hope that things might change.

After a few days Hall was allowed to wear the hospital uniform, and was taken, chained by the wrist to an orderly's wrist, to be walked in the grounds like a dog. 'There were other men outside, too. They were privates, and non-commissioned ranks, all wearing the hospital uniform blues. Some were sitting on the grass, staring. Some walked to and fro across it, not talking, simply staring. Some muttered to themselves. Not one spoke to another. Some just stood, some were shaven, some had sores, some had V.D., advanced V.D. They were mad, stark staring mad. They would scream in the most awful, ghoulish manner. Such sounds I shall never forget.'

For the psychotic, syphilitic inmates, they were the sounds of a gothic, Dantean hell in a Hampshire field, uttered by ambling, shuffling nightmare figures in what looked like a provincial park. Only when he was visited by his parents was Hall removed from Netley, and transferred to the Bethlehem Royal Hospital at Beckenham, Kent, where the regime was more benign, and where, three months later, he was discharged, purged of his insanity – an insanity that D Block had done little to cure.

*   *   *

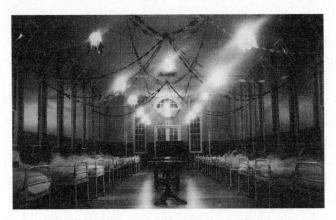

The only known photograph of the inside of D Block in operation; the main ward, Christmas 1937. The blurred shapes indicate that the beds are occupied.

When R. D. Laing was working at a mental hospital in Scotland in the early 1950s, a doctor brought in a tray of biscuits to the psychiatrists' lounge. They had been made by women patients. The doctors refused to eat them. '[They] were afraid of catching schizophrenia', wrote Laing. 'Who knows? It might be contagious, like herpes...' Far from being a contagious disease, Laing believed that madness could actually enhance human experience; that through it, the self could be recreated anew, as if reborn. 'Madness need not be all breakdown', he wrote. 'It may also be breakthrough.' Laing rose from a dysfunctional middle-class Glaswegian family to become the most charismatic and controversial practitioner of psychiatry in post-war Britain. He believed that disorders such as schizophrenia were rooted in the events of family history. In the Fifties and Sixties, with hospitals full of institutionalised people like my Uncle Cyril, Laing sought to free them from their prisons, to overturn accepted notions of madness and its treatment. In the process he moved from theorist to mystic and performer, introducing romanticism to a rational science. The anthropologist Joan Westcott likened him to the Trickster, a mythological figure 'who deliberately transgresses social conventions and is able to assume animal forms or change its sex at will'. In Jungian terms, wrote Daniel Burston, the Trickster represents our 'shadow side', 'a relentless and often shocking truthteller, who gives voice to disturbing truths most of us repress'; he also signifies 'an arrest in development . . . An eternal adolescent whose antipathy to authority and convention renders it difficult or impossible for him to enter into the normal flow of life.' Others thought Dr Laing ought to have joined the mad rather than set them free.

In the turned-on, tuned-in Sixties, Laing would become a rock star by default, criticised for glamorising insanity yet championing the dispossessed and the countercultural by virtue of his chosen field and his 'oppositional identity'. He was against 'the demonic side of science . . .' wrote Burston, 'in its bland erosion of our sense of solidarity with one another and other species by rationalizing cruelty and indifference'. In 1951, such cruelty and indifference – and the conflict of his own romanticism with institutional rationality – were to become vividly real for the young doctor. Aged twenty-three and just out of medical school, Laing was conscripted and posted to D Block.

Little had changed at Netley's asylum since Roger Hall's incarceration there thirteen years previously. Sensitised to issues of mental health by the phenomenon and treatment of shell-shock in the First World War, military psychiatry had been keen to find physical cures for such problems; more especially because the Freudian 'talking cure' was still regarded with some suspicion, and seen as of little use to the long-term mentally-ill. Most shell-shocked soldiers had recovered within nine months enough to rejoin society; others, suffering from serious mental disorder or psychosis, were dispatched to civil asylums, such as the thirty-three-year-old private in the Royal West Surreys evacuated from France to Netley in September 1918, who had been 'normal' until six weeks before, when he 'heard his mother had thrown herself out of a window'. Now he complained of 'some sort of electricity wireless' in his head and nine months later, 'still very delusional', was committed to an asylum.

During and after the war military mental hospitals were

criticised for their treatment of soldiers – in 1920 the magazine *Truth* had exposed 'obscene methods of torture', a 'general atmosphere of brutality' and overcrowding in some hospitals. The issue aroused strong public feelings, suspicions which were encouraged by the closed nature of the military asylums and the physical cures they employed. In such a culture, rigorous, tangible action was preferable to the 'talk, talk, talk' of analysis. As recently declassified documents show, D Block treated mental patients using increasingly experimental methods, often more enthusiastically than its civilian counterparts. A military hospital, after all, was less open to public scrutiny – although D Block was annually reviewed by the Board of Commissioners, the heirs of the nineteenth-century Commissioners in Lunacy.

Their report in 1927 found that 'the cases of different psychoses fell into the same group and followed the same course as in civilian life'. Then they had recommended open-air verandahs as 'a most valuable aid to the treatment of mental diseases' in their experience. A subsequent report noted that three patients had attempted suicide, 'two by means of strangulation with the tape from their trousers, and one by pushing his head through the window of the acute ward'. But these incidents were played down, and the unit was presented as a progressive institution: 'Our visit satisfied us that D Block, Netley, continues to be conducted in a highly efficient manner and that the security, treatment and welfare of the patients received there are fully provided for.'

In 1928 a new extension was built at D Block, a Quanset hut-like building with a semi-circular roof. This contained a nineteen-bed ward which would be given over to a new and apparently miraculous physical cure from the European home of psychiatry, Vienna. When treating a diabetic drug addict in 1927, Dr Manfred Sakel discovered that the accidental overdose of insulin he had administered had not killed his patient as he feared, but had instead cured her craving. Sakel began to experiment with insulin in other forms of mental disturbance, and developed a technique in which patients would be given an overdose of the drug to send them into a profound coma – followed by death if the process was not halted by the introduction of glucose solution by a tube into the stomach or a vein. When they came round they were calmer, and better able to accept psychiatric counselling.

'Deep insulin treatment' was introduced to Britain in 1936, and like electro-convulsive therapy – refined by Sakel's Italian associate Ugo Cerletti and in use four years later – it was widely used in psychiatric hospitals where 'it had deservedly a revolutionary impact' on sufferers from schizophrenia and manic depression, although no one was quite sure how it worked. The authorities at Netley's asylum, ever keen for such progressive physical treatments, embraced insulin treatment as part of their arsenal of cures which already included malaria therapy (used to treat 'general paralysis of the insane', terminal syphilis), hydrotherapy ('in the form of continuous baths'), 'continuous narcosis' and later ECT and leucotomy (lobotomy) – the heirs of the 'electrical therapy' and *überrumpellungsmethode* of Yealland and Kaufmann. The enthusiastic use of such therapies in D Block was a symptom of the desperate need for new treatments in psychiatric medicine, an attempt to catch up with the progress of its physical counterpart. Around the time that Laing was posted to Netley, the Board of Commissioners reported that 'the number of patients who are given the benefit of this treatment [insulin] at Netley is probably larger than in the great majority of civil mental hospitals in this country'.

During the Second World War, D Block had treated the sufferers of combat fatigue. Although aware of the problems of the last war, the military authorities deliberately downplayed the notion of 'war neurosis', reasoning that in this manner they would minimise the number of soldiers (from a largely conscripted army) affecting mental illness. The war saw another remarkable role for D Block's staff, too: in 1943, shortly after his abortive 'peace flight' from Germany to Scotland, doctors from Netley were sent to examine Rudolph Hess, then being held in a house, Mytchett Place, near Aldershot (where he would attempt suicide by jumping over the banisters). It was another of Netley's persistent myths

313

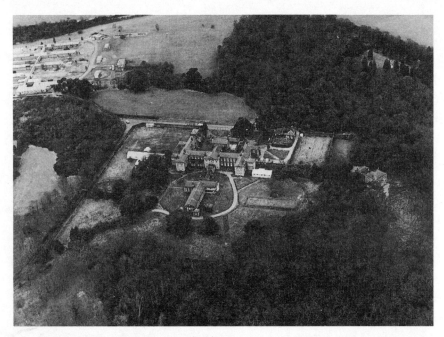

A post-war aerial view of D Block, showing the 1908 and 1928 extensions, the 'spider' hospital (left-hand corner), and military cemetery (right)

that Hess was actually brought to D Block, perhaps to effect the plan to hypnotise and return him to Germany programmed with the assassination of his Führer.

After the war, in an attempt to dispel its image, D Block had become 'P' Wing ('P' for 'psychotic'). 'The change of name has recently taken place', noted a report in 1949, 'as it was felt that officers returning to their units might be at a disadvantage if it was realised that they had been treated in "D" Block which was widely known throughout the Army as a centre for patients suffering from mental illness.' Its neighbour, the spider hospital, E Block, had also been turned over to psychiatric care, and was now known as PN Wing; 'PN' standing for 'psychoneurotic'. Yet despite such attempts to update itself, Netley retained its forbidding identity, still overshadowed by its brick walls, a formidable barrier to the outside world.

On his arrival at Netley, Laing discovered that his first duty was to attend the patients in the insulin ward. The drug was administered at six in the morning. Over the next four hours, the dosage was increased steadily, until the patients went into 'deep comas and sometimes epileptic fits. The policy was to put it in at a level at which epileptic fits were liable to occur, but to avoid them if possible', noted Laing. 'Backs could break.' Because the drug made its subjects hypersensitive to light, the entire ward was blacked out, turning dawn into twilight. In this profound gloom, the staff could move about only by means of lights strapped to their foreheads and surrounded by shiny metal reflectors. Working like a miner at the coalface of madness, Laing attended his patients in their state of suspended animation; it was his responsibility to return them to consciousness. It was as if they had to be taken near to death to be brought back to life, to be resurrected like their shell-shocked and re-educated D Block predecessors. Here too the therapy seemed to achieve remarkable cures, through the relief of survival and the sheer shock of what the patients had gone through. Exorcised of their evil spirits, their psychiatrists had become witch doctors, and their medications *muti*, sympathetic magic.

'Around ten o'clock, we poured quantities of 50 per cent glucose into the patients through stomach tubes', wrote Laing. 'We hoped we had got the tube into the stomach rather than the lungs' – it was difficult to tell with a patient in a coma. Pressurised drips were used on veins which had virtually disappeared, having burst from thrombosis; missing their target in the dark, needles would instead inject glucose solution into the tissues. Such mishaps seemed only a step away from Netley's infancy and its ill-trained nurses. Fumbling in the dim light of the torches on their heads, the doctors 'might have to take a scalpel to "cut down" and stick a needle into something one just hoped was not an artery or a nerve'. Ten years later, David Stafford-Clark would note that 'Even in the best hands mortality from irreversible coma was a danger', and that 'insulin has been virtually abandoned in most clinics . . .' It is clear that Laing was shocked by what he saw at Netley. To his generation, coming to terms with the appalling truths of the war, these therapies from 1930s Austria and Italy, with their eugenicist undercurrents, must have appeared little better than the experiments carried out by Nazi doctors on human guinea pigs.

Throughout his time at Netley, Laing kept a diary, scribbling down in a small notebook accounts of his reading, his influences, his emotions and his dreams in an existential commonplace-book. In it he allowed his recent memories to intrude on the reality of his present. Sequestered on this isolated site with its huts and high walls, he recalled his time in Paris, 'Marijuana cig. low dives in Montmart . . .' [sic]; scenes from films – 'The last few shots in <u>All Quiet on the Western Front</u>, Emile Jannings in the <u>Blue Angel</u>. The egg smashed on his head'; and the philosophers he was reading, 'Darwin, Kierkegaard . . . Nietzsche, Pascal, Freud, Ellis, Betr. Russell . . .' Through this book of himself, Laing traced his journey into Netley's enclosing world.

R. D. Laing – Personal Comment 1952.
2/2/52 Age 24 R.V. Netley Lt RAMC Sunday Night. Drunk . . . The essence of what it is that I seek to achieve by drunkenness is still unrevealed to me.
8/2/52 Sunday morning – every day is a reprieve every day is an other chance. The world is infinitely forgiving: infinitely cleansing.

The world may have been forgiving, but Netley had the infinite capacity to depress Laing, who turned more and more to alcohol after work. A few days later, he wrote, looking forward to his discharge:

Perhaps in 2 years time I shall read these lines with a wan seasoned smile on my face. Will my brain tolerate two years of pickling? What irreversible brain changes will develop. A subtle change has overtaken me. I am very drunk as I write this and yet here I am coherent, articulate, coordinated, fluent: and not over garrulous. It must be a simple thing to gain self-mastery; but why? Why should we? Why not get drunk: why not commit suicide? Suicide is the end of pleasure as well as of pain.

Reading the case histories he assembled while at Netley, it is easy to see why Laing would have felt this way, even had he not been reading Camus; dealing day by day with the extremes of the human condition made him question his own state of mind. From Laing's own papers, his private accumulation of psychotherapeutic evidence, come manila files stuffed with typed official RAMC forms, the personal narratives of Netley's post-war patients.

Most were young men, conscripts doing their National Service, many from deprived backgrounds. 'Browned off' with life and often in trouble with the law, the lives of these Fifties tearaways had been disturbed by war, and tipped from ordinary adolescent worries into mental instability by conscription and the insti-tutionalisation of military service. Their stories are updates on the historical pathology reports of the nineteenth-century hos-pital: where those case histories of tuberculosis and syphilis were products of compressed populations and primitive health care, the twentieth century epidemic was of mental disorder, symptom of a disturbed century.

One young man was admitted to Netley in 1951 from BMH (British Medical Hospital) Singapore via *Empire Fowey* with a diagnosis of schizophrenia; his was a typical story. 'On the ship his talk was incoherent and his behaviour violent and impulsive', noted Laing. 'Shortly before arrival in Singapore he started to urinate and defecate in his cell. In Singapore Military Hospital he was very nearly inaccessible and degraded in his habits with no sense of personal hygiene. He seldom finished a sentence. He constantly reiterated the phrase. "I am the King. I am the f— King".' Laing observed that the man 'stared vacantly into space, and was completely out of touch with his environment. A few ECTs did not produce significant improvement . . . The opinion of the Psychiatrist at Singapore was that he was definitely psychotic . . .' A diagnosis of 'schizophrenia simplex' was concluded, and the man was recommended for discharge.

Such bureaucratic judgements of Solomon run through the files, counterpointed by a table drawn up by Laing, a terrible graph of botched and successful suicide attempts with ties, aspirins, broken bottles and safety pins, resorted to by desperate young men. There are sad letters from mothers asking for their sons to be kept from doing harm to their own bodies, and perhaps most affecting of all, vivid personal testaments from the patients themselves, rambling like their minds in biro scrawled over blue notepaper. There's a sense of futility about these witnesses to human pain, lamentations set down in useless words which could not begin to evoke their suffering; as though they were trying to voice the pain that their dumbstruck predecessors had been unable to express as they paraded in front of the film cameras; as though their painful essays were extensions of those silent movie captions. And just as those figures had dissolved into the ether, so on the whim of their superiors could these men vanish into the psychiatric system, or be discharged into the 'normal' world. To Laing, their experiences had to amount to something more than the deadened state of an insulin coma or an electro-convulsed mind; perhaps that is why he preserved them.

Netley was still receiving casualties from mainland Europe and especially Germany, much of which remained occupied by Allied troops, many of them national servicemen working among a population which blamed them for the fact that cities such as Berlin and Hamburg were now mere mountains of rubble. One soldier was admitted from the military hospital in Hamburg where he had been diagnosed as a paranoid schizophrenic and had received insulin treatment with no success. His symptoms were 'unspecific, unsystemised querulous complaints against practically everything. Also "very bad nerves"; – "no appetite" "feels dizzy", and weak when people look at him . . .' For days the man ate only tiny amounts of food, 'and then only if someone takes a sample of it before his eyes. He believes that the Sister

318

and all the other patients want rid of him. He has said that he would be better dead and repeatedly says that there can be no improvement in his condition. The whole cast of his thought and action is grossly paranoidal though his delusions are not systematised. He does not appear to be hallucinated except perhaps for taste.' Laing's diagnosis was paranoid schizophrenia; the patient's fate, to be transferred to a civilian mental hospital 'under certificate'.

Like Laing himself, these were young men coming to terms with a post-war world, and their place within it. Another man, acquitted of the manslaughter of his best friend, nonetheless believed he had killed the man and was haunted by his ghost. For such patients, sodium pentothal, the 'truth serum' used by the Americans, was prescribed to bring the source of their dysfunction to the surface, hauling it up from the darkness below. One soldier would vomit after every meal; another would refuse to move, defecating where he crouched. Many cases seemed hopeless, pathological; others appeared more the result of moral judgements than medical conditions. One twenty-five-year-old private, admitted for 'heavy drinking and homosexual practices', was thought by his Medical Officer to be 'genuinely interested in curing himself . . .' The man had served in the Middle East from 1944–8: 'At this time he was not drinking so heavily, nor did he practise much homosexuality.' But when he returned to the Middle East in 1949, 'he was drinking heavily', wrote Laing:

> After a number of drinks he always came round to looking for another homo. He said he never was really at a loss to find partners. He was inclined to be violent also when drunk and for this he got into some trouble but never for his homosexual practices except when involved in fights with other homos over a common love-object. He began to live two lives – at night, and during the day . . . Once he went to his MO complaining of 'nerves' in the hope that he would be referred to a psychiatrist whom he could tell but this manoeuvre did not come off.

On examination the man was described as 'Lean, lithe build; brown skin; golden hair. Physical habits normal...' He maintained that 'he has not been marked off by other people as a "homo" or branded as a "Nancy boy". Through the day he is alright. After a few drinks he becomes frankly homosexual. He plays both active and passive roles.' Concluding that the man was 'a psychopath type III with other abnormal elements in his personality', he was 'recommended for discharge and downgraded to Pulheems Category M2 (two) S8 (eight)'.

Then regarded as a psychiatric disorder, according to one orderly working at Netley around Laing's time there, homosexuality was a case for treatment in itself:

> Some of them admitted to it to get out, quite frankly, whereas lots of them, they didn't want to get out ... but they were found out, and of course they were discharged. Sometimes a chap would be so distressed, he could be suicidal. They tried, very often, to wean them off it a bit. They used to show them pictures of women, and men, and give them electric shocks. But again, that wasn't being cruel, 'cos if a chap was young, and just a bit, you know ... But if a chap's blatant about it, if he was caught in the local bog or whatever, he was discharged with a criminal record as opposed to a medical one...

Another of Laing's patients believed a gang had 'interfered with him by telepathy' and that 'Jews, Freemasons, nurses and doctors plotted to send him mad...' Like some First World War hysteric or Arnold White and Pemberton Billing with his Black Book, he saw enemies everywhere. 'He believes himself to be "psychotically affected by the Free Masonic way of life" by "ventric sound radiation attracting the lunar nerves" acting through "the free body field"', wrote Laing, intrigued by the man's fantasies. 'The Free Masons are an organisation dedicated to exercising power over other people. "No one can be an Officer without being a Free Mason" "They have been doing this for over 300 years" etc etc.' The patient would be ill-rewarded for his subversive revelations of world domination. Diagnosed as seriously paranoid schizophrenic, he was transferred with 'all available medical documents and escort of two' to Netley from Catterick. His eventual fate, like that of the other lives enclosed in these manila files, is unknown.

Perhaps the most extraordinary of all the stories was that of a man born in the north of Britain whose father, a fisherman, had drowned at sea, and whose mother had 'died of "grief" 6 months later'. One of his brothers had been killed at Arnhem; a sister had died in an air raid. The patient had been transferred to Netley from Cambridge Military Hospital where he had tried to hang himself with a strip of blanket while under arrest for petty theft in the guardroom. Examined by Laing, he claimed 'that he masturbated 5/6 times a day for years. Affirms extensive association with prostitutes and that he has been himself a homo-sexual prostitute. Confesses to almost every perversion. Married in July 1951 and has one child. Claims he loves his wife, but she is cold, "enjoys masturbation better".' As part of his therapy, the man was asked to write an account of his life – although given its neatly-written and self-dramatising fervour, perhaps he volunteered the story himself.

The soldier began by declaring that his favourite job was clean-ing the mortuary at the Cumberland Infirmary when he left school. During the war he received a shrapnel wound in his head at Dieppe, and was taken prisoner of war. Freed in 1945, he re-enlisted and was posted to Germany. Like the Germans made to view concentration camps in order to demonstrate their reality, young men serving in this shifting, destabilised landscape were suddenly made aware of the reality of total war and its aftermath; perhaps the experience disturbed Laing's patient's mind, or at least brought to the surface incipient instability. In Germany, like his Victorian predecessors and many of his peers, the man contracted syphilis. He went absent without leave, and when recaptured, was badly treated in prison, and suffered a nervous breakdown after being beaten up by the military police. Like Roger Hall, he escaped again and hid in the snow 'underneath an old pig trough while the search party looked for me'; there he became frozen to the ground and couldn't move for eight hours. Once again he was recaptured, escaped, and this time was given shelter by a prostitute from whom he contracted gonorrhoea. Moving across war-torn Germany, evading the military police, he fell in with a pair of absentees from the US army; together they drank hooch which temporarily blinded him.

After further misadventures and brushes with military law, the man found himself back in Britain, working in another mortuary. 'I especially like suicides, I had quite a lot of them down there', he wrote. 'I used to try and imagine what went through their minds before they killed themselves, and I used to wonder what it was like.' His CV seemed that of someone destined to do damage to himself; yet presented with such a history, Laing's assessment was unsympathetic. Still part of the establishment he would later disavow in a manner yet more anarchic than his patient's, Laing evidently did not like the man or his lack of contrition. 'He is facile and full of himself; no genuine repentance. Asked why he stole from the Q.M. stores, said "My wife had no sheets and cutlery. She had to have them. You would have done the same. I was caught. I'm always unlucky".' Laing diagnosed a 'psychopathic personality with emotional abnormality ... Recommended to be boarded and discharged.' Discharged, doubtless to follow a similar life all over again, to end Heaven knows where. Neither the army, nor its psychiatrists, could do much with such men: there were limits to their social responsibility.

Nor could a lieutenant in the RAMC afford to be sentimental. It was Laing's responsibility to 'downgrade' out of the Army on psychiatric grounds those soldiers unwanted by the service. This apparently rigorous bureaucratic process was in fact quite arbitrary, and seemed to be directed towards the supply of men required by the services: one month they sent ten per cent back and discharged ninety per cent; another, the proportions would be completely reversed. 'The Korean war was on. Manpower, conscription, morale presented problems. Malingering could become a major issue, if one wanted to become too fastidious.' It was Britain's Vietnam, and as in the United States a decade later, 'A lot of soldiers seemed to be prepared to go to almost any lengths to get out.' It was as though the regime at Netley was designed to deter malingerers rather than cure the genuinely ill. It seemed matters had hardly changed since 1914. And in this archaic, punitive atmosphere, closed off from the outside world, Laing's own sense of subversion would foment.

If Laing's papers show that the inmates of Netley were at last being given a voice, they also raise the question of whether anyone was listening. For most of the time, those patients who were not plunged into darkness, comatose on insulin, were condemned to a waking silence, as though someone had perverted the strictures of Cistercian monks and applied them to this twentieth-century isolation. It was the barely-contained silence Roger Hall had remembered as his fellows exercised in D Block's walled garden; the silence of their own madness made worse by its manic interruptions.

Netley's rules forbade the staff from talking to the patients, or encouraging the patients to talk to them; only doctors could address the inmates. The entire process of psychotherapy in D Block was carried out in the third person. To Laing, this seemed a new and unnecessary torture, a thumbscrew of alienation: 'No patient was expected to speak to a member of staff unless spoken to. Talking between patients was observed, reported and broken up. Pairing off was prevented. Friendship was not forbidden because psychotics are incapable of it. But they might form a *folie à deux*: difficult to destroy clinically, but still clinically interesting if the worst came to the worst.' It was a bizarre development on 'persuasion': a one-sided therapy in which the 'talking cure' was done to military order. It was in effect a gag which made the mad manageable.

'As a lieutenant expected to enforce these commands, I was

of course not subject to them myself', wrote Laing; he became their voice, a voice of dissent. 'I asked the patients on insulin about their hallucinations and delusions. One of them had the interesting delusion that he was humped out of bed in his drugged sleep in the middle of the night, dragged out of the ward and beaten up somewhere by two men in Army uniforms. Another patient came up with the same delusion. An interesting case of communication without words: telepathic *folie à deux*. Then a third patient came up with the same delusion . . .' Shortly after, a corporal and private on night duty were court-martialled, convicted, and given a dishonourable discharge with two years' hard labour. (As Laing was recording this anecdote, the telephone rang: a man on the other end told him about his father, a private in the Army who had been diagnosed schizophrenic and was made to clean the lavatories with a razor blade, 'until Lieutenant Laing put a stop to it'.)

After his stint in the insulin ward, Laing was assigned to 'a neurotic-psychopathic-alcoholic-battle-neurosis-anything-goes-miscellaneous ward'. The tools at his disposal included 'pre-tranquillizer drugs – barbiturates, chloral-hydrate, paraldehyde, electric shocks, "modified" insulin, straitjackets, "padded cells", injections, tube-feeds, amytal abreactions, antabuse, hypnosis. The army espoused vigorous, "muscular" treatment for its psychiatric casualties and patients.' One evening when Laing was on night duty, he heard a manic patient raving inside a padded cell; he ordered an injection to be administered if the man did not quieten down. But before it was given, Laing had the cell opened, and sat down to listen instead. After half an hour, the patient calmed down and didn't need the sedative.

It was Laing's 'moment of epiphany'. For the next few nights he stayed longer, 'until I was almost "hanging out" during the night with him in his padded cell. I felt strangely at home there, lounging on the floor.' Rather than analyse, Laing just listened. 'At first I could <u>almost</u> understand him, I could <u>almost</u> follow. He was very fast. He was in a padded cell because he had knocked himself out by taking a running jump, head first, at a brick wall.

He could be anyone he cared to be merely by snapping his fingers ... Most of the time he was a gentleman catburglar and safe-blower in Manhattan or London or anywhere ...'

The eighteen-year-old son of a prostitute and an army officer, the patient had been forced into the army by his father; as a result he suffered 'severe anxiety states' and psychosis. Laing became the man's 'companion' in his fantasies, 'a sort of Sancho Panza to his Don Quixote ... His padded cell had become a refuge for me and his company a solace ... He was flying around in his mind, like a bird ...' Laing believed in his ability to save the man, like Shelley before him, who wrote in 'Julian and Maddalo' (based on his discourses with Byron in Venice) of a madman, the Maniac, whom they found in a Venetian asylum:

> ... I imagined that if day by day
> I watched him, and but seldom went away,
> And studied all the beatings of his heart
> With zeal, as men study some stubborn art
> For their own good, and could by patience find
> An entrance to the caverns of his mind,
> I might reclaim him from his dark estate ...

Laing saw many such men petrified by fear in Netley's padded cells; to him it seemed uniquely a disorder of his time. 'What was going on here?' he asked himself. 'What sort of thing was this? It was quite unlike *encephalitis lethargica* and the stuff neurologists see.' (Laing had witnessed victims of the 1920s epidemic in Glasgow, still frozen in their paralysed bodies thirty years later.) He observed another army officer, aged twenty-eight, who stayed in the middle of his cell day and night, naked, wide-awake, quivering, as though his body image blurred with the disturbed image of his mind. He ate nothing, and relieved himself on the floor. Jabbering 'in fast *ratatatatats* like bursts of machine-gun fire', his speech echoed round the room 'so that he is under continual machine-gun fire from all around, even ... the ground.'

'*Completely* terrified', the naked officer pounced like a feral cat on anyone who tried to enter his cell. Worried he would soon die of exhaustion, the staff had him sedated and force-fed. But some could not be kept from harm: the desperate would end their torment by hanging themselves in the shower block. Others escaped into the woods to be found with their throats cut, or drowned themselves in the reedy ponds in the valley below, pathetic victims of their illness.

To Laing, the whole notion of an asylum seemed to be a question of social control rather than psychotherapy. Like Charles Myers and W. H. Rivers before him, he had been drafted into the military to apply civilian psychiatry to the victims of war and martial discipline; and like them, he was both fascinated and appalled by what he found, and by what he was expected to do. He responded by reacting against the system, and by using it to further his own lines of research. Laing's experiences at Netley in the Fifties were crucial in forming his revolutionary theories, carried out in consciousnesss of recent history. When he considered that the human race had disposed of perhaps one hundred million of its 'fellow normal men in the last fifty years', he concluded that humanity seemed to be suffering from one mass psychotic episode; in such a world it was easy to believe that the mad were sane, and vice versa. 'Sanity is determinism and totalitarianism', Laing wrote in his Netley diary. 'It is death to the soul and the end of freedom. Against this self-justified tautology, this invincible and inevitable self-rectitude, the romantic revolt takes its origin.'

Laing's revolt was against the twentieth century's 'sublimated pursuit of power, or the hegemony of reason'; the same reasoning that led to its totalitarian states and their perversions of social Darwinism. It was as though Laing's arrival at Netley coincided with the culmination of two centuries of industrial alienation; the same pressures against which the romantics and the goths had reacted (and which had reached a perverted denouement in Germany). Here, in this clinical prison on a Hampshire field, with an empire rapidly deconstructing around him, Laing's

326

'romantic revolt' was expressed in evidence of what fellow psychiatrists would call his 'oppositional identity'. Once he was standing with a fellow doctor when an RAMC major walked by. 'Don't you salute majors?' the man barked. 'If they are nice majors', Laing somewhat camply replied. He was reprimanded for his civilian insolence: 'You're in the army now.'

As a witness to the human suffering at Netley, Laing was concerned that he had become complicit in it. It was a uniquely post-war crisis: 'It became clear to me that I was involved with the puzzle of human misery, and one of the things that deeply disturbed and puzzled me was why the world we live in was such a miserable, cruel and violent place.' He continued to read existentialist texts, including Camus' *Le Mythe de Sisyphe*, an essay on hopelessness which seemed to reflect the state of Netley's inmates: 'It seems to me the final absurdity is that he remains in his place of torture, and anguish, and despair', wrote Laing; Netley's patients had no choice.

To Laing, it was obvious that D Block's imposed silence produced men exhibiting mutism or deafness, as if they too were complicit in the process; men who had shut themselves off from the world in response to its tyrannies. The trauma that had sent them to Netley was real enough, but once there, its institutional regime – its brick walls, barred windows and padded cells – served only to send them deeper into the silence to which they had consigned themselves. Rather than curing its patients, Netley was making them madder.

Laing left Netley after a year. In 1958 he wrote his first book, the existential-influenced *The Divided Self*, which drew partly on his experiences there. Its intent was to see the sanity in lunacy, but in the process Laing himself underwent a transformation, from psychiatrist to media celebrity. His 'therapeutic community', Kingsley Hall, a former church in London's East End, became a sort of libertarian Bedlam where Sixties celebrities visited its most famous inmate, Mary Barnes, a former nun who walled herself in her room as a dirty protest anchoress, smearing herself with her own excrement and painting with it.* Dubbed an 'Acid Marxist', half-pop star, half-guru, Laing later became a lecturer at the Anti-University of London, founded in Shoreditch in the spirit of the 1968 riots in Paris and which offered Francis Huxley's tutorials on dragons, Yoko Ono on art, and his own studies in 'inner space in Greek, Christian and Egyptian mythologies'.

Laing died suddenly of a heart attack in 1989. There is no record of his having returned to Netley, nor of his having witnessed Netley's ghosts, although while he was there, an exorcism was carried out in the main hospital to rid it of its Grey Lady. But after his friend's death, Bob Mullan, a film-maker and psychology lecturer, saw Laing at a tube station and in a newsagent's in London: 'I recognised him and then he was gone . . . there was no mistake. It was him. Yet I am neither mad nor am I an incurable romantic.' Like the ghosts of Netley, Laing's spirit refused to rest.

---

* Fifty years earlier, 'The Unseen', one of Arnold White's essays in *The Views of Vanoc* (1911) had referred to 'the case of Mary Barnes' in whom 'no fewer than ten distinct and separate personalities were revealed', including 'a blind imbecile' who could 'draw admirably', even though 'Mary Barnes (the normal A) could never draw at all'.

The World is Infinitely Forgiving

It is not wise to find symbols in everything that one sees.
It makes life too full of terrors.

OSCAR WILDE, *Salome*

W hen my now-married brother moved into a house next
to the hospital, with its railway line running at the end
of his garden, his elderly neighbour spoke of the soldier-patients
who used to stand over the tracks: solemn, staring figures, awaiting their moment. Some escapees were considered dangerous
enough for the whole village to be put on alert, and were pursued
by a doctor and a pair of burly white-coat-clad orderlies. But as
my brother noted laconically, their quarries were usually found
drinking in the Station Hotel.

Like the main hospital, the asylum was beginning to show a
'steady and progressive deterioration in the decoration and
fabric. There are now leaking roofs, rotten floors, and crumbling
plaster in many parts of the building.' Yet it continued to expand
in pursuit of physical and sometimes experimental therapies:
soon after Laing left, a new insulin ward was commissioned, and
the visiting inspector 'was interested in a biochemical laboratory,
with much new equipment, where work with irradiated iodine

is being carried out . . .' Meanwhile, PN Wing specialised in alcohol and drug abusers and short-term patients such as the singer Terry Dean who, like Elvis Presley, was called up for National Service at the height of his fame. Suffering from a nervous breakdown, his arrival at Netley created a local sensation – the equivalent of a modern celebrity checking into a dependency clinic – not least for the young National Servicemen employed in the hospital, Laing's contemporaries like Ed Parker, who preserved photographs of his fellow workers including a snap of 'Cpl Attwood – My Friend?' in a substantial quiff and suede shoes and a dandified army uniform.

In the late 1950s, anti-psychotic drugs began to supersede insulin and leucotomy, and by the Sixties, as Laing was exploring his LSD alternatives to psychiatry, the latest advances in psychotropics (dubbed 'chemical straitjackets') came to Netley, along with a more enlightened regime. The two blocks were renamed again, Victoria House and Albert House, and the bars were removed from the old asylum's windows. Colonel R. Davies, the new commanding officer, announced 'I'm going to have the high wall knocked down as well, if I can.' 'Occasionally a patient walks out for there are no walls to keep him in', he told a local reporter. 'When a patient goes missing first a check of the block is made, then the grounds and then if he has yet to be found the local police are informed as well as the Military Police, Naval Patrol and the police force near the absconder's home town.' The same report noted that 'Recent trouble spots have produced many casualties. Terrorist action in Aden and recent riots in Northern Ireland are two trouble spots where the bad living – and dying – conditions have taken their toll of man's mental stability.' Colonel Davies concluded that 'this place is absolutely perfect for rehabilitation. I don't think there is a better place for our sick servicemen in Britain.'

But by the late Seventies, Netley's psychiatric function had run its course. Like its vanished older cousin, it too was deemed old-fashioned and out of date, and in 1978 the buildings were closed down and the patients moved out. The last remnant of

Netley's once-great hospital site had fallen empty, its clamorous existence silenced yet still echoing with its past. It also presented a temptation to trespassers, and one summer's afternoon Peter and I broke into the compound.

The asylum lay at the end of one of the hospital's abandoned tarmac roads, the back lane from the main hospital to the rear gate set in the high brick wall. Beyond was a Victorian landscape: cedars in dark strata, gravel paths obscured by docks and rusty brown sorrel, the once close-cropped lawn now a hayfield of dry summer grass. Ahead stretched the asylum itself, the sun pouring in through its windows.

In an extension on one side of the building a door stood half-open. Inside were a pair of deep iron baths standing side by side; the taps had stopped running long ago. The floor was covered with broken glass and scraps of paper, dry and dusty. Everything was light and still. I did not know then that this hut-like structure had housed the insulin ward, with its darkened rooms of comatose patients once patrolled by Laing.

A green- and cream-painted corridor led into the heart of the asylum. Pushing through doors half off their hinges, we moved through the building, past other, bigger rooms. At the end of another corridor was a row of cells. A sort of cloister ran in between them and the older extension beyond, allowing a glimpse of the sane world outside – or at least, the walled enclosure of D Block's grounds. In retrospect, what affected me most – what frightened and thrilled me – was the atmosphere of abandoned functionality and imposed order, a potent mix of institutions: medical, military and psychiatric. It felt like the sort of place from which it was not easy to escape, even now. There were alarm bells at regular intervals along the walls, and thick prison-like doors inset with elliptical peep-holes. Each cell was lit by a solitary window, set too high to allow a view; the walls were thickly padded as though covered with enormous mattresses, their seams split and the stuffing spilling out like a ripped teddy bear.

As the sun flooded the cell with a light that must have seemed

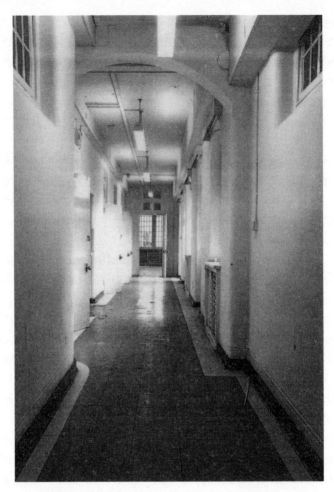

Abandoned D Block corridor, late 1970s

cruelly bright to its inhabitants, Peter shut the door on me. The momentary sense of panic and claustrophobia was intense. The walls muffled all sound, as though I were in a calico-lined submarine. It wasn't dark, but there was a finality to the loss of light, a diminishment that was somehow exciting; a sense of deprivation, but of security, too. Our macabre game was cut short by the sudden appearance of a sorely-tried security guard in the far corner of the field. He shouted, rather half-heartedly, as we ran off through the long grass, too far away to catch.

After that the asylum seemed to haunt my dreams, as if I'd picked up something from those brief seconds of entrapment in the padded cell. I imagined myself in a strait-jacket, sitting in the corner of the tiny room, obsessively rocking – although this may have been an image from a rock video as much as it was reincarnation. Later my brother, who knew one of the security guards, reported that etchings had been found on a first floor window, scenes of Victorian soldiers and masted ships scratched into the glass. The same guard once saw a light and a face in an upstairs window, only to discover that the room had been bricked up. D Block still seemed haunted by that face at the window, as though the film of its shell-shocked inmates were being replayed through its etched glass.

Soon afterwards the spider hospital was razed to the ground, its concrete worthless and unsalvageable, the foundations bull-dozed to form a great modern earthwork that could yet contain its bones. All that was left were its driveways, the disconnected nervous system of its function and history. The grass pushed up through the crumbling asphalt, and ornamental firs, planted to give it human scale, grew out of shape, overgrown with brambles and ivy. In the undergrowth, emerging out of the earth like splinters out of skin, came bits of crockery, broken bottles and brown teapots stamped with the stigmatic arrow mark of Government property; and among them a cache of unlabelled phials containing what looked like iodine, as though the traces of medical experimentation had been hurriedly buried in these green fields.

D Block remained intact, still the stuff of rumours – the most alarming, to local residents, that it was about to be turned into a prison. In the summer of 1980, only weeks after Peter and I had trespassed in the asylum, the developers moved in. The twentieth-century extensions were demolished, returning the building to its original form. Its corridors were knocked into the wards and the courtyard glazed over in an enthusiastic embrace of Eighties post-modernism with white metal beams and toughened glass designed to resemble the superstructure of a ship. The asylum was appointed as a training centre for the Hampshire Constabulary. Rooms that were secure wards now housed policemen; the grounds became as neat and tidy as a civic park.

But the brick wall which resisted Colonel Davies's reforms remained, a long, unscalable reminder of benevolent tyranny which did not fall, as other walls did, in the last decades of the twentieth century. The arched windows looking out on the lawn still seem to reflect the ghosts of the past, as though, like the abbey's *lux nova*, they might project scenes from the asylum's history, modern images of the Day of Judgement. Inside the building the inmate-etched window panes are on display, their outsider art scraffito of fusiliers and sergeants, birds and horses, warships and castles, a bottle and a glass all signed in multiple by 'P White, 47th Regt.'. Lit from behind by a fluorescent strip like an advertising hoarding, they are a votive offering to the building's unquiet spirits, a talisman of the constabulary's stewardship.

Upstairs, along a pseudo-nautical gangway that looks down

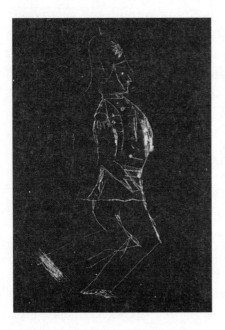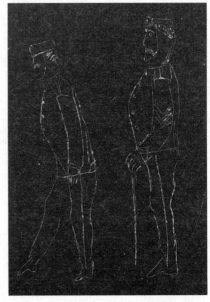

on the canteen area as though from the deck of a liner, is a police museum, a faintly comic collection of truncheons, helmets and handcuffs. In one glass case, however, is the photograph of a shiny Webley revolver and a shrine-like display dedicated to its owner, 'the Monocled Mutineer': Percy Toplis, the Great War outlaw. A fugitive from the rebellion against the martial horrors of the Etaples training camp, Toplis left the underclass of deserters behind the front lines,* and back in England reinvented himself as an officer, an English Jay Gatsby in a gold monocle. Sent as a souvenir to the Hampshire officer who first arrested Toplis, the lens itself still sits next to its jeweller's box, a potent relic of his insurrection; a bold usurpation of class, subverting its aristocratic hauteur into an arrogant symbol of rebellion.

Next to the monocle are a pair of photographs, the before and after of this modern Jekyll and Hyde. One shows Toplis posing in his appropriated officer's uniform: tunic, jodhpurs and boots, a wide Sam Browne belt over his shoulder, austere hair swept back over his handsome face. The other, his police mugshot, has the mutineer in a flat cap, unshaven and on the run. Alongside is a catalogue of the items found in the deceased's possession, a sad laundry list of suit, shoes and underwear (one blue sock, one brown) and, in a brown paper parcel, a tin of Vaseline and 'one injection tube'. Visitors to the police museum are informed of Toplis's crimes: serial offender, convicted thief and rapist, a man

---

* 'These men lived . . . in caves and grottoes under certain parts of the front line', wrote Osbert Sitwell. 'They would issue forth, it was said, from their secret lairs after each of the interminable checkmate battles, to rob the dying of their few possessions . . . and leave them dead. Were these bearded figures, shambling in rags and patched uniforms, and pale with a cellar dampness . . . a myth created by suffering among the wounded, as a result of pain, privation and exposure, or did they exist? . . . At any rate, the story was widely believed among the troops; who maintained that the General Staff could find no way to deal with these bands until the war was over, and that in the end they had to be gassed.'

of bad stock – what Arnold White would have called a degenerate. Yet Toplis's friend maintained that in another generation he would have been regarded as an 'intellectual socialist'. Even now, under these glass cases in Netley, the struggle for the secret history of war is still being fought.

Below the museum, policemen and women in black and white bustle about the modern interior bright with pale wood and puce upholstery. But the place cannot dispel the history charged in its bricks: the west wing has a cold, 'eerie' air, and people are reluctant to linger there after dark. Next door, in the building which was once the commanding officer's home, techniques are practised for the interrogation of terrorists, and police dogs prowl in kennels outside. In a mocked-up city street recruits are trained in the assertion of public order, ready to face the modern heirs of the striking masons and shanty-dwellers who protested the hospital's construction a century before; while new fir saplings hide a hangar-like firing range filled with weaponry, breaking the mid-week quiet of the park with ominous booms and thuds.

It seems appropriate that D Block and its memories should remain closed off from public scrutiny. The overgrown woods that surround it retain an atmosphere of the darkness that was within, the demons which they now seek to keep out. Sinuous ivy fingers the Victorian mortar, and nettles and deadly nightshade skirt the walls. They could almost be the remnants of a lost civilisation, a memory of the site's Roman occupation, the outpost of an older empire.

After the dead of winter, bluebells thrust up from their Sargasso Sea of leaves, competing with croziers of lime-green ferns. Under the tree-filtered light the blue haze turns the woods into a coral reef, a scene from a hyper-real Pre-Raphaelite painting. *Hyacinthoides non-scriptus*, Britain's national flower, blooms on St George's Day; an ancient symbol of solitude and regret named after the handsome Spartan whom Apollo accidentally killed, and whose blood produced the flowers as it seeped into the earth. And as Flanders poppies symbolise scarlet tunics and the blood of the trenches, so these mauve bells seem to echo the blue of hospital undress. Netley's monks used the flowers to treat leprosy, and they have been found to contain a compound effective against tuberculosis. But such curative powers are countered by superstition: it is bad luck to bring bluebells into the house, and a child who picks them alone in a wood will never be seen again.

Strewn across the muddy path are the wilting stems of abandoned blooms. The stilled sounds draw you in deeper, 'glad to the brink of fear', a sensation of being watched. A cloud passes over the sun, chasing its shadow through the trees. Under the ivy and barbed-wire bramble lies more hospital litter: old jars, bits of brash white sanitary ware, and a thick bottle, its neck snapped to a jagged edge with one word – 'Imperial' – still legible in raised letters on the green-brown glass.

From beginning to end, the hospital's lanes led its inmates, swallowing them up, engulfing them in Netley's all-encompassing culture. For those whose grip on life was faltering, the proximity of the military cemetery, tactfully sited at the furthest point of the grounds, was a salutary *memento mori*. In wartime cortèges assembled every afternoon to the mournful Dead March, processing along a raised causeway through the woods at the furthestmost end of the site to culminate in a repeating loop of the Last Post.

The construction of this modern earthwork in the ancient woodland valley was a considerable undertaking for Netley's nineteenth-century landscapers, heirs of the barrow-makers' skills as they moved tons of earth to create steep banks. Now held together by the tenacious roots of tall beeches, the sides fall away to overgrown gullies where iron-stained streams rush through brick conduits to the sea. Rising above this wilderness was a route which took up where the railway tracks left off, a final connexion in the inexorable journey that began with a train to the Front and ended in a Hampshire wood.

Even now this green corridor has the air of a mythological

passage, a movement from dark to light. At its end the tunnel-like lane suddenly opens out into a tranquil, tree-protected space, an immaculate arboretum. In turf cut close as a number one crop grow monkey puzzle trees from Chile, Corsican pines and dark Victorian yews. This is the most beautiful part of the grounds, reserved for itself. It sinks in its own time, quiet enough to hear birdsong, just as its occupants once heard birds sing at dawn.

Here are the hospital's lost souls, marking its history in grave-stones. Three thousand five hundred lie under these rolling hills, as though heaving with their dead. Walter Edwin Willis, died in 1894 aged thirty, 'most patient in affliction'; William Goater, twenty-seven in 1882, died 'having survived his return from the Egyptian Campaign only a few days'; Charles Gumbley, 'passed away May 23rd 1892', his memorial 'erected by his sisters Emily and Kate'. Three of the stones mark men drowned in South-ampton Water; and another, a sergeant of the Royal Garrison Artillery 'who met his death by falling from the troopship "Sici-lia" in Southampton Docks'. And remembered in the strange reversed characters of Cyrillic are three seamen of the Tsar's navy, brought to Netley as victims of disease on an official visit to Southampton in 1873.

Until the First World War, headstones were paid for by

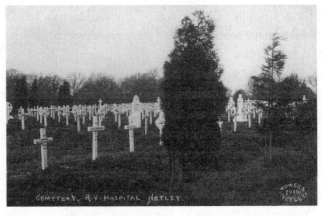

Netley Military Cemetery, c.1920

338

relatives, and so more than half of Netley's interred went unnoticed above ground. Then came the pathetic temporary wooden crosses which carried the memory of the war dead into the 1920s, like the little crosses and poppies still placed here every November. Erecting a central monument, a fit setting for crimson wreaths on grey stone, the Imperial War Graves Commission introduced a democracy of the dead: regulation two foot eight inch Portland slabs, inscribed with the global reach of modern war: 'E. Mbenyesi, South African Native Labour Corps, Died 25 August 1917'; and the unclaimed enemy, '*Ein Deutscher Soldat*', each an unknown soldier. But most of these neat stone rows remember young Englishmen whose loss was a mystery to those who loved them: 'Rfn. C. G. Vincent 18th Hants Regt. Died Jan 9th 1916. Aged 19. He Tried To Do His Duty. Greatly Missed By His Comrade Jack.'

It was in November, the month of remembrance, of falling leaves and fireworks, of silent clouds of poppies and notes in a wooden box on the church altar, that Peter died. He was my oldest friend; we'd kept in touch since school, our separate lives drifting apart yet still connected. In that strange week, I picked up a book on Wilfred Owen. But it wasn't until a year later that I realised that the anniversary of Owen's death was Peter's too.

That morning I'd cycled out early, just after dawn, to fetch a newspaper. At a crossroads close to our house was a large red-brick house trees, set back from the road and surrounded by yew and holly trees which also hid a pair of plain-fronted and even older-looking villas. They were Victorian relics stranded on a stretch of land somehow overlooked by developers; the fact that a well-used road ran directly in front of them seemed to accentuate rather than detract from their remoteness from the modern world. Occasionally you'd see an old-fashioned car backing out of a drive and on to the busy road, but this was a rare sight; whoever lived there seemed as reclusive as the houses themselves, hidden behind their high, dark hedges.

A notice was pinned to the white pailing fence that protected the larger of the houses. Out of curiosity I swung back and stopped to read it. In dispassionately-typed legalese, it announced that the buildings were due to be demolished.

Pushing through the gate – which promptly collapsed – I propped my bike against an overgrown laurel. The house was already in ruins, its roof removed and open to the sky, indecently exposing old bedroom wallpaper as if someone's underwear drawer had been turfed out in public. Bricks had tumbled down the chimneys and out of their fireplaces, caught in freeze-frame as the house imploded. In the skeletal roof whitened laths filtered the early morning sun. The site looked like a piece of installation art; gutted and turned inside-out, its innards on show to all-comers, a blatant mockery of the family home it once was. It was a cruel, heartless sight, as though a pogrom had been visited on an English suburb. A smouldering bonfire and the faint impression of brick dust hanging in the air diffused the light; a mist hovered around the deconstructed building and its grounds.

On one side of the house stood a large garage with an attic space above it. Its roof had entirely fallen in, exposing bare wooden fishbone rafters and allowing the cold morning light of autumn to fall on what it had contained. An old ladder was propped up against the beams, leading nowhere. The floor was entirely covered in mounds of rubbish, all of a colour, vaguely that of mud: neutral, primeval, the stuff of which other things are made. What lay there appeared to be rotting down into the earth: rusty tools, broken chairs with heraldic, shield-shaped backs; a soaking wet greatcoat, navy blue gym shorts and other pieces of unidentifiable uniform; a gas mask, its flat blank lenses cracked and vacuous like the eyes of a dead fish. But the pile was mostly made up of books. Hundreds and hundreds of books. Technical texts, school books, religious tracts, pulp fiction from the 1920s with lurid covers advertising their sensational tales, French grammars and German dictionaries, old editions of Shakespeare and Victorian novellas, all tumbling from broken shelves on to the garage floor, their sum total of European culture brought down by the predations of the English climate. I picked up a brown soaking wad of pages from the pile. A name, Permain, was written in faded ink inside; the book was dated 1830. I picked up another: again, the same name. And another, dated 1826, and another, dated 1763. It seemed inconceivable that I should find an eighteenth-century book lying in a heap of rubbish in Sholing. This collection of generations had survived world wars and the social changes of two centuries only to perish in a sodden mass strewn across a garage floor, rapidly being reduced to compost.

I moved around the ruined house and through its grounds, littered with kitchenware, enamel pans and a huge 1950s fridge dragged out from the kitchen by the contractors. I imagined brutal men in hard hats engaged in the sort of pillage which even then was going on in parts of Europe's dark heart. A tall conifer, its elderly branches sagging with age like an ancient spinster, stood in the middle of the lawn; the frost was beginning to be burnt off the grass by the rising sun. I had already been there more than an hour, but time seemed suspended in the autumn mist. Picking my way across the tufty grass of a lawn uncut for years, I pushed through a gap in the laurel hedge at the end of the grounds.

It was almost shocking to find another pair of houses there: unseparated twins, similarly decrepit, similarly in the process of demolition. And here, among all the rubbish of useless hardware, shattered slates and broken timbers, was another pile of papers and books. They'd been pushed into a bonfire-like pyramid, apparently ready to be burnt, though now too wet for any match to take. I knelt to look through the heap of old music and pulp fiction: *Goal*, depicting a handsome footballer of the 1930s, his curly blond Flash Gordon hair swept back from his forehead with a girl at his side looking imploringly into his stern blue eyes; a brochure for the Union Castle line from Southampton to South Africa, and with a 1950s postcard from Cape Town to one of the house's inhabitants, written at a time when apartheid's blond champions went unsanctioned by the world. Beneath them

341

were more books, with the family name – Jacob – inscribed inside. Perhaps they were Jewish. There was a yellow-jacketed Gollancz book from the Thirties, *Catholic Conversions*, edited by Father D'Arcy, the socialist priest who steered Evelyn Waugh and Edith Sitwell in the direction of Rome. On the cover was a list of contributors, among them Noël Coward's friend Sheila Kaye-Smith and Oscar Wilde's betrayer Lord Alfred Douglas, the man who took the Old Bailey stand at Noel Pemberton Billing's trial to declare that his former lover had been 'the greatest force for evil in Europe in the last 350 years'.

These piles of rubbish from the evidently literate, even intellectual households spanned more than a century of history; they summed up a hundred years of English life. From the stolid nineteenth-century respectability of religious texts, to Edwardian sheet music of pop songs; from Twenties paperbacks of Edgar Wallace novels with murderous Chinese mandarins clutching stiletto knives, to the *Weekly News* with a strap line announcing 'Mussolini says no Heil to Hitler' and inside blurry sepia photographs of Japanese atrocities carried out on Chinese peasants; from Victorian pattern books of corsets and bloomers, to Fifties women's magazines bright with the colour of lipstick. I picked up a damp page of typescript; it was apparently part of a novel and evidently written in the Forties: 'When Hess becomes a Paderewski, and he a Stalingrad of new and youthful appearance, then will the old ones dance, eh, my pretty?... I am for Stalin. Such a beautiful figure and such a tremendous show of it...' Perhaps the writer was a musician too, maybe a teacher; notebooks had scribbled musical notations, and sketches of Nancy Astor and Edith Sitwell. Other exercise books contained notes for another book, and grotesque doodles of weird human and animal figures, the product of a vivid, if not intoxicated imagination caught up in greater events yet sequestered in this suburban backwater.

Yet none of this was as strange as the fragment of newspaper that lay underneath:

Daily Sketch, Friday August 20, 1915
ANOTHER PIRATE ATTACK ON WOMEN AND
CHILDREN
*Huns Torpedo And Sink A White Star Liner Close To Where
The Lusitania Went Down.*

Above the headlines ran news of the sinking of the *Arabic*
('No lives lost, no thanks to Tirpitz'); below was a photograph
of the ship, and a portrait of a woman in a shirtwaist and plaited
hair: 'Stella Carol, the famous singer, and her husband were on
the boat.' Scribbled in ink above the picture was the reason for
the paper's preservation: 'I heard her sing on the Soton Pier.'
On the other side of the page, among the rest of the war news
– 'German Wedge In Russian Lines'; 'Writer's Description of
Zeppelin Bombs On A Prison' – another headline reminded the
tabloid readers that while Armageddon might be upon Western
civilisation, Society carried on regardless.

THE PRETTIEST WAR-BRIDE – *Mr. Asquith's Niece
And Her Eight Pretty Bridesmaids.* PREMIER AND SIR
E. GREY AT THE GLENCONNER WEDDING.

A year previously, in the mythic summer of 1914, Sir Edward
Grey, the Foreign Secretary, great lover of birds and reluctant
proponent of war, had stood in his office in Whitehall, turned
to Lord Glenconner and said, 'The lamps are going out over
Europe. We shall not see them lit again in our lifetime.'
  Only one other page of the paper had been saved: a centre-page
spread of photographs: 'The Glenconner Wedding: Yesterday
Clare Tennant married Adrian Bethell.' And there, at the bottom
of the report, stood the pages, dressed in pseudo-medieval garb –
'costumed à la Edward VI., in bright geranium red, with fillets of
dull gold on each merry, curly head, and silver belts'. The taller of
the pair smiled slyly, if not winsomely out of the ancient news-
print: Lord Glenconner's nine-year-old son, Stephen Tennant.

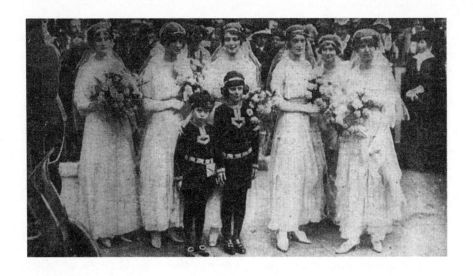

Two generations after that picture was taken, I had become obsessed with another photograph of Tennant as an androgynous Bright Young Thing posing in his Silver Room, wearing a wasp-waisted pin-stripe suit and his brother's leather flying jacket over his shoulders, as if in an ironic gesture to the war that had gone before; a war against which his lover, Siegfried Sassoon, had protested. The image seemed to sum up a sense of subversive glamour; it held me with the power of an icon. Tennant had ended his days in eccentric reclusion in his Wiltshire manor, where I would visit him, bearing orchids and chocolates and Beaton's photograph. That afternoon he had spoken to me in an archaic voice echoing down the century. With my audience at an end, I was left alone in his manor house, the wind whistling through the windows and doors, the dead leaves of autumn drifting against them.

Now I stood here, in another autumn, looking at another picture. The other figures in the grainy, heavily screened photograph looked like indistinct, historic ghosts. Not Stephen. He had life, an ironic, self-amused vitality; a feyness which rose above the dreary fates of those around him. He seemed to be smirking at himself, and at me, and at the history that lay in tatters around my feet.

*   *   *

In the years after its demolition, the hospital grounds lay fallow while the authorities decided what to do with them. As I left school for college, Netley's parkland stood empty and unpossessed; even then it was proposed not to allow the land to be opened up for public use; that it should still remain 'out of bounds'. Finally, in 1980, with the foundations of the hospital levelled and turfed, the site became a country park. The imperial had been municipalised.

Yet like an eighteenth-century landscape planned for future generations, Netley's grounds continued to grow to maturity, even without the buildings they were meant to beautify or obscure. In acre after acre stretching back from the sea, only Mr Page's trees remain: solemn and dark at the edge of paths, silent sentries guarding the corners of empty fields full of memories, as if, when the building was demolished, its memory was displaced to the land around it; as if the lost memories of its shell-shocked soldiers had returned to haunt these fields and woods. In their peacefulness they seem to recall war: evergreen, living monuments, as though they alone remember its past. The lanes around D Block's high walls seem freighted with solitude, overhung by trees, stopping abruptly where structures should have been: the isolation hospital, the stables, levelled ruins subsumed by vegetation, their function lost to history. Every trace of the hospital, strewn across its site as though by an enormous explosion, becomes a relic: a moss-covered piece of masonry, bits of rubble in the grass, a rusting gas lamp gaunt and broken like a tree struck by lightning, once a meeting place for lovers under the shadow of Netley's towers and turrets.

In their wilder tracts the grounds are still coursed by footpaths, which authority could not, in the end, erase, as though the very ancientness of their use was embedded in the earth, these bolt holes and hiding places, cutways for rabbits munching grass in the late afternoon sun and the foxes that hunt them. There is a sense of peace here, a haven from the suburbia around. Like Netley's abbey, the site's past protects it from encroaching subtopia; and like the abbey, its new identity still deceives. Few of its users know it, but parts of this parkland on which they walk their dogs are still under military control, still subject to military regulations drawn up in the Second World War.

The two hundred acres which for a century were 'out of bounds' may have been opened to the public – like some Communist state whose barbed wire had suddenly been pulled down – but there remains something shadowy about the blind red-brick back of the officers' quarters rising against the dark green of the pines; or the low metal five-bar gates painted in military black and white stripes; or the railway lines discernible in the gravel and turf, their resolute metal iron smooth from the carriage wheels which carried their mortal load, resonant with the history at Europe's heart, a darkness which reverberated even in this corner of England. Yet the hospital's demolition also heralded the end of an era in which the authority of the institution and the state went unquestioned. Perhaps its absence is also a symbol of a greater freedom, a greater hope.

At four on a weekday afternoon, the factory siren sounds, as it did when I was a boy, and the workers cycle home through the park, along a lane where the inmates of D Block were once sent on their Sunday route march. A miniature steam train chugs through the old railway embankment, and the gravel paths resound to the crunch of baby buggies rather than spinal carriages and wheelchairs. Caravans and camper vans occupy the fields where the hutted hospital stood. In its third century of existence, a place built for regeneration is devoted to recreation; to kite-flying and football, jet-skis and yacht clubs.

Yet there are physical reminders of what was here. The grandeur of the officers' mess, with its twin campanile, survived bids from the local television station and a proposal to turn them into sheltered housing for the elderly, but succumbed to the inevitable expensive apartments with sea views. Stripped of the vines which once covered its stucco, presumably the damp which endangered the health of Dr Moorehead and spawned fungus on his wallpaper has been cured. The observatory that stood in front of the building, where amateur astronomers could watch Orion progress across successive winter skies, has vanished, but the YMCA hut, built in 1940 and furnished in a hundred different woods from around the world – an arboreal version of the hospital's Victorian museum – now houses the park offices, a café and a hall hired out for wedding receptions. The rows of red-brick bungalows built in the 1870s as married quarters now house policemen and women, while down the overgrown path of Gas House Lane lie the remnants of the hospital incinerator and laundry, its tall chimney now levelled. The electricity generator has been turned into a day nursery, and the sentry boxes have disappeared from the entrance gates, but at low tide you can still see the rotting stumps of the 300 foot jetty constructed in 1855 to bring Queen Victoria ashore.

What happened to all those people, the disappeared of Netley, scattered in its diaspora? I imagine them all walking across the empty green fields in their uniforms and blue pyjamas and open-backed gowns and cross-emblazoned aprons like a Stanley Spencer resurrection, returning to a place which no longer exists. Or like the soldier reported missing at the Battle of Loos in 1915 only to turn up twenty years later as a white-haired vagrant, having been discharged with a head wound from a German prisoner of war camp in 1921 and sent to 'a mental hospital at Southampton' from which he wandered England, 'a man without a name, or memory'.

Netley's scattered survivors return to the site to retrieve their memories: the local man who remembers an idyllic stay here in the Forties, treated for a chest complaint; the American nurse who had fun as a teenager there during the war. Standing in its non-existent shadow on a sunny summer's afternoon, an elderly gentleman asked where the hospital was; he had been stationed there during the war. 'It was a lovely place', he said; he could not believe it had gone. It is almost unbelievable that the hospital should no longer exist – as unbelievable that it ever did. Like Zallinger's mural, with its colossal dinosaurs walking the earth, the absence of the building's own hugeness, its own myth, makes its disappearance all the more improbable. Like the dinosaurs, its size was the source of its demise; like the Empire it served, the hospital was torn apart by history itself.

And by some bizarre freak of circumstance or plot, its history has vanished. There are practically no official documents to record what went on in the building. No surgical reports, no doctors' notes, no inventories or timetables, no pathological specimens stored away in jars, no publications to document the triumphs and tragedies of its medical care. Nothing beyond a handful of papers which survived, entirely by chance, and the photographs and postcards which provide missing pieces of an incomplete jigsaw, pictures without words. The silence of the archives resonates over the years. It determines the power of the hospital's memory, the reason for its place in my imagination. It is as if the vastness of the undertaking itself is matched by an equally vast vacuum which no amount of old photographs can fill.

Empty since 1958, since England's colonies began their final disintegration, the hospital, like the Empire, had never been operative in my lifetime. Perhaps that, and the fact that I have no distinct memory of the building, makes it all the more powerful, and my version of its history more obsessive: as if its history was actively being rerun ahead of me, the hospital itself leading me on. It suddenly becomes clear that my attempt to rebuild the hospital is an attempt to reclaim my own past; perhaps even to reinvent it. Netley's ruins are still witness to the reveries of Thomas Gray, to a teenage Noël Coward entertaining the troops, and to Stephen Tennant, flying south for the winter as I pass along corridors I never walked.

In 1998 a reunion was held on the centenary of the presentation of the Victoria Cross to Private Vickery and Piper Findlater. Royalty seldom came to Netley now; instead, the veteran members of the RAMC were greeted by a message from The Queen Mother read by the Lord Lieutenant of the county at a service in the Royal Chapel. Outside various marquees housed displays – 'Subject to Operational Commitments' – by the Army

Medical Services ('Ward Scene'), the Royal Navy/Fleet Air Arm ('Aeromedical Evacuation in Bosnia'), and the US Air Force ('Display by Flying Ambulance Surgical Trauma Team'). For one brief day, the military had returned to reclaim Netley from the mountain bikers and dog-walkers.

In one tent, a bright-eyed black woman from Washington serving with the US Medical Corps was showing visitors a photograph album assembled by a nurse who'd served there during the Second World War. Alongside tourist-like snaps of the New Forest and a bombed Southampton, there were pictures of the woman and her friends larking about in the grounds fifty years previously, when the Americans had last come to Netley. It was odd to see the hospital from across the Atlantic – it suddenly seemed both glamorous and dark, rather like the woman showing me the photographs, her uniform that much more tailored than her modern British counterparts: the young boys sweltering in their ill-fitting caps wishing they were kicking a ball about in the park; the young girls prim in their flat shoes, daydreaming of discos and platform shoes. The day's proceedings ended with the Last Post and a proud march past of a handful of veterans in the unnaturally hot spring sunshine, then everyone went on their way. In the final years of the twentieth century, as what Netley was and what it meant slipped out of mind and slowly away, there was nothing more to keep them here.

Out in the open, down by the sea, the park returned to the normality of the sunlit afternoon, overlooked only by the chapel tower like a gnomon on a giant sundial, casting its shadow, silently marking time. Inside the building a new hospital museum has been created out of the sacred space. Wall displays tell its history in blown-up photographs; old glass cases contain medals and uniforms; and showroom dummies in hospital undress stand in stiffly for the congregation that once sang hymns from their pews, overhung by regimental standards. One figure lies wounded on a wheeled stretcher, overlooked by a mimetic Queen Victoria with pity in her plastic eyes.

349

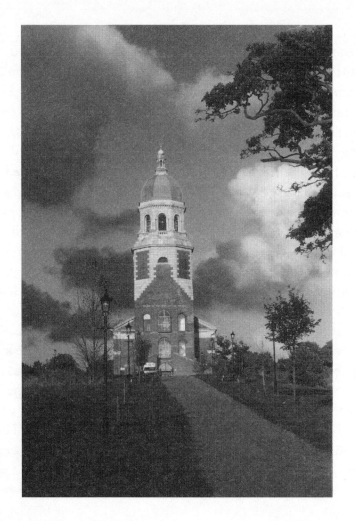

Some older men and women stand reading the captions, some remembering. But most young visitors don't linger long here. The place still has the hushed air of a church when the sun is shining outside, and perhaps they find it uncomfortable, all that history of illness and war, the cabinets with their medical instruments and khaki bandages, the spooky mannequins; the lady on the desk speaks of footsteps in the empty building. Instead they climb the iron stairway to the chapel's belfry, past arches once connected to quarter-mile long corridors but which now end in nothingness, a clean break with the past, as if to wipe away all that pain.

At the top of the building, emerging breathless from the gloom into the light, they are rewarded with a panoramic view of the waterside scene, arranged under the dome like a camera obscura. Southampton Water shimmers in the sun as passenger ferries and container ships drift into view; a flock of geese race the airliners high over the New Forest's purple-grey horizon. Further down the water, beyond Fawley's metal spires, yachts with bright-coloured sails flutter round the Isle of Wight, a promise of freedom and leisure.

From their eyrie the visitors survey this placid tableau, watching the children run about below. For them history is the stuff of the dark wooden cabinets and old postcards; but for me it is the memory of a military hospital and the shadow of its foundations in the turf.

Epilogue

. . . So, while the light fails
On a winter's afternoon, in a secluded chapel
History is now and England

T. S. ELIOT, *Four Quartets*

———

The succession of suburban stations passed by the grimy train window, white witnesses to my exile. I was just seventy miles from home, but I felt as abandoned as I had when I'd first gone to school back in Southampton. Now that seemed impossibly homely and far away compared to this benighted place.

The damp of autumn pervaded the air as though tainted by the dark-flowing river at the end of the road, its willows trailing their branches like girls' hands from a punt – a mock Oxbridge idyll in this suburban hell. In the lost world of 1976, the tree-muffled streets of Teddington were England set in aspic; a pre-modern world of mock-Tudor and wrought iron. The wooden ticket office and the little row of shops by Strawberry Hill station – newsagent's, grocer's, off-licence – served a community of commuters glad to leave the 5.15 from Waterloo, to stroll home and shut the door on London.

An hour or so later, I'd make the journey in reverse, taking another train into the centre of the city at night. Richmond, Mortlake and Putney passed by, protected from metropolitan wickedness by prophylactic privet. As the train shunted towards town, the landscape changed and hardened. There were fewer trees and more buildings; not the semis of Twickenham or gentrified villas of Barnes, but higher, taller, dirtier buildings, soiled by the city and its dark past, the history ingrained in the stone and brick. By Battersea's high-rises one long brick wall had been covered in successive generations of graffiti, from *Led Zep* through *Skinz* to the magic four letters of rebellion, *Punk* – the same letters I carved into the wooden door frame of the railway compartment.

The train reached the heart of the capital, rejoining the river, now wide and black and anonymous after its own suburban journey. I walked over Waterloo Bridge, the sodium street lights skimming the sulky, mysterious water. In the early dark of late autumn, the Thames seemed both repellent and magnetic, its hypnotic waters eddying and swirling round the bridge's stanchions. I followed the morning route of Eliot's hurrying commuters now safely back home in Middlesex. Ahead, in Covent Garden's wasteland, the streets around the market were devoid of flowers and people, a dead space still in the process of colonisation. I moved on through narrower streets hemmed in by tall buildings, lifeless after hours; past empty offices and disused warehouses with rusty cranes and chains hanging above like instruments of torture. Merely being there after dark was a statement of decadence: no one in suburbia, and certainly not in Southampton, went out on a Monday night.

On Neal Street's shabby strand I joined a queue. In front of me stood girls in plastic macs and fishnet stockings; thin boys with bleached blond hair and biker jackets were talking in a drug-like drawl as though they were both speeded up and slowed down at the same time. It may have been a dirty backstreet in a forgotten part of London, but it was suddenly and impossibly glamorous, the sort of glamour I'd only ever imagined from the New York gossip columns of *Rock Scene*, as though its flashlit photos of David Johansen, Ava Cherry and David Bowie had been brought to life.

I felt the excitement rising like a drug within me; it was as though some connexion had been made. Downstairs in the sweaty basement, past Johnny Rotten standing stare-eyed and obstreperous across the narrow rat-run corridors, The Vibrators were performing in their platform boots and lurex trousers, trying to look like the New York Dolls. In the shadows at the back of the room others were waiting for their man. In the darkness of this scuffed-up, squatted cavern, anything was possible. There was no pit between stage and floor; like a medieval mystery play or a chivalric tournament, nothing stood between audience and participant. There was little to distinguish the one from the other: just a shower of spit and sweat and ear-crunching amphetamine noise. It was a place in which you could feel entirely at home yet at the same time threatened, and threatening.

By day I made another pilgrimage, this time to the far end of the King's Road where the smart shops petered out into council estates. The name seemed suitably apocalyptic: World's End, a hubristic gesture of contempt for the suburbia beyond. Gripping the cuffs of my Oxfam mohair jumper, I plucked up courage to enter the door on the kink in the road. The shop window was opaque and devoid of display, save for a single blue fluorescent strip and a steel plaque announcing 'Seditionaries: Clothes for Heroes'.

This was the blank generation's blank façade, the antithesis to Strawberry Hill's suburban shops. Inside the walls were covered in gigantic upside-down photographs of blitzed London, and from scaffolding poles hung tribal uniforms of expensive tartan straps, chrome D rings and screenprinted muslin. Two or three girls lounged round the till, chewing gum, but, unlike the snotty assistants nearer Sloane Square, their indifference seemed disposed to accept me as a member. Other customers might have been shoving the merchandise up their jumpers for all they cared, as they chatted over the counter and drawled into the phone like Warhol superstars. I made friends with Tracy and Debbie, and syphoned my grant to finance a shirt emblazoned with an inverted crucifix and the word *Destroy*; a punk equivalent of

354

St Veronica's cloth or the Turin Shroud, its overlong sleeves fastened with hooks and rings like a straitjacket from D Block.

Thus armoured, back at college I ran the gauntlet of the bar with its beer-swilling, trouser-dropping rugby players and their choruses of 'Sweet Chariot'. I knew they were condemned to middle-age and mortgages, while my future dream lay in some fantastic cellar beneath the streets of Piccadilly where David Bowie, Lee Miller and Oscar Wilde would be lounging at the tables with telephones, Gîtanes and glasses of absinthe to hand, while Nöel Coward, Siouxsie Sioux and Bryan Ferry took turns to perform the cabaret.

Leaving home had been as inevitable as London was my destination. My birthplace offered provinciality, Little Chef meals and couples in parked cars turned unalterably towards the view as they sipped tea from vacuum flask tops. London promised glamour and escape. But now I was escaping it in turn. Netley's gothic imagining – from the fantasy of its abbey to the reality of its hospital – seemed to embody my past, my own search for identity. It had become a place of solace – but also a place in which to exorcise that past.

The last winter of the century seemed washed out with wind and rain. The weather had conspired to cover the phenomena of a millennial year obscuring eclipses, shooting stars and unusually bright moons in thick grey cloud which sent yet more rain, falling in sheets straight from the sky to the ground, as if the sky itself were falling down, as if Ruskin's premonitions of storm-clouds and plague-winds had come to pass. Under Waterloo's station canopy grey light fell on underground entrances swallowing the new commuters arriving from Esher and Europe. Slowly, our train pulled in the opposite direction out into the daylight and past collapsing buildings, 1970s tenements new-built when I passed as a punk, now being torn down barely two decades after their hard-shouldered construction.

History had stopped, to be reset with the station clock, like the Revolutionary calendar, back to year zero. The past was behind us and the centuries stood back to back; a tangible sense of inevitability as the fireworks exploded and showered the night air with descending embers, the scent of gunpowder drifting in the aftermath. There was no going back now: the past was being rewritten by the future, its immense yawning emptiness filled by slowly falling stars.

The unreal city slipped past the window, tugging at the landmarks of memory: the dome of the Imperial War Museum, a verdigris echo of Netley's chapel and once the home of Bedlam; in his house nearby Blake saw a vision of an angel 'stand in the sun and move the universe'; the central platform of Clapham Junction on which Wilde was kept one rainy afternoon, reviled and spat at by his fellow passengers on his way to Reading Gaol; and that same graffitied wall in Battersea, now almost obliterated by tags just as suburban train windows have been updated with more scrawl, cut into the glass like the asylum's etched windows.

Imperceptibly the inner city cedes to Metroland and New Malden, where I had once stood waiting for the train to London, hair sprayed gold and slicked back in imitation of the idol I was at last to see. For his 1976 *Station to Station* tour, David Bowie had arrived at Victoria, refusing to travel by plane, driven through the concourse in an open-top car like the head of a decadent state come to seize power, his coke-thin frame greeting admirers (mysteriously conjured up and assembled behind crash barriers) with an open-palm wave construed by the press as a fascist salute. The androgyne's return was as stage-managed as the rest of his alien existence. A day or so later, in a cavernous Wembley Empire Pool hall more fitted to hockey matches, the audience were shown the surreal hallucination of Buñuel's *Un Chien Andalou*, collectively shivering on cue when a pig's eye was slit open with a razor. Moments later the screen rose and the relentless, exciting engine of the title track began, the Thin White Duke throwing darts in lovers' eyes, and another railway journey from suburban Kent via Siberia and Berlin to the industrial grey of the TransEurope Express for Ralf and Florian to meet David and Iggy.

The train moves on through comforting rows of white villas backed up to entangled embankments over which bags of petrified cement are tipped into a nomansland of ghostly silver birches. The accretion of outhouses and conservatories crawl past, an endless corridor of suburban acres, suddenly broken by the sun's rays through grey-lowering clouds. For an instant God's brief benediction shines as though from a medieval illumination, and in an act of transformation only England can accomplish, the train crosses the county border into Hampshire, and home.

Under the subdued English sky the fields fall away to the gentle valley where Alix and I once looked out to see cows and ponies grazing obediently like toys. 'I'm looking at the little one sitting by the fence', she said, with a four-year-old's acuity as the stilled idyll – gabled farm cottages, blue-smoking chimneys, a manor house at the end of a tree-lined drive – was suddenly transcended by a leaping, magical hare, a witch's familiar to conjure it all away. 'And this green pastorale landscape, were to me/ More dear, both for themselves and for thy sake!'

At Winchester station, the train stops to draw breath; people wave friends and family goodbye, unabashed by the public exposure of their love. The station lies low in its wooded ravine, serving a country town and a now expanded commuterdom. Once my journey back to London was arrested down the line; there'd been a 'fatality' at Winchester. It was mid-morning, the sun was shining, the businessmen were in their suits. Our lives had been interrupted by someone else's despair. Grumbling, we boarded a bus outside Eastleigh station, which would take us to Basingstoke to enable us to continue our journey there.

But rather than driving up the bland canyon of the motorway, we took another route, as if the bus driver were reluctant to subject his human load to the horrors of the arterial autobahn. Instead we drove through narrow lanes and villages with woody, watery sounding names, through those places I'd never see, 'each glimpse and gone for ever'. Slowly the chatter of the businessmen and their phones fell silent, cowed by the beauty of the country-side through which we were passing. Every day this land unfurled by their window; it was as if only now, taken out of their routine, they actually noticed it.

From the top deck I saw the B roads of my youth swing beneath us, the old routes of family holidays: a dense wood underlain by an even denser carpet of bluebells; driveways and farm tracks, the scent of may and silage wafting in through the bus windows, which were occasionally brushed by the upper branches and leaves of trees, caressing us as we passed. It was as though the entire detour was an atonement for that anony-mous death in Winchester's station gully; an hour out of time and into another green world.

Finally the bus arrived among the ziggurats of Basingstoke, an outpost of Silicon Valley set above the trees like a *Star Wars* city, its high buildings breaking the skyline and surrounded by scrubby fields. As we waited for the train to take us into London, I looked across to the facing platform, where I had stood the night before my father died.

That day I'd been to a grand wedding in the grounds of a moated Jacobean manor. It was high summer, bakingly hot; there'd been jousting in the fields, and a dark-haired knight had won. In the early evening I left the party and its guests and flowers under the filtered light of the marquee on the lawn, to return to Southampton, and stood beneath an illuminated poster hoarding: it was advertising a football magazine, and Robert Lee of Newcastle United knelt on the turf, legs apart, arms outstretched, as if in an ecstatic saintly communion. The accumu-lated heat of the day was seeping up from the tarmac and in from the countryside beyond the station's wrought iron gates.

That night, back at home, the bedroom lamp casting a yellow-orange glow as though the sun were setting inside our house, I watched as the nurse put my father to bed. His body, so like mine, now resembled an Egon Schiele drawing; a *memento mori*, just as I walk like him, drink my tea and eat my cake like him, my sister says. The following evening, as he lay calm and unmoving in bed, I left him for the last time. On the way to the bus stop, at the bottom of our road where I had once turned to see lightning strike, a car slowed and pulled up behind me. There were four lads inside. One in the back wound down his window and called, ''Ere mate.' As I turned, expecting to give directions, he said, 'Fuck off!', and they drove off, laughing.

That summer night the train back to London pulled through another sunset, the burning sky on one side of the tracks, the lush green of the watermeadows dark on the other. Back in my flat, the red light was flashing on the answerphone. I rang my brother back at home. Dad had died an hour or so after I'd left. And as I'd left, kissing him for the first time in thirty years, I thought I heard him call out my name – although he had been comatose for days – the single syllable drifting down the stairs, the stairs down which I had tumbled on the first day I came to that house.

As the delayed train for London pulled into Basingstoke, the spell of our country detour seemed broken at last. I remembered again the evening I'd left my father, the train back to London. It seemed now, and for ever after, I would be completing that journey.

As we drew nearer the capital, I could feel its oppression descend on me, the polluted air which gave me a twenty-four-hour headache everytime I returned to the city. Next to me an elderly man with a Brummie accent was regaling an overtanned youngish man with his account of the Winchester 'jumper'. He speculated on the victim's sex; on the way the train had picked up speed as it left the platform; how the driver had been taken away 'shell-shocked' for 'counselling'; naming what had been unnameable, providing details I didn't want to know.

I tried to blot out his voice, but he carried on. As we approached Clapham, he pointed out a building. 'You've heard of Bedlam? That's it. That's where the Queen Mother's sisters were kept. She never knew until one of them died.' From his coat pocket he pulled a rolled-up cap, unfurled it and put it on, tugging it precisely into place over his silver hair. 'I put this on when I go into London', he said, 'because of all the grit in the air from the air conditioning.'

He went on to describe his new shower, the platform on to which we were drawing, the red lights that were showing; it all came pouring out, indiscriminately, leaping from subject to subject until I began to think he might be an inmate from Bedlam himself.

Beyond Winchester's downs, in whose folds Owen saw his fallen comrades, we move through a languid landscape overcast by the long shadows of the year's beginning. Cars funnel southwards through a chalk gash cut into the hill, while the train races a river that brims as though someone had left the tap on. Drawn into the city, past yellow lights of other lives glimpsed through suburban windows, past sewage works and petrol stations and Osborne Road, my birthplace razed for another bypass but still overseen by its monkey puzzle trees. The buildings halt long enough to allow a wide-angled view of the river, curling sluggishly past a pair of gothic cormorants that balance on either end of a floating plank. Then, in a last transformation, the train plunges into a tunnel cut under the city and emerges out the other side, on to the platform of Southampton Central.

The tannoy announces 'Sholing' and 'Netley' and I board the local train, dawdling round the river bend, past the boatyard where in the years before the First World War Noel Pemberton Billing built 'boats that fly rather than aeroplanes that float', and called his company 'Supermarine' to sound modern, exciting and new. Billing's future vision saw a sky full of his inventions, but there's little left to show for his efforts now, only the rusting hulk of a boat which looks as though it might have carried Fitzcarraldo up the Amazon or Conrad up the Congo, and soon the sea will swallow this shore and the rest of Hampshire in turn, leaving only its hills standing above an English Atlantis as the water washes over cathedrals and car-parks 'all gone under the sea'.

Southern England will sink as if overburdened by its population, Nature's revenge on Man's hubris for daring to steal its acres from the sea. The drained land on Western Esplanade, now the home of hotels and giant shopping malls, will be reclaimed again; coral will grow on the decaying remains of Toy 'Я' Us, and tresses of giant kelp will sway over the Novotel's concrete stumps. Sandbags on suburban garden walls will attempt to keep the sea at bay just as Canute once tried to turn the tide at Southampton's shore, and Spike Island will be an island once more.

Leaving the sea behind, the train climbs the hill inland, along a track built to serve Netley's hospital, and in a last effort, pulls into Sholing station.

To the monks of Netley Abbey, time was contemporaneous, fluid, cyclical. For them, as for St Augustine, memory was 'the present of things past'. Things happened forever in years varied only by seasons which could mean plenty or hardship; harvest and spring, summer and fallow following each other into infinity. The world was ordered by religion, and they looked back and to the side, rather than ahead; time belonged to God, not Man. Rulers and plagues, famines and wars came and went, but for them the notion of the past, present and future was expressed in typology, in which the events of the Old Testament symbolically foreshadowed those of the New. Time itself was a gothic image.

The age of the machine would bring the regulated measure of clocks and watches rather than sundials on church towers, and a sense of progress towards 'glorious goals'; a sense of time which the Romantics would subvert, seeking to turn it around by force of imagining alone. For them, Netley's gothic ruins stood as a kind of time machine, travelling back to the mystical stasis of the medieval age. In my imagination I too sought to turn the past around: the present was preordained; the future was another matter.

Back in my suburban bedroom on a tinny tape recorder, David Bowie sang about the five years stuck on our eyes, and at the Classic cinema in Southampton's High Street, *2001* promised a cybernetic dictatorship. As I lay in my narrow bed by the window, while Bowie drifted in white space, a sci-fi Dietrich in powder-blue suit and make-up singing 'Life on Mars', I dreamed of UFOs landing in our back garden, scanning the dark skies in my head for phosphorescent craft about to conquer the world. But the future did not descend from outer space. It arrived as if by train, materialising in out-of-town stores and transported down suburban telephone lines, to be retailed as adjuncts to genetically reinvented identities of the future, colour-coded like the spines of my *Junior World* encyclopaedias and their pictures of shiny plastic atomic models, images of the past and future collected in the century's attic. And in a Somerset field, Mark and I watch an ageing Thin White Duke ripple his fingers for the mice in their million hordes as the fires burn in front of him and the stars shine behind until they all go out.

The trees have grown tall around the house now, masking it from the road, filtering out the modern world and the distant murmur of traffic on a weekday morning. But the fog horns still sound from Southampton Water, where the sea mist is dense, muffling all noise and slowing the progress of its shipping. Low echoes drift in from the far shore; a sudden wash breaks on the beach. Invisible in the mist, anything could be passing by: a container ship of the Grimaldi line, heirs of the 1338 raid, or the ghost of a White Star liner; a barge dredging gravel, or a troopship bound for the Western Front; a submarine or a sea monster, swimming sinuously out to the ocean beyond.

Southern England suffered badly in the great storms of the century's end. Secondhand winds from Jamaica and yet more lustrous tropical islands swept up the Solent, whirling trees about like chaff, creating vast crop circles. Down at Netley, the new country park was devastated, losing a quarter of its trees; the gracious elms of the main avenue had already been destroyed by Dutch elm disease in the early 1970s. The view from Nurse Luker's window would be very different now.

But just as the hospital's demolition had liberated this space, so the falling of its trees let in new light, and regeneration began again. The bluebells in D Block's woods spread their colony and the natural world reasserted itself, healing its own scars, closing over old wounds. Now the parkland is quiet and placid, open to the sun, warming the skin. Time is still suspended here, but it is now free; like the lull between leaving school and leaving home: a long hot summer, caught between adolescence and adulthood, between freedom and duty, a heightened sense of what was and what could be. And as the tide drifts in and out, so does your past and future, ebbing and flowing with your dreams, looking across the still water to the light as the sun sets, always ahead on some future journey.

Here, where the blunt stone stump of the hospital's pier falls abruptly away, my journey ends. I realise there's nothing there, nothing beyond its sawn-off end. No Roman barges, no plague ships, no stately ocean liners and no sea serpents; only old car tyres standing upright in the mud, and the ghost of myself. And endless sea, grey-green glittering sea the same the world over, the same water lapping the same shores, watched by the same people. It is only our dreams that are different.

The tide is high; the water buoys me up in its swell. And as I swim out to sea, Netley recedes behind me, floating away like an island.

It's a beautiful place; nothing ever happened here.

Acknowledgements

Mark Ashurst and Michael Bracewell are between them the spiritual and intellectual godfathers of *Spike Island*; their support and good counsel has been immaculate and unfailing. I have also relied on Neil Tennant for his insight and Linder Sterling for her inspiration, while a summer filming with Adam Low focused many ideas for me. Hugo Vickers, as ever, provided sound advice. But perhaps most importantly, I have drawn on (perhaps raided is a more accurate word) the collective memories of my brothers and sisters – Lawrence and Stephen, Christina and Katherine – and, above all, the recollections and experiences of my mother, Theresa. Without her love, patience, practicality – and cups of tea – this book could never have been written.

My agent, Gillon Aitken, and Lesley Shaw and Emma Parry at Aitken Associates were indefatigable on my behalf. But the end product of *Spike Island* ultimately owes itself to the faith and trust of Christopher Potter and Andy Miller's sympathetic and intuitive editing. I am also grateful for Rachel Connolly's copy editing, Carol Anderson's proof reading, Chris Shamwana's design work and Ed Miles's photography. Thanks, too, are due to Sarah White and Kate Balmforth for efficiently escorting the book to publication.

The tantalising nature of Netley's hospital and its paucity of records meant that my attempt to reconstruct it relied on sometimes slender leads. Patrick Kirkby, the assiduous historian at the Royal Victoria Country Park, put me in touch with Lin Dowdell and Nigel Wood, whose extensive collection of Netley ephemera has helped to illustrate the book. I also have Patrick to thank for other illustrations in the book and, together with David Rymill at the Hampshire Record Office, for the plans that embellish the endpapers. On my daily pilgrimages to the hospital site, Peter Leslie at the Royal Victoria Country Park, and Yvette Scorey at the Royal Chapel Heritage Centre, were always enthusiastic and helpful, and together with the rest of the staff at the RVCP, are stalwart custodians of the hospital's memory and the flourishing open spaces that have taken its place.

I must also thank Will Eaves at the *Times Literary Supplement* for publishing my first attempt to write about Netley – an article which was in effect the genesis of this book; Jennie Gray of the Gothic Society for indulging me in another essay in *Udolpho*; and Fiachra Gibbons for commissioning a third piece on the hospital which appeared in *The Printer's Devil*.

Back in London, Helen Wakley at the Wellcome Institute produced box after box of fascinating material and answered my endless e-mails. In Glasgow, David Weston and Jack Baldwin guided me to the Laing papers at the Glasgow University Library; the staff of the Public Record Office at Kew and the Hampshire Record Office in Winchester were exceptionally helpful in producing arcane documents. Elaine Fisher at the British Red Cross showed me more material from their archives – including my grandmother's First World War VAD record. Lt-Colonel John Darroch and Sheila Orchard at the Royal Hampshire Regiment also helped with information and photographs of my grandfather's war service. Robert Longmore wrote to me of his own grandfather, and allowed me to quote from Sir Thomas's papers; Judith Perkins wrote of her aunt, Esther Helen Audrey Luker, and allowed me to quote from her diaries. Captain Peter Starling, curator of the Army Medical Services Museum, Aldershot, granted me permission to quote from the RAMC Muniment Collection. Jon Wynne-Tyson allowed me to quote from the estate of Esme Wynne-Tyson, his mother. Brenda Phillips passed an expert eye over the chapters dealing with the early years of the hospital. And I am particularly grateful to Allison Derrett, Assistant Registrar at the Royal Archives, Windsor;

quotations from Queen Victoria's Journal are used by the permission of Her Majesty Queen Elizabeth II.

I am indebted to many other persons, institutions and organisations. In Southampton: the staff of the local studies collection at Southampton Central Library; Woolston Library, Bitterne Local History Society, St Mary's College, the *Southern Daily Echo* archive and Sholing Cycle Centre. In London: the Contemporary Medical Archives Centre at the Wellcome Institute; Anthony Richards, Archivist, and the staff of the Imperial War Museum; Terence Pepper, curator of photographs at the National Portrait Gallery; the Guildhall Library; the Barbican Library; The Lindley Library, RHS; The British Architectural Library, RIBA. Elsewhere: Bob Cox and the Hampshire Constabulary Training and Support Headquarters, Netley; Susan Evans and the National Monuments Record, Swindon; Cork City Museum; and the Medway archives, Rochester.

I would also like to thank James Jameson and the Netley Historical Society; Peter Owen, Helen McPhail and Philip Guest of the Wilfred Owen Association; Keith Alexander and Jane Mayes at the BBC; Sean Mackenzie, Luke Cardiff, Godfrey Kirby and Louis Caulfield on the Pevsner shoot; Jon Savage; Janet Street-Porter; James Chatfield-Moore; Sam Goonetillake; Florence Goonetillake; Nigel Larcombe-Williams; Mike Jay; Professor Jon Stallworthy; Hui-Yong Yu; Dr Pamela Ashurst and Ron Ashurst; Rob Holden and Claire Eastman; Andrew Eastman; Jane Preston; Michael Holden; Madeleine Groves; Sheila, Terry and Clare Goddard; and my young friends Alix, Oliver, Harriet, Jed, Jacob, Lydia, Poppy, Cyrus and Max.

Philip Hoare, Southampton, January 2001

Illustration Credits

Notes

Bibliographic note: all texts used are cited in the source notes.

Abbreviations used:

BL: British Library, London
BRC: British Red Cross archives, London
CMAC: Contemporary Medical Archive Centre, Wellcome Institute, London
HRO: Hampshire Record Office, Winchester
IWM: Imperial War Museum archives, London
PRO: Public Record Office, Kew
RA: Royal Archives, Windsor
RAMC: Royal Army Medical Corps Muniment Collection at the Wellcome Institute, London
RCHME: Royal Commission on the Historical Monuments of England, Swindon
RVCP: Royal Victoria Country Park archives, Netley

Prologue

1 'each would make . . .' Nikolaus Pevsner and David Lloyd, *The Buildings of England: Hampshire and the Isle of Wight*, Penguin, 1967, p. 350
2 'the best hard . . .' Major General A. MacLennan, OBE (Retd), *History of Netley*, unpublished manuscript and related papers, RAMC
2 'blue pointing mortar . . .' *Terms of Contract and Specification for the Erection of the Royal Victoria Hospital at Netley*, Eyre & Spottiswode, 1856, RAMC, CMAC
3 'Passengers by Cape . . .' *Daily Telegraph*, 12 February 1898

5 'a museum of appliances...' Colonel Kenneth MacLeod, 'Netley', *Caledonian Medical Journal*, RAMC 485, CMAC, p. 379

5 'the implements by which...' *Paul Brothers' Guide to Southampton*, 1900, SCL

6 'the bodies of foetuses...' Sir William Aitken, *Descriptive Catalogue of the Pathological Specimens contained in the Museum of the Army Medical Department, Netley*, Vol. I Harrisons & Sons, 1892

6 'distinguished surgeons...' Joan Howard, *Fort Pitt*, Medway Archives, Rochester, p. 5

'rather a gruesome sight...' *Navy & Army Illustrated*, 19 March 1897, Vol. III, No. 33, p. 216

6 'for those not accustomed...' *Paul Brothers'*

8 'imps of darkness...' Steve Connor, *Independent*, 24 August 1999

Spike Island

15 'What greatness had not...' Joseph Conrad, *Heart of Darkness*, Penguin, 1982, p. 7

15 'the hill...' William Whitlock, Introduction, John Paynter, *Memories of Old Sholing*, Sholing Press, Southampton, 1991, p. 20

16 'one of the great signature...' Richard Mabey, *Flora Britannica*, Sinclair-Stevenson, 1997, p. 230

17 'all chained...' Margaret Spence, *Hampshire and Australia, 1783–1791, Crime and Transportation*, Hampshire Papers Issue No. 2, Hampshire County Council, December 1992, p. 10. For remarks on the derivations of Spike Island, I'm indebted to John Holt's essay, 'Spike Island' (Paynter, p. 137); and to my former history master, James Jameson.

17 'official Siberia...' Robert Hughes, *The Fatal Shore*, Harvill Press, 1986, p. 162

18 'From th' emerald...' Niall Bruncardi, *Haulbowline, Spike and Rocky Islands*, Éigse Books, Fermoy, Co. Cork, Ireland, 1982, p. 43. Bruncardi records two remarkable inhabitants of Spike Island: the explorer Colonel P. H. Fawcett who was stationed there before the First World War and who would vanish without trace on his 1925 expedition into the Brazilian jungle in search of a fabulous lost city

(thus inspiring Evelyn Waugh's *Handful of Dust*); and Ellen Organ, an artillery man's daughter who in 1908 acquired a religious following as 'Little Nellie of Holy God'. In her 'brief stay on earth', Nellie's 'perception of and love for the Real presence induced the Church authority to allow her to receive the Eucharist at the age of four and a half years'. (Bruncardi, p. 49)

20 'prettily set in a pine . . .' Pevsner, p. 593
23 'He ran round . . .' John Paynter, *Bygone Days of Sholing*, Sholing Press, Southampton, 1984, p. 25

In a Lonely Place

34 '. . . The shores fringed . . .' *Visitors' Descriptions: Southampton 1540–1956*, Southampton Corporation/Camelot Press, 1961, p. 24, quoting A. G. L'Estrange, ed., *The Life of Mary Russell Mitford*, Bentley, 1870, Vol. I, pp. 207–8
35 'Atlantic Pulse' *Tide Tables 2000*, Associated British Ports, Southampton
35 'A seaport . . .' Alfred Temple Patterson, *Southampton: A Biography*, Macmillan, 1970, p. 2
35 'the sea-reach . . .' Conrad, p. 5
37 'and his equally benevolent . . .' William Cobbett, *Rural Rides*, Dent, 1967, Vol. II, p. 478
38 'To those who like . . .' *ibid.*, p. 470
39 'Netley Abbey ought . . .' *ibid.*, p. 473
39 'Natan-leaga . . .' William Howitt, *Ruined Abbeys and Castles of Great Britain and Ireland*, Alfred Bennett, 1864, pp. 93–4
40 'to satisfy . . .' Gill Holloway, 'Roots of Woolston', *Woolston and Sholing: A Series of Extracts, Notes and Personal Reminiscences, with an Historical Introduction*, Local Studies Group, Southampton, 1984, p. 8
40 'crowded with Normans . . .' *The Southampton Annual*, 1900, SCL
40 'to be of considerable . . .' *The Victoria History of the County of Hampshire* (1903), University of London, 1973, Vol. III, p. 297
42 'of horror . . .' David Robinson, ed., *The Cistercian Abbeys of Britain: Far from the Concourse of Men*, Batsford, 1998, p. 25
42 'lonely, wooded . . .' *ibid.*, p. 25

42 'they make a solitude . . .' *ibid.*, p. 26

42 'What are these fantastic monsters . . .' William Anderson, *The Rise of the Gothic*, Hutchinson, 1985, p. 87

43 'crypto-pagan . . .' *ibid.*, p. 87

43 'new light' Michael Camille, *Gothic Art*, Weidenfeld & Nicolson, 1996, p. 28

43 'the strange blue . . .' Anderson, p. 30

43 'window of Heaven', Camille, p. 54

43 'free warren . . .' MacLennan

44 '8s of their usual . . .' *Victoria History*, Vol. II, p. 148

45 'the town suffered . . .' *John Bullar, Historical Particulars Relating to Southampton*, T. Baker, 1820, p. 23

46 'forasmuch as manifest sin . . .' John Hare, *The Dissolution of the Monasteries in Hampshire*, Hampshire Papers No. 16, Hampshire County Council, September 1999, p. 3

47 'a man the most famous . . .' Cobbett, Vol. II, p. 190

48 'The Queenes Maiestees . . .' Bullar's 1818 *Guide to Southampton*, p. 26, 'by an entry in the register of St Michael's parish, Southampton', HRO. Tradition held that monarchs returning from France would stay overnight at Netley, before moving on to Winchester.

48 'other offices' *Victoria History*, Vol. III, p. 476

49 'sold the whole . . .' Broome Willis, *ibid.*

49 'for the purchase . . .' K. A. Ford, *Netley Abbey Village*, Kingfisher, Southampton, 1990, p. 7

49 'not to be instrumental . . .' Ford, *ibid.*

49 'somewhat Jesuitical . . .' Howitt, p. 95

49 'tore off . . .' *Victoria History*, Vol. III, p. 476

49 'in an exertion . . .' *Guide to Southampton*, 1796, HRO, pp. 95–6. The young son in Walpole's *The Castle of Otranto* is killed by a falling statue; a similar death from tumbling masonry features in Heine's gothic tale, *The Abbey in the Woods*.

50 'the accident had . . .' Howitt, p. 95

50 'ruins, ivy, owls . . .' A. J. Sambrook, 'Netley and Romanticism', *Netley Abbey*, Department of the Environment guide, 1976, p. 25

50 'Enclosure like a Buonaparte . . .' David Wright, ed., *The Penguin Book of English Romantic Verse*, 1976, p. xvi

52 'In fact they are...' W. S. Lewis, ed., *The Correspondence of Horace Walpole*, OUP/Yale, 1973, Vol. XXXV, pp. 249–51

52 'His taste...' Timothy Mowl, *Horace Walpole: The Great Outsider*, John Murray, 1996, p. 7

53 'apostrophised...' Hughes, p. 159

54 'With our own island...' Katherine Turner, ed., *Selected Poems of Thomas Gray, Charles Churchill and William Cowper*, Penguin, pp. xvi, 77

54 'all the beauties...' W. S. Lewis, ed., *The Correspondence of Horace Walpole*, OUP/Yale, 1948, Vol. XIV, p. 83

55 'I wished for you...' *ibid.*, p. 58

55 'On the arrival...' Lewis, ed., *The Correspondence of Horace Walpole*, Vol. XXXV, p. 249

56 'at Mr. Vining's...' Paget Toynbee and Leonard Whibley, eds., *The Correspondence of Thomas Gray*, OUP, 1935, Vol. II, p. 843

57 'pregnant with poetry...' Sambrook, p. 24

58 'providing its owner...' Robert Harbison, *Deliberate Regression*, André Deutsch, 1980, p. 66

58 'greatly improved...' Sambrook, p. 22

59 'an immense garden...' Richard Holmes, *Shelley: The Pursuit*, HarperCollins, 1994, p. 460

59 '*THE RUINS OF NETLEY ABBEY*...' Guide, 1765, HRO

60 'It is fortunate...' *Guide to Southampton*, 1796, HRO, pp. 94–5

60 '*Within the sheltered centre*...' William Sotheby, 'Ode, Netley Abbey; Midnight', pamphlet, HRO, p. 25

61 'Dear sir...' William Pearce, *Netley Abbey, an Operatic Farce*, W. Woodfall, 1794, HRO

63 'Should danger...' 'William Shield's operas', Guildhall Library

63 'sympathies with the...' Stanley Sadie, ed., *The New Grove Dictionary of Music and Musicians*, Macmillan, 1980, pp. 254–5

63 'a pretty successful...' National Portrait Gallery archives

64 'Composed...' 'Wm Shield's operas', Guildhall Library

64 'the most famous...' Sambrook, p. 26

64 'persecuted virtue' Rev Richard Warner, *Netley Abbey, A Gothic*

Story in Two Volumes, Southampton, Printed for the author by T. Skelton & Sold by G. Law, Ave Mary Lane, London 1795, BL, p. 190

65 'Few people . . .' *Guide to Southampton*, 1796, HRO, p. 91

65 'by being calm . . .' Isaiah Berlin, *The Roots of Romanticism*, Chatto & Windus, 1999, p. 6

66 'a large . . .' Holmes, p. 31

66 'ruinous and full of owls' Thomas Love Peacock, *Nightmare Abbey*, Penguin, 1969, p. 42

66 'mystery was his . . .' *ibid.*, p. 44

67 'Southampton is . . .' Daniel Defoe, *A Tour Through the Whole Island of Great Britain*, Penguin, 1986, p. 154

67 'Bathing has generally . . .' *Guide to Southampton*, 1796, HRO, p. 67

68 'interested spectators' Patterson, p. 41

68 'walked long by moonlight . . .' *Correspondence of Horace Walpole*, Vol. XXXDV, p. 249

68 'This place is still . . .' *Correspondence of Horace Walpole*, Vol. XIV, p. 58

68 'the rougher elements . . .' Patterson, pp. 52–4

69 '*Extract of a letter* . . .' *The Times*, 5 August 1786

70 'This place . . .' *ibid.*, 15 July 1788

70 'If Southampton has decreased . . .' *Guide to Southampton*, 1781, Guildhall Library

70 'and many gentlemen . . .' Patterson, p. 44

70 'dotty' 'This suggestion is offered for what it is worth to the editor of Murray's Dictionary, and all others interested in philology', John Lane, introduction, Count de Cartrie, *Memoirs of the Count de Cartrie*, John Lane/Bodley Head, 1906, p. xxv. Cartrie worked for Dott for a few months to pay off his debt before moving to Itchen, between Sholing and Woolston. The story – translated from Cartrie's memoirs discovered in a Torquay bookshop in 1904 – evaporates in 1800 when, having left Southampton, he takes passage for Hamburg and is left there, waiting for a passport.

Itchen was then the home of the 'wicked' Marquis of Lansdowne, who lived in a gothicised villa, Peartree House (later home of Henry Shrapnel, inventor of the explosive shell), and who in 1804 built a

Fonthill-inspired gothic castle in Southampton. Lansdowne would become landlord to the Austens. Itchen would also lay claim to two legendary youths: a teenaged Napoleon Bonaparte, said to have lodged there with the family of the captain on whose ship he was travelling; and Richard Parker, the sixteen-year-old cabin boy whose cannibalisation by his shipmates after the wreck of the *Mignonette* in 1884 created a sensation in late Victorian England. Parker's memorial still stands in the churchyard of the seventeenth-century Jesus Chapel – itself partly built using stone from Netley Abbey – on Peartree Green.

71 'We hear that...' Deirdre Le Faye, ed., *Jane Austen's Letters*, OUP, 1997, p. 123

71 'young women...' *ibid.*, p. 157

71 'As they drew near...' Jane Austen, *Northanger Abbey*, Minster Classics, 1968, p. 216

71 '.... Northanger turned up ...' *ibid.*, p. 188

72 'Never was there...' Deirdre Le Faye, Kent County Archives

73 'holy mother Guillotine' Cartrie, p. 238

73 'The *reading public*...' Peacock, p. 68

74 'Of all the ridiculous...' Cobbett, *Rural Rides*, Vol. I, p. 56

74 'national style' Megan Aldrich, *Gothic Revival*, Phaidon, 1994, p. 93

74 'On Mondays...' Sambrook, p. 26

75 'Wall'd up...' R. H. Barham, *The Ingoldsby Legends*, Frederick Warne, 1891, pp. 293–7

77 'retreat for retirement' Pevsner, p. 512

77 'slowly, but surely...' *Visitors' Descriptions*, *p. 29*, quoting 'Provincial Society, Southampton', *The Whitehall Review*, 9 March 1878

78 'an answer...' Camille, p. 9. Conversely, Jonathan Meades has declared that the Gothic Revival was principally a way of 'making the secular sacred' for an age of flux which sought to root itself by reference to a medieval past. (*Victoria Died In 1901 And Is Still Alive Today*, BBC 2, 7 January 2001). In the mid-nineteenth century 'Battle of Styles', gothic architecture was favoured by Conservative politicians, and Italianate by Liberals. The classical Italianate represented progressive rationality and reason; gothic, reactionary superstition and atavism. That the two co-existed is deeply symbolic of a schizophrenic epoch.

78 'The place has been . . .' *Punch*, 1861, quoted *Southampton Times*, 19 July 1862

78 'The visitors and tourists . . .' Howitt, p. 97

78 'Horace Walpole, in his days . . .' *ibid.*, p. 96

79 'obsession with black skies . . .' John Batchelor, *Ruskin*, Chatto & Windus, 2000, p. 289

80 'medieval court' Phoebe Stanton, *Pugin*, Thames & Hudson, 1971, p. 190

80 'A pale sky . . .' Rhonda K. Garelick, *Rising Star*, Princeton University Press, 1998, pp. 48–9

80 'People's sense of beauty . . .' Humphrey Jennings, *Pandæmonium: The Coming of the Machine as Seen by Contemporary Observers*, André Deutsch, 1985, p. 355

81 'In 1828 the ruins . . .' Pevsner, p. 348

81 'The visitor, seated . . .' Howitt, p. 91

82 *n* 'the whole yearly cost . . .' MacLennan, RAMC. Guillaume's book on Netley was published by Forbes & Webb in 1848.

Pray Stop All Work

89 'You might as well . . .' Lytton Strachey, *Eminent Victorians*, Chatto & Windus (1918), 1979, p. 146

89 'It will be . . .' *Hampshire Independent*, 24 May 1856

90 'to prevent . . .' J. R. Fairman, *Netley Hospital and its Railways*, Kingfisher, Southampton, 1984, p. 10

90 'light up . . .' MacLennan, RAMC

90 'Lord Winchester . . .' Queen Victoria, journal, 20 May 1856, RA

90 'A considerable . . .' *Hampshire Independent*, 24 May 1856

91 'We walked a short . . .' Queen Victoria, journal, 20 May 1856, RA

91 'tried the stone . . .' quoted *Illustrated London News*, 17 December 1966

92 'a gun exploding . . .' Queen Victoria, journal, 20 May, 1856, RA

92 '. . . After which . . .' *ibid.*

92 'one of the most imposing . . .' *Hampshire Independent*, 24 May 1856

93 'the soldiers at . . .' Queen Victoria, journal, 20 May 1856, RA

93 'Her Majesty . . .' *Hampshire Independent*, 24 May 1856

93 'returned at once . . .' quoted *Illustrated London News*, 17 December 1966

93 'nightingales sing charmingly in . . .' Queen Victoria, journal, 20 May 1856, RA

93 'malodorous sewers . . .' John Holder, *The Story of a Great Military Hospital & Royal Victoria Country Park*, Hampshire County Council, p. 4

94 'Are these really . . .' MacLeod, p. 379

94 'The Queen is very anxious . . .' MacLennan, RAMC

94 *n* 'a dreary piece . . .' *Illustrated London News*, 9 March 1861

95 'it would be . . .' Introduction, *REPORT ON THE SITE, Etc., of the ROYAL VICTORIA HOSPITAL, near Netley Abbey, Presented to the House of Commons by Command of Her Majesty*, Harrison & Sons, 1858

96 'numerous advantages . . .' *ibid.*, p. 40

96 'a pestiferous marsh . . .' *British Medical Journal*, 1857, quoted Sylvia Turtle, 1991, RVCP, p. 4

96 'Three miles above . . .' Fairman, p. 15

97 'entirely surrounded . . .' *REPORT*, 1858, p. 41

98 '109 acres . . .' *ibid.*

98 'very anxious' MacLennan, RAMC

98 *n* 'It possesses a bold façade . . .' *The Lancet*, 9 May 1868. Netley embodied the ongoing 'Battle of Styles' of the Whigs versus Tories. In 1857, the Liberal Palmerston instructed Gilbert Scott to reconfigure his gothic designs for the Foreign Office in an Italianate style, while Prince Albert's designs for Osborne drew on Barry's Italianate Trentham Hall in Staffordshire (1834–49). In the 1860s a 'compromise Italianate style' was decided upon as a solution to the stylistic debate (as endorsed by Albert for the South Kensington museums). With 'its round-arched red-brick buildings [owing] something to contemporary German fashions', it is characteristic that this compromise should have been used at Netley. (David Watkin, *English Architecture*, Thames & Hudson, 1979, pp. 162–4)

99 'as though a Venetian . . .' quoted *Hampshire Magazine*, June 1980

99 'deep gratification' Sir Henry W. Acland, *An Address Delivered at Netley Hospital*, pamphlet, 1887, BL, p. 7

99 'when we are . . .' MacLennan, RAMC

99 'effluvia' *Report*, 1858. On 2 April 1856 it was reported that Chamberlayne was disinclined to sell the extra land because of local opposition to the hospital, but in August he was discovered to have let 20 acres of the required land to Captain Brady of Peartree as a brickfield for £10 an acre. Chamberlayne was suspected of trying to extort money from the Government, and 'the matter was resolved by applying compulsory purchase under the Defence Act 1842 and the Ordnance Board Transfer Act 1855'. (Fairman, p. 11)

100 'enormous importance . . .' Berlin, p. 30

100 'that great drama . . .' Friedrich Nietzsche, *On the Genealogy of Morality*, 1887, quoted Michael Neve and Mike Jay, *1900*, Penguin, 1999, p. 93

100 'I stand at the altar . . .' Elspeth Huxley, *Florence Nightingale*, Weidenfeld & Nicolson, 1975, p. 150

100 'This is one more . . .' Strachey, p. 145

100 'God spoke and . . .' Huxley, p. 16

101 'Superintendent . . .' *ibid.*, p. 71

101 'What a comfort . . .' Stella Bingham, *Ministering Angels*, Osprey, 1979, p. 50

101 'he found easy . . .' Huxley, p. 153

101 'She put before us . . .' Prince Consort, diary entry, 21 September 1856, quoted Cecil Woodham Smith, *Florence Nightingale*, Constable (1950), 1996, p. 265

102 'accidentally released . . .' Woodham Smith, p. 276

103 'whenever the hospital . . .' *The Builder*, 20 September 1856, pp. 510–11, RIBA library. Having published Mennie's plans in its edition of 23 August 1856, a month later the magazine had turned on Netley's shortcomings, finding particular fault with 'the placing of the baths and the "latrines" together, and the position of the latter between side wards . . . We speak with the results of actual experience before us, and we trust Mr Mennie will take it into consideration . . .' (20 September, p. 511). A subsequent editorial of 24 July 1858 attacked the 'ill-advised reports of the Netley committee, which mainly serve to show great want of acquaintance with the subject'. (p. 493)

103 'a pipe to conduct . . .' *The Builder*, 13 June 1857, p. 341, quoted RCHME, NBR: 100128

103 'susceptibilities' Woodham Smith, p. 276

103 'She knew her power . . .' Strachey, p. 150

103 'It seems to me . . .' Woodham Smith, p. 276

104 'highly objectionable . . .' Fairman, p. 13

104 '*clay*, or rather *brick earth* . . .' *REPORT*, 1858, p. 7

105 'question 10,025', *REPORT*, 1858, p. 7

105 *n* 'she had never seen it . . .' Strachey, p. 168

106 'that the means . . .' Report, 25 May 1857, PRO WO 33/A

106 'military medical education . . .' MacLeod, p. 382

107 'that one of the first problems . . .' T. R. W. Longmore, letter to author, 14 September 2000

107 'the authority for . . .' *REPORT*, 1858, p. 8

108 '*brick earth*' *ibid.*, p. 153

108 'You are all right . . .' *Southampton Times*, 26 October 1861

109 'and the occupiers . . .' *ibid.*, 14 December 1861

109 'The patient . . .' Florence Nightingale, letter 9 September 1858, quoted MacLennan, RHMC

109 'I have been down . . .' Florence Nightingale letter to Sir John White, 4 June 1857, Greater London Record Office, courtesy Patrick Kirkby, RVCP

110 'to avoid the fulfilment . . .' RCHME, NBR: 100128

110 'a notable defeat . . .' Woodham Smith, p. 332

110 'The entire staff . . .' *Southampton Times*, 6 December 1862. The first patient was admitted to Netley on 11 March 1863. (Fairman, p. 16)

110 *n* 'to each ward . . .' *The Lancet*, 9 May 1868, p. 592

In The Very Best Style

112 'Standing in the midst . . .' Lieutenant-Colonel John Graham, *The Navy and Army Illustrated*, 19 March 1897, p. 208

114 'extinguished . . .', Fairman, p. 16. In 1885 'a concession of access . . . by carriages' was made to the owners of Hamble Cliff, the gothic villa on the headland beyond the hospital (built in 1806 using mullions

salvaged from an older gothic building in Southampton). (MacLennan, RAMC) Its grandiose stable block – still standing, and often mistaken for part of the hospital site – was presumably built, in the 1880s, as a result.

114 'we are sure . . .' *Gardener's Magazine*, Vol. II, 1835, p. 60, Lindley Library, Royal Horticultural Society. William Bridgewater Page (1790–1871) was the proprietor of the Southampton Botanic Gardens, formerly the Old Spa Gardens, in the town; his nursery stood on what were then the town's outskirts at Hill.

114 'pump' *The Lancet*, 3 May 1868, p. 592. The article noted that because the windmill was set 'in a hollow in the very lowest part of the hospital grounds', it turned only 'under the inspiration of a south-west breeze'. As it claimed these seldom came in summer – when the pool was most needed – the facility was rendered less than useful. 'The water-supply to the hospital is, in fact, altogether inadequate, and is one of those fatal blunders for which our military engineers are so notorious.' (pp. 592–3)

115 'have been moved . . .' *A Brief History of the Royal Victoria Hospital*, article, SCL

115 'one of the earliest . . .' *Southern Evening Echo*, 7 March 1955

116 'down a steep hill . . .' Interview with Mr Norton, 3 October 1966, MacLennan, RAMC

116 'At Divine Service . . .' RVCP display

118 'severe censure . . .' MacLennan, RAMC

118 'difficult, depressing . . .' Woodham Smith, p. 277

118 'A corridor passes . . .' MacLeod, p. 380

119 'In the year 1878 . . .' Sir Arthur Conan Doyle, *A Study in Scarlet*, OUP, 1993, p. 15

120 'Drill before breakfast . . .' MacLeod, pp. 384–5. Noting 'the dinner excellent and moderate in price' in the officers' mess and the wide range of games and facilities available, *The Lancet* commented in 1868 that 'in fact, the life of an army medical candidate at Netley is rather a thing to be desired'. (9 May 1868, p. 593)

121 'present at the . . .' Royal Chapel pamphlet, June 1965, MacLennan, RAMC

121 'bloody fields . . .' *Illustrated London News*, 12 October 1895

122 'clear, precise ...' Longmore obituary, SCL

122 'I sometimes meet ...' Simon Daniels, *Enemies at Peace*, Eastleigh, 1993, p. 70

123 'I love the English ...' Stephen Taylor, *Shaka's Children: A History of the Zulu People*, HarperCollins, 1995, p. 193

124 'My, how they do ...' *ibid.*, p. 215

125 'the concept of killing ...' *ibid.*, p. 234

125 'The projectile ...' Longmore Papers, LP 33–4, RAMC 1139

127 'Dear Mr Longmore ...' *ibid.*, LP 33/5

130 'Case of Capt. Strange ...' *ibid.*, LP 32. Longmore was made Honorary Surgeon to the Queen in 1868 and knighted, at Osborne, on 30 July 1886. His son recalled one royal visit to Netley, when he was sent running down the corridor to fetch a bottle of whisky from the black bag of the hospital pathologist, Sir William Aitken, for the Queen's equerry, John Brown. (H. F. Longmore, *Southern Evening Echo*, 8 December 1966.) Longmore died in Swanage in 1895 and was brought back to be buried at Hamble churchyard. He was survived by his widow, Lady Longmore who, clad in black Victorian mourning, lived on at The Paddock, Woolston, until 1921.

131 'History of Disease ...' Pathology Reports, RAMC

133 'of interest ...' Pathology Reports, RAMC

133 'two rupees ...' Casualty Returns: Royal Victoria Hospital, Netley, PRO WO 25/3260

133 'When admitted ...' Pathology Reports, RAMC

'1171: Three sections ...' Aitken, *Descriptive Catalogue*, Vol. I, pp. 323, 215

133 *n* 'the constantly sick ...' RAMC 446/26. One of Netley's unofficial facilities was at least one local brothel in the village, euphemistically named 'Rose Cottage'.

134 'Our troopships ...' *Navy & Army*, 19 March 1897, p. 208

A Remarkable Improvement

135 'We look down ...' RVCP display

136 'tells me he wishes ...' Anne Summers, *Angels and Citizens: British Women as Military Nurses 1854–1914*, Routledge & Kegan Paul, 1988, pp. 70–1

136 'It was *preferred* . . .' Huxley, p. 30

136 'to discourage the men . . .' Turtle, p. 6

136 'women, as a rule . . .' Summers, p. 71

137 'no *door* . . .' *The Builder*, 23 August 1856, p. 457. The magazine added that 'as there is no fireplace, the orderly [or nurse] will be interested in looking to the fire and comfort of the ward for himself, as well as for the patients'. (*ibid.*)

137 'cannot and do not . . .' Summers, p. 108

137 'Superintendent-General . . .' *ibid.*, p. 72

138 'shut his eyes . . .' Huxley, p. 99

138 'Without her . . .' *ibid.*, p. 143

138 'What a twelvemonth . . .' *ibid.*, p. 132

139 'silently receiving . . .' Summers, pp. 92–3

140 'state of the nursing . . .' *ibid.*, p. 73

140 '. . . My impression . . .' *EVIDENCE Taken before COMMITTEE OF INQUIRY AT NETLEY HOSPITAL*, Eyre & Spottiswoode, 1869, PRO WO 33/20. In 1868 *The Lancet* declared 'The lady superintendent, though no doubt a well-intentioned person, is the *bête noire* of the establishment' and that 'the public should enquire why a whole public establishment is sacrificed to please a lady of aristocratic connexions'. (9 May, 1868, p. 593)

144 'which was beyond . . .' Turtle, p. 6

144 'impossible for any . . .' *EVIDENCE*, PRO WO 33/20

144 'Sisters are required . . .' Edward Lugard, ed. *Regulations for the Nursing Service at the Royal Victoria Hospital, Netley*, 1870, BL

145 'had to provide evidence . . .' Bingham, p. 115

145 'Hospitals were made . . .' *Regulations* . . . , 1870, BL

145 'impropriety . . .' Turtle, p. 6

146 'with 8 nurses . . .' Queen Victoria, journal, 12 August 1879, RA

147 'Remember when you . . .' Bingham, pp. 115–16

147 'each sister . . .' *ibid.*, p. 111

147 'so much prized . . .' *Navy & Army*, 19 March 1897, p. 209

150 'nervous at the thought . . .' Queen Victoria, journal, 8 May 1863. Until his death in 1861, Albert had made annual visits to Netley, whose towers were visible, by eye glass, from those of Osborne, across the Solent.

150 'The first public act . . .' *The Lancet*, 16 May 1863, p. 560. Victoria made a total of twenty visits to Netley.

150 'without doubt the moon was uninhabited' Queen Victoria, journal, 8 May 1863, RA. Playfair (1818–1898), 1st Baron Playfair of St Andrews, born in Meerut and later Liberal MP and postmaster-general. He had been Gentleman Usher to Prince Albert, and served on the committee for the Great Exhibition. A man of wide-ranging scientific interests, Playfair corresponded with Faraday, Babbage, Charles Barry and the astronomer Sir John Herschel. Playfair's prescient proposal on chemical weapons 'was considered inadmissable by the military authorities, who stated that it would be as bad a mode of warfare as poisoning the wells of the enemy. There was no sense in this objection . . .' maintained Playfair. 'Why a poisonous vapour which would kill men without suffering is to be considered illegitimate warfare is incomprehensible.' (Wemyss Reid, ed., *Memoirs and Correspondence of Lyon Playfair*, London, 1899, p. 160). Playfair was an advocate of vivisection and compulsory vaccination, and therefore an exemplar for Almroth Wright (*see below*). Having investigated the disease which caused the Irish potato famine in the 1840s, he engaged Netley's renowned Dr Parkes, whom he presumably met on this visit, to work with him on the Cattle Plague Commission in 1865.

151 'very hot . . .' Queen Victoria, journal, 12 August 1879, RA

151 '. . . It was very touching . . .' *ibid.*, 29 November 1882

152 'It is really very wrong . . .' *ibid.*, 20 August 1881

152 'Her Majesty's visit . . .' unsourced press cutting, 19 February 1895, Lt-Col. William Dick, 'Literary Notes' album, RAMC

153 'Heroism often went . . .' *Southern Evening Echo*, 2 August 1985

153 'I'm afraid I do not . . .' MacLennan, RAMC

154 'assisted by her . . .' *Daily Telegraph*, 12 February 1898

155 'present all the patients . . .' *Brief History*, p. 6

156 'words that thrilled . . .' Address by Lt-Col. M. H. Burge, D Block ceremony, 14 May 1999

157 'Oh, another . . .' *Hampshire Chronicle*, undated cutting, 1898, SCL

157 'I was on the point . . .' Queen Victoria, journal, 14 May 1898,

quoted 'Programme of Events', Royal Chapel, Netley, 14 May 1998, RVCP

158 'What a contrast . . .' *Navy & Army*, 19 March 1897, pp. 208–9

163 'on operations . . .' Dick, RAMC

166 'On the different forms . . .' CMAC GC/70

166 'feminine mind . . .' Michael Holroyd, *Bernard Shaw: The Pursuit of Power*, Chatto & Windus, 1989, p. 160

166 'a woman who . . .' Almroth Wright, *Alethetropic Logic*, p. 231, quoted Zachary Cope, *Almroth Wright: Founder of Modern Vaccine-therapy*, Nelson, 1966, p. 140

167 'plucked' Leonard Colebrook, *Almroth Wright: Provocative Doctor and Thinker*, Heinemann, 1954, p. 45

168 'the medical arrangements . . .' MacLeod, p. 388

168 'late night . . .' Holroyd, p. 161

169 'I believe . . .' *ibid.*, p. 162

169 'to carry out . . .' Colebrook, p. 67. For the lead on Wright's dubious experiments in South Africa, I'm indebted to Dr Jacalyn Duffin's programme notes for *The Doctor's Dilemma*, Shaw Festival, Toronto, 2000.

170 'and then used . . .' Holroyd, p. 164

170 'cooked' *The 'Cooked' Statistics concerning Anti-Typhoid Inoculation Used during the Recruiting for the Great War*, British Union for the Abolition of Vivisection, pamphlet, 1914, BL: 'Sir Almroth Wright, the maker of the particular brand of anti-typhoid vaccine which is now being so blatantly advertised in the Press, in the same manner that vaccination against small-pox used to be extolled, has recently contributed two letters to *The Times* in praise of his own production. These letters contained some very curious statistical errors, which were pointed out in letters to the Editor – which, needless to say, were not allowed to appear . . .' After the war Wright continued to pursue his medical and ethical theories. He was married twice, having been separated from his first wife, who later returned to him seeking a cure for her facial cancer. Despite taking her to the Radium Institute in Paris, he could not save her. Wright himself died in 1947.

171 'as if a magic lantern . . .' T. S. Eliot, 'The Lovesong of Arthur Prufrock', line 106

171 'Of the scientific . . .' undated cutting, Dick, RAMC

173 'hospital undress' *Daily Telegraph*, 12 February 1898

173 'a remarkable improvement' Fairman, p. 52. As long ago as 1858 Sydney Herbert's Commission had recommended a branch line to serve the hospital. What is now the Southampton–Portsmouth line had been laid in 1866 specifically for that purpose, although it left a half-mile gap between Netley station and the hospital itself.

Enter His Gates with Thanksgiving

175 'As I stood . . .' H. V. Morton, *In Search of England*, Methuen, 1984, p. 29

177 'an unexpected climax . . .' A. J. P. Taylor, 'War by Time-Table', *From the Boer War to the Cold War*, Hamish Hamilton, 1995

181 'at the massacre . . .' pamphlet, Royal Chapel, June 1965, Mac-Lennan papers, RAMC

181 'excellently protected promenades . . .' *Daily Telegraph*, 12 February 1898

182 'badly designed and useless . . .' *Southern Evening Echo*, letter, 3 February 1966

182 'future emergencies . . .' RVCP display

183 'Doecker' press cutting, BRC

183 'presented as a sort . . .' 'The following inscription is to be read on the frontal walls: "Transportable Baracke des Central Comité der deutschen Vereine vom rothen Kreus. Berlin. Oktob: 1899" (undated press cutting, SCL). The site had already been developed with a series of cottage bungalows, built in 1878, as a later press cutting noted, 'for the accommodation of wives and families of soldiers who are inmates of the hospital. Before these cottages were erected the poor wives of invalids had perforce to live in the back slums of Southampton, several miles away, exposed to the temptations of that rowdy seaport. The then chaplain of the garrison, the Rev. Mr Ponsonby, was the local secretary of the fund, and the donors were the people of the United Kingdom, who were roused to action by appeals from Mr Ponsonby . . .' (Dick, RAMC)

183 'The Welsh hospital . . .' transcription, 9 February 1915, BRC

185 'the pad on which ...' Hughes, *Fatal Shore*, p. 161

185 'Many new huts ...' Capt. Esler, typescript, IWM 74/102/1

186 'industrial island machine' caption, Tate Modern

187 'and if there had ...' Reminiscences of Lady Gaddom, BRC T2/GAD

187 'there were other...' Andrew Bamji, 'Facial Surgery: The Patient's Experience', in Hugh Cecil and Peter H. Liddle, eds., *Facing Armageddon: The First World War Experienced*, Leo Cooper, 1996, quoting from Anon., *Diary of a Nursing Sister on the Western Front 1914–1915*, Blackwood & Sons, 1915

188 'one of the grimmest...' Bingham, p. 157

188 'Its arrival was ...' Lady Gaddom, BRC T2/GAD

188 'but sometimes ...' Bingham, p. 139

189 'I cannot believe ...' Harold Owen and John Bell, eds., *Wilfred Owen/Collected Letters*, OUP, 1967, p. 470, by permission of Oxford University Press

190 'equipped' postcard caption, HRO

191 'V is for Vaccine ...' Album, July 1917, BRC 1464/11914

191 'we seemed to have ...' Netley British Red Cross Magazine, April 1918, HRO

192 'were a little upset...' *Southern Evening Echo*, 2 February 1967

192 'and their Suite' Netley British Red Cross Magazine, June 1918, HRO

193 'As your turn ...' *Times* cutting, undated, CMAC

193 'Are we Downhearted?...' postcard caption, Lingwood Netley Hospital Archive

Remembrance Day

196 'Footfalls echo ...' T. S. Eliot, 'Burnt Norton', *Four Quartets*

196 'rounds were exchanged' Lieutenant-Colonel John Darroch (Retd), Royal Hampshire Regiment Museum, in conversation with the author.

208 'Here at last ...' J. B. Priestley, quoted *Southern Daily Echo*, 13 September 1999

208 'Once off that...' Priestley, quoted Gordon Sewell, 'Southampton in the Twentieth Century', in J. G. Morgan, ed., *Collected*

Essays on Southampton, Southampton County Borough Council, 1961, p. 96

D Block

216 'And this also . . .' Conrad, *Heart of Darkness*, p. 7
216 'Accommodation is provided . . .' *Navy & Army*, 19 March 1897, p. 209
216 'A short distance . . .' Dick, RAMC
217 'A small creek . . .' Extracts from the *British Archeological Association Journal*, June 1867, HRO. Such hoards are usually buried at a time of unrest or violence, prompting speculation the Netley find may have been the result of a raid or battle during the later years of Roman occupation.
217 'military lunacies' Patrick Kirkby, 'Netley Military Asylum', HRO 92M91/8/2/10
217 'moral management' Bob Mullan, *R. D. Laing: A Personal View*, Duckworth, 1999, p. 40
219 'was under the impression . . .' *Southern Evening Echo*, 29 May 1973
220 'Sir, Having received . . .' RAMC 1185, CMAC
221 '. . . The Military Lunatic Asylum . . .' undated press cutting, Dick, RAMC
223 'To-day we fly . . .' Arnold White, *The Views of Vanoc: An Englishman's Outlook*, Kegan Paul, 1911, p. 147
224 'From this time . . .' Richard Slobodin, *W. H. Rivers*, Sutton, 1997, p. 55
224 'on the class of nerve cases . . .' CMAC GC/137
226 'On arrival from overseas . . .' *The Lancet*, 27 May 1916, p. 1074–5. The two establishments demarcated degrees of neurosis and psychosis: 'D Block, Netley – All cases of acute mental disorder arising in soldiers overseas were transferred to this section . . . At the same time a Neurological Section was formed in the main Hospital Building, Netley, the chief object of which was to permit the removal from the convoys arrived at D Block from overseas of all cases which the medical officers there considered did not require supervision of a special kind,

as some cases had so far recovered on arrival at Netley as to be deemed suitable for treatment in a Neurological rather than in a Mental Section.' (*ibid.*, p. 1074)

227 'hysterical gait' Dr Arthur Hurst, FRCP and Dr J. L. M. Symns, with the Royal Army Medical Corps, the Medical Research Committee and Netley (Hampshire) and Seale Hayne (Devon) Military Hospitals, *War Neuroses*, 1917. Royal College of Physicians/ Wellcome Trust. 22 mins; 16mm film. Hurst and Symns reported on 'The Rapid Cure of Hysterical Symptoms in Soldiers in *The Lancet*, 3 August 1918, noting such cases as the private suffering from a 'nose-wiping tic'. The 'kinematograph record ... was done at 10 am on Jan. 23rd ... He was then treated by active persuasion and re-education ... the improvement was so rapid by 12 o'clock another kinematograph record was taken ... He was not only able to walk quite well, but could actually run.' (p. 140)

228 *n* 'he had been strapped ...' Ben Shephard, *War of Nerves: Soldiers and Psychiatrists 1914–1994*, Jonathan Cape, 2000, p. 77

230 'a method of exploration' *ibid.*, p. 119

230 'During the night ...' William McDougall, *Outline of Abnormal Psychology*, New York, 1933, pp. 289–92

233 'From the earliest days ...' Hurst and Symns, *The Lancet*, 3 August 1918, pp. 139–41

233 '*Persuasion ...*' *REPORT of the WAR OFFICE COMMITTEE of ENQUIRY INTO 'SHELL-SHOCK'*, HM Stationery Office, 1922, pp. 128–30, RAMC 739/19

235 'wave of sentimentality' Shephard, p. xix

235 'the machine gun ...' *ibid.*, p. 137

236 'to the all-powerful will ...' *ibid.*, p. 309

236 'that many of Hurst's ...' *ibid.*, p. 80

238 'denied and laughed ...' Neve and Jay, p. 160

238 'it is not generally ...' A. Simpson, *Hot Blood and Cold Steel*, Tom Donovan, 1993, p. 92, quoting Philip Gibbs, *Realities of War*, Heinemann, 1920

238 'their evil hour ...' Siegfried Sassoon, *Sherston's Progress*, Faber & Faber (1936), 1960, pp. 88–9

239 'in a block ...' Shephard, p. 75

239 'Hanwell ...' White, p. 281

240 'large % utterly useless . . .' RAMC 446/18

240 'but not out of . . .' *ibid*. In *The History of the Great European War* (W. Stanley Macbean Knight, Caxton, 1919) a plate captioned 'German Prisoners Entering the Cages' notes, 'A careful study of the faces of many of these German soldiers will show that they present aspects of the unmistakably "degenerate" type; they contrast badly with the clean, alert British soldier.' (p. 194)

240 *n* 'cult of Wilde'. The case was heard by Justice Darling who was himself named as one of the 47,000, and who would subsequently preside over the post-war enquiry into the executions for cowardice. For more on this example of war hysteria, see Hoare, *Wilde's Last Stand*, Duckworth, 1997.

242 *n* 'quickly smothered . . .' Alexandra Ritchie, *Faust's Metropolis*, HarperCollins, 1998, p. 285

243 'The men had heard . . .' Mabel Lawson, *Suburbs of Southampton: Book IV 'Woolston and Sholing'*, Southampton, p. 23

243 'All the men . . .' *ibid*., p. 38

244 'light wounds . . .' Daniels, p. 136

245 'It is a fact . . .' *ibid*., p. 133. See also Daniels MS, IWM K.90/

246 'At the same time . . .' Donald A. Parr, *Web of Fear: Ghosts of Hampshire and the Isle of Wight*, Breedon Books, 1996, p. 98. Netley continues to produce similiar stories: the 'Grey Lady' is still reported, in places as far apart as Netley's military cemetery (as a flitting grey figure moving across the gates) and Weston Shore, where it recently scared a young angler one evening; while the nearby Victorian houses, opposite the castle's lodge, were considered so haunted that before their recent conversion to flats, an exorcism was carried out. Along the road, by the abbey ruins, drivers have seen spectral lights processing across the lane, causing their engines to stall. Such reports from Netley's gothic twilight – along with those of ghostly chanting and other manifestations – would be entirely familiar to Thomas Gray's lusty ferryman.

247 'Friday 11 February 1916 . . .' Esme Wynne, diary, courtesy of Jon Wynne Tyson.

247 'The cot cases . . .' Netley British Red Cross Magazine, April 1918, HRO

248 'Fisherman's Spring' *ibid*. The 'porch' was built in 1877 by the

Hon. Eliot Yorke, MP, who lived at Sydney House, a 1790s villa designed by Sir John Soane, along the shore from the hospital. The structure itself is now only visible in bits of red brick rubble and rotting wood embedded in the cliff, although fresh water still flows through it and out to the sea.

248 'Impressions in a Great War...' Netley British Red Cross Magazine, May 1918, HRO. Esme Wynne would herself become a Christian Scientist after the war.

249 'We sailed down...' Vera Brittain, *Testament of Youth*, Gollancz, 1978, p. 293. Brittain's dread was due to the fact that she had been told that *Britannic* had been built as a sister ship to *Titanic*.

249 '... My mind was unperturbed...' Siegfried Sassoon, *Memoirs of an Infantry Officer*, Faber (1930), 2000, p. 36

250 'The Voyage'...' *Owen/Collected Letters*, p. 470

250 'neurasthenia (143)...' PRO 44908, WO 138/74, website

250 'at the edge of the world' Jean Moorcroft Wilson, *Siegfried Sassoon*, Duckworth, 1998, p. 243

250 'the illusory War Films...' Jon Stallworthy, *Wilfred Owen*, OUP/Chatto & Windus, 1974, p. 170

251 'drawing plans...' *ibid.*, p. 174

251 'a city dominated...' *ibid.*, p. 178

251 'lay in holes...' *ibid.*, p. 182

253 'I shall have...' *Owen/Collected letters*, p. 470

253 'Dearest of Mothers...' *ibid.*

254 'a kind of wizard...' Shephard, p. 62

254 'the "Welsh"...' *Owen/Collected Letters*, p. 471

254 'the key to many...' *Owen/Collected Letters*, p. 508

254 'There is little abnormality...' PRO 44908, WO 138/74 website

254 'perhaps the most...' *Owen/Collected Letters*, p. 471

254 'this excellent concentration camp...' *Sherston's Progress*, p. 23

255 'a Harrow boy...' Stallworthy, p. 268

256 'Why hast thou...' Introduction, *REPORT ... INTO 'SHELL-SHOCK'*, RAMC 739/19

256 'the world is suffering...' Shephard, p. 143

256 '*Behaviour Characteristics...*' *REPORT ... INTO 'SHELL-SHOCK'*, p. 183

257 'I have been reading . . .' *ibid.*, p. 182

257 'in the course . . .' *The Lancet*, 26 February 1916, p. 475

257 'Dr Read defined . . .' *REPORT . . . INTO 'SHELL-SHOCK'*, p. 21

261 'was changing . . .' Brittain, pp. 496–7

Towards a Better Britain

263 'Before a building . . .' W. H. Ausell, *Towards a Better Britain*, RIBA, 1943, p. 2

265 'warm and as usual . . .' *Southern Evening Echo*, letter, undated cutting, RAMC

265 'How long do you think . . .' *ibid.* The south coast was a popular site for such sanatoria. In 1878 'The National Cottage Hospital for Consumption and Diseases of the Chest on the separate principle' was built at Ventnor in the Isle of Wight, next to Appuldurcombe, one of the intended sites for Netley's hospital. It too boasted Victoria as its patron, and like Netley, spread out in a great linear development, but this time took advantage of the resort's 'Undercliff' and its micro-climate by building individual verandahs for its inmates (its founder, Arthur Hill Hassall, believed patients should be kept apart in single rooms), giving it the appearance of so many semi-detached villas. Dr T. A. Ross, renowned for his work on war neurosis, was consultant there before working at the Cassel Hospital, Penshurst, Kent, where he too would treat Stephen Tennant. The Cassel was partly founded by Henry Head as a place where 'all that had been learned in the bitter experience of wartime might be used in dealing with neuroses among the civilian population', and had been financed by the millionaire Sir Ernest Cassel after he was shown Arthur Hurst's clinic at Seale Hayne. (Shephard, p. 162)

266 'The Commanding Officer . . .' MacLennan, RAMC

267 'littered with soggy . . .' *ibid.*

269 'had largely crumbled . . .' Patterson, p. 187

269 'The strongest feeling . . .' Robert Cook, *Southampton: Britain in Old Photographs*, Sutton Publishing, 1996, p. 49

269 *n* 'the aerial holocaust . . .' Shephard, pp. 174–5

269 *n* 'clinics emptied...' Anthony Beevor, *Mail on Sunday*, 8 October 2000

271 'What <u>have</u> I done...' Miss E. H. A. Luker, diary entry, 18 November 1943, IWM

271 'not sorry to see...' *ibid.*, 10 January 1944

272 'mostly suffering...' Roberta J. Norton Henry, 'Memoirs of a Psychiatric Nurse', RVCP

273 'When we reported...' Navy Nurse Sara E. Marcum Kelley, RVCP

274 'Treatment for combat fatigue...' Roberta Henry, RVCP

275 'pampered' Ben Shephard in conversation with Jeremy Paxman, *Start the Week*, BBC Radio 4, 23 October 2000

275 'Most patients talked...' Roberta Henry, RVCP

276 'The new aesthetic...' *Towards a Better Britain*, pp. 134–7

277 'comprehensive view...' *Daily Telegraph*, 12 February 1898

277 'Mesopotamian Oil Wells' *Memoirs of an Infantry Officer*, p. 202

278 'The first view...' *The Times*, 11 February 1956, quoted *Visitors' Descriptions*, p. 36

279 'It was frequently...' Mrs F. Skinner, letter, *Southern Evening Echo*, 5 February 1966

280 'male patients...' *Southern Evening Echo*, 4 December 1958

282 'shocker' *ibid.*, 31 January 1956

283 'Y' *ibid.*, 27 June 1963. At the Public Record Office, only one file, DT 33/2055 is yet to be released (closed until 2008), and deals with inspectors' reports on the hospitals in 1948. At the Hampshire Record Office, one file, concerning a suicidal/escape caution ticket issued at D Block, 23 July 1949, remains closed until 2025.

287 'a name of Gothic...' Patrick Wright, *The Village That Died For England,*, Jonathan Cape, 1995, p. 172

287 'form effective landmarks...' Pevsner, p. 599

287 'a monster of a building' *ibid.*, p. 350

290 'had Florence Nightingale's plans...' *Hampshire Telegraph*, 5 March 1970

290 'the demolition contractor...' John James Stott, HRO 92M91/5/85

291 'reported to be . . .' *Southern Evening Echo*, 10 September 1966

292 'Thus next year's new car . . .' Press release, 16 September 1966, Southern Daily Echo Library

294 'Uniform or Lounge Suit' invitation, Southern Daily Echo Library

His Dark Estate

299 'My Days & Nights . . .' Alexander Pope, quoted Richard Davenport-Hines, *Gothic*, Fourth Estate, 1999, p. 39

302 'Everything suddenly . . .' C. A. E. Moberly and E. F. Jourdain, *An Adventure*, ed. Joan Evans (1911), Faber, 1955, p. 33. De Sade reference from Anthony D. Hippisley Coxe, *Haunted Britain*, preface, Pan, 1975, p. 10

302 'slowly turned . . .' Moberly and Jourdain, p. 41

303 'the best authenticated . . .' A. J. P. Taylor, review of Lucille Iremonger, *The Ghosts of Versailles*, undated cutting, *The Observer*, 1957

303 *n* 'a dinotopic refuge . . .' W. L. T. Mitchell, *The Last Dinosaur Book*, University of Chicago Press, 1998, p. 188

305 'You'll be sent . . .' Mark Le Fanu in conversation with the author, 3 October 1997

305 'I used to lie . . .' Roger Hall, *Clouds of Fire*, Bartley Brothers, 1975, pp. 13–17

307 *'Extracts from Netley . . .'* HRO 92M91/1/1/4

308 'I was placed . . .' Hall, pp. 18–21

310 '[They] were afraid . . .' R. D. Laing, *Wisdom, Madness and Folly: The Making of a Psychiatrist, 1927–1957*, Macmillan, 1985, p. 154

310 'Madness . . .' Daniel Burston, *The Wings of Madness: The Life and Work of R. D. Laing*, Harvard University Press, 1996, p. 1

311 'normal . . .' Shephard, p. 157

312 'obscene methods . . .' *ibid.*, p. 157

312 'talk, talk, talk' *ibid.*, p. 209

312 'the cases of different . . .' Board of Commissioners' Report, 12 June 1928, PRO MH 95/34 RVH

312 'two by means . . .' *ibid.*, 22 July 1932

313 'it had deservedly . . .' David Stafford-Clark, *Psychiatry To-day*, Pelican (1952), 1963, p. 203

313 'in the form of . . .' Board of Commissioners' Report, 1931, PRO MH 95/34 RVH

313 'continuous narcosis' *ibid.*, 1943

313 'the number of patients . . .' *ibid.*, 18 December 1956

314 'The change of name . . .' *ibid.*, 10 August 1949

315 'deep comas . . .' *Wisdom, Madness and Folly*, pp. 90–91

315 'Even in the best . . .' Stafford-Clark, p. 203

316 'Marijuana cig: . . .' 'Personal Comment', Laing Papers, uncatalogued at time of research, Glasgow University Liberary

317 'Browned off' *et seq.*, *ibid.*

320 'Some of them admitted . . .' Maurice Williams, interview with author, 6 March 1998

320 'interfered with . . .' Laing papers, Glasgow University Library

323 'The Korean war . . .' *Wisdom, Madness and Folly*, pp. 94–5

323 'No patient . . .' *ibid.*, pp. 92–4

324 'moment of epiphany', Mullan, p. 53

324 'until I was almost . . .' *Wisdom, Madness and Folly*, p. 95

325 'severe anxiety . . .' John Clay, *R. D. Laing: A Divided Self*, Hodder & Stoughton, 1996, p. 46

325 'a sort of Sancho Panza . . .' *Wisdom, Madness and Folly*, p. 96

325 '. . . *I imagined that* . . .' P. B. Shelley, 'Julian and Maddalo', quoted Holmes, p. 456

325 'What was going on . . .' *Wisdom, Madness and Folly*, p. 97

326 '*Completely* terrified . . .' ibid. One source maintains that suicides were found face down in the shallow water, having tied their own heads down with the reeds.

326 'fellow normal men . . .' Mullan, p. 113

326 'Sanity is determinism . . .' Adrian Laing, *R. D. Laing: A Biography*, Peter Owen, 1994, p. 51

326 'sublimated pursuit . . .' Burston, p. 199

327 'Don't you salute . . .' Clay, p. 45

327 'It became clear . . .' *ibid.*, p. 44

327 'It seems to me . . .' Mullan, p. 54

327 'therapeutic community'. Kingsley Hall, a gaunt two storey building with high arched windows, had been run by the Lester sisters since before the First World War as a practical exposition of their beliefs,

with a soup kitchen, chapel, and 'sanctuary room' for runaways. In the late 1920s it was an international centre for militant pacifism; in 1931, while attending a conference on India, Mahatma Gandhi had lived for ten days in a wooden shed on its roof, along with a goat to provide him with milk.

328 *n* 'the case of Mary Barnes . . .' White, *Views of Vanoc*, p. 146

328 'Acid Marxist' Mullan, p. 133

328 'inner space . . .' *ibid.*, p. 109

328 'I recognised him . . .' *ibid.*, p. 4

The World Is Infinitely Forgiving

329 'It is not wise . . .' ed. R. Aldington, *Oscar Wilde: Selected Works*, Heinemann, 1946, p. 332

329 'steady and progressive . . .' Board of Commissioners' Report, 23 September 1953, PRO MH 95/34 RVH

329 'was interested in . . .' *ibid.*, 10 June 1955

330 'Cpl Attwood . . .' John James Stott, HRO 92M91/5/85

330 'I'm going to . . .' *Hampshire Telegraph*, 5 March 1970. Shephard compares the embrace of largactil in the mid-1950s to the introduction of penicillin in general medicine, a 'miracle drug' which 'made it possible to clear the asylums'. (p. 364)

334 'P. White, 47th Regt.' display, Netley Force Support HQ. Reviewing the conversion of D Block in 1988, *Architect's Journal* noted 'It is hard not to wonder at the lavishness of this fully equipped police headquarters. The capital expenditure for law and order is self-evidently outpacing that for education; Hampshire county architects, renowned for school design work, now have their hands full with buildings for law and order. This is the reality of Mrs Thatcher's third term.' (Gillian Darley, *Architect's Journal*, 20 July 1988, p. 34)

335 *n* 'These men lived . . .' Osbert Sitwell, *Laughter in the Next Room*, Macmillan, 1949, p. 6

336 'intellectual socialist' William Allison and John Fairley, *The Monocled Mutineer*, Quartet, 1986, p. 14

337 'glad to the brink . . .' Ralph Waldo Emerson, 'Nature'. In *The Golden Bough*, published just before the First World War, Sir James

Frazer described the cults of Adonis and Attis (who committed suicide by castrating himself while tied to a pine tree) and the belief that their blood propitiated the harvest and stained the flowers of the field: 'In the summer after the battle of Landen, the most sanguinary battle of the seventeenth century in Europe, the earth, saturated with the blood of twenty thousand slain, broke forth into millions of poppies, and the traveller who passed that vast sheet of scarlet might well fancy that the earth had indeed given up her dead.' (*The Golden Bough*, Chancellor Press, 1994, p. 340.) In 1916 Wilfred Owen dedicated 'A New Heaven' to an unknown soldier 'on Active Service', 'Though still we crouched by bluebells moon by moon' (the lines continue, '– Let's die home, ferry across the Channel! Thus/ Shall we live gods there . . .') (Stallworthy, ed., *Collected Poems*, p. 59.) A year later, in Easter 1917, Sassoon approached the Western front feeling as though he were 'interfused with some sacrificial rite which was to celebrate the harvest'. (*Memoirs of an Infantry Officer*, p. 118)

342 'the greatest force . . .' Hoare, *Wilde's Last Stand*, p. 152

342 'When Hess becomes . . .' found manuscript, Spring House. At the time of writing, the site has been redeveloped for housing, and its trees felled.

347 'a mental hospital . . .' Harold T. Wilkins, *Mysteries: Solved and Unsolved*, Odhams, 1958, p. 171

Epilogue

352 'So, while the light fails . . .' T. S. Eliot, *Four Quartets*

356 'stand in the sun . . .' Peter Ackroyd, *Blake*, Sinclair-Stevenson, 1996, p. 195

357 'And this green pastorale . . .' William Wordsworth, 'Lines Composed . . . above Tintern Abbey', *Penguin Book of English Romantic Verse*, p. 113

357 'each a glimpse . . .' Robert Louis Stevenson, 'From a Railway Carriage', *A Child's Garden of Verses & Underwood*, 1913

360 'boats that fly . . .' Adrian B. Rance, ed., *Sea Planes and Flying Boats of the Solent*, Southampton University Industrial Archaeology Group/Southampton City Museums, 1981, p. 5. From the turn of the

century until the 1960s, Southampton Water was officially designated as an aerodrome. After the war Billing continued his career as inventor and quixotic politician, while the company was taken over by his partner, Hubert Scott-Paine, who developed speed boats piloted by his friend T. E. Lawrence. Supermarine's Woolston works would go on to develop the Spitfire, designed by R. J. Mitchell.

360 'all gone under . . .' T. S. Eliot, 'East Coker', line 99. This chapter was written before the winter floods of 2000–1, and the increased coastal erosion, which has sent the mature oaks growing above the Fisherman's Spring slowly collapsing on to Netley's beach.

361 'the present of things . . .' Camille, p. 83

361 'glorious goals', Berlin, p. 107

INDEX

References in italic indicate illustrations

'A', Private 'B', 163

Aberfan, 28 & *n*

'Abide With Me', 212

abreaction, 227, 231, 236, 324

Aden, 196, 330

Adonis, 396

'Age of Reptiles, The', 303, 303 *n*, *304*

Aitken, Sir William, 133, 165, 370, 381

'Akaba', 24–5, 300

Albert of Saxe-Coburg and Gotha, Prince Consort, 90, 91, 94 *n*, 153, 304, 382–3; & origins of Netley Hospital, 94–5, 99,110, 149–150; designs Osborne, 93, 377; death of, 148, 150, 382

Aldershot, 313; Military Tattoo, 215

Aldrin, Buzz, 206

Alexandra, HM Queen, 192

Alice (film), 285–6, *286*

Alice, Princess Andrew of Greece, 83

Alice in Wonderland, 119, 251, 285–6

Alix, 357

Allan, Maud, 53, 240 *n*

All Quiet on the Western Front, 316

Alma, Battle of, 121

Amazon (river), 360

Amballa, 196

American Civil War, 122

American Hospital (Netley) *see* E Block

Anderson, Inspector General A., 115

Anderson, Corporal, 228

Anderson shelter, 26, 214

'Angels of Mons', 246

Anne, Nurse, 141–2

Antiquities of England and Wales, 58

Anti-University of London, 328

apartheid, 341

Apollo, 336

Apollo XI, 206

Appuldurcombe, IOW, 96, 391

Armstice, The, 255, 257

Armstrong, Neil, 206

Army Medical Department, 95, 136

Army Medical School, 101, 120–1, 122–3, 150, 165, 168, 220

Army Medical Services, 349

Army Nursing Service, 139

Army Special Investigation Bureau, 282

Arnhem, battle of, 321

Ashley, Private, *228*

Assurance Medical Society, 224

Asquith, Henry Herbert, Earl of Oxford and Asquith, 343

Astor, Nancy, 342

Atlantic Gulf West Indies Refinery (Fawley), 277

Atlantic Pulse, 35

Atlantis, 360

Attis, 396

Attwood, Corporal, 330

'Auld Lang Syne', 63

Austen family, 70–72,

Austen, Jane, 67, 70–2; *Love and Friendship*, 71; *Northanger Abbey*, 71

Austen, Fanny, 72–3
Ausell, W.H., 263
Author's Club, 248
autognosis, 234
Avon (river), 39

Babbage, Charles, 383
Bacon, Francis, 232
Baden-Powell, Lord, 83
Balaclava, battle of, 121
Balfour, Arthur James, 1st Earl, 166
Balmoral, 101, 103
Barham, Reverend Richard Harris, 75–6; *Ingoldsby Legends*, 75–6
Barker, Granville, 166
Barnes, Mary, 327–8, 328 *n*
Barry, Sir Charles, 98 & *n*, 377, 383
Barry, Charles, 98 *n*
Basingtoke, 357, 358, 359
Bath, 199
Battersea, 353, 356
Beard, George M., 224
Beaton, Sir Cecil, 53, 344
Beatrice, HRH The Princess, 124
Beatson, Inspector-General G. S., 143
Beaulieu, 41, 48
Bedlam (lunatic asylum), 223, 232, 327, 356, 359, 360
Bell, Dr Joseph, 122
Belsen (concentration camp), 233
Benedictines (religious order), 41
Bentley, Richard, 52, 53
SS, *Berengaria*, 208
Berlin, 131, 195, 261, 318, 385
Berlin, Isaiah, 65
Bethell, Adrian, 343
Bethlehem Royal Hospital, Kent, 309
Bevois Mount, Southampton, 55, 60
Billing, Noel Pemberton, 240 *n*, 285, 320, 342, 360, 397
Bimbo, 25

Birch, Eugenius, 115
Birmingham, 199, 250, 359
Bitterne, (*see frontispiece*), 31, 70, 200, 212, 214, *201*
Bitterne Grove (The White House), 70; *see also* St Mary's College, Southampton
'Black Book', 240 *n*, 285, 320
Blake, William, 65, 356
Blavatsky, Madame Helena Petrovna, 237
'Blind Peter', 47, 58, 73
Bloemfontein, 167, 168
The Blue Angel, 316
Board of Commissioners, 312, 313
Boer War – see South African War
Borley Rectory, 302
Bosnia, 349
Botany Bay, New South Wales, 17–18, 185
Botany Bay, Sholing, 17–19, 185
Bouchoir, 250
Bournemouth, 77, 115, 172, 199; pier, 172
Bowie, David, 22, 83, 353, 355, 356, 361–2; *Ziggy Stardust*, 83; 'Five Years', 83; *Station to Station*, 356; 'Life on Mars', 362; as Ziggy Stardust, 83; as The Thin White Duke, 356, 362; as Thomas Jerome Newton, 22
Bradford, 200, 202, 204, 205–209, 211–12
Brady, Captain, 378
Brighton, 77, 115, 172; pier, 172; Royal Pavilion, 93
Bright Young People, 69, 344
SS *Britannic*, 249, 390
British Archaeological Association Journal, 217
British Army Psychiatric Unit, 305; *see also* D Block
British Medical Hospital, Singapore, 317, 318
British Medical Journal, 96

British Union for the Abolition of Vivisection, 384
Brittain, Vera, 249, 261, 390
Broadlands, Romsey, 103
Brönte family, 205
Brown, 'Capability' Lancelot, 277
Brown, Reverend James, 56
Brown, John, 381
Brown, Dr William, 234, 251, 254
Brunel, Isambard Kingdom, 3–4, 179
Brunton, Mary, 73
bubonic plague, 45–6, 67
The Builder, 103, 378
Bunüel, Luis, 356; *Un Chien Andalou*, 356
Buonaparte, Napoleon, 50, 375
Burdett-Coutts, W., 168
Burston, Daniel, 311
Byron, George Gordon, Lord, 325

'C', Lance Corporal, 163
Cadland House, 277
Caine, Caesar, 248–9
Calcutta, India, 300
Calshot Castle, 56
Camberwell, London, 242 *n*
Cambridge Military Hospital, 321
Camus, Albert, 317, 327; *Le Mythe de Sisyphe*, 327
Canute, King, 361
Cape Town, 341
Cardiff, 156, 199
Carol, Stella, 343
Caroline of Anspach, Queen of George II, 70
Carroll, Lewis, 217, 286; *see also Alice in Wonderland*
Cartrie, Comte de, 70, 302, 374
Cartwright Hall, Bradford, 205
Cassell, Sir Ernest, 391
Cassell Hospital, 391
Catholic Conversions, 342
Catholicism, 27, 32, 78, 84–5, 136, 181, 246, 263, 301, 342, 371

Cattle Plague Commission, 383
Cenotaph, Southampton, 212
Cenotaph, Whitehall, 259
Cerletti, Ugo, 313
Cetshwayo ka Mpande, 123–4, 125, 151
Ceylon (Sri Lanka), 158
Chamberlayne family, 36, 80, 82 *n*, 84, 187
Chamberlayne, Tankerville, 80
Chamberlayne, Thomas, 98, 99, 378
Chamberlayne, William, 36–8, 61, 65, 77, 98, 109
Chandos, 2nd Duke of, 68
Chaplin, Charles, 194
Chatham, Kent, 93, 94, 100, 217
Chelsea Hospital, 89
'Chelsea Pensioners', 279
Chester, Colonel, 221
cholera, 96, 105 *n*, 133
Chopin, Fredrich, 53; *Marche Funebre*, 53
Charley's Aunt, 247
chemical warfare, 190, 383
Cherry, Ava, 353
Chester, 280
Christian Science, 249, 390
Chronicles of Narnia, 301
Churchill, Charles, 54
Churchill, Sir Winston, 202, 270, 276, 305
Church Path, Sholing, 20–22, 37
Chute, John, 52, 56, 68
Cistercians (religious order), 41–6, 51, 54, 58, 80, 81, 95, 110, 136, 137, 181, 225, 323, 337
Civic Centre, Southampton, 209, 210
Clapham Junction, 356, 359
Clare, John, 50, 53 *n*
Clarke, Sir James, 96, 101
Clarke, Sister, 139
Classic cinema, Southampton, 362
Clausentum (Roman Southampton), *see frontispiece*; 39, 217, 301

Clements, Miss, 26–7
Clow, Private, 154
Campaign for Nuclear
  Disarmament (CND), 212, 280
Cobbett, William, 27, 47, 65, 75,
  208; *Rural Rides*, 36, 37, 38, 39,
  74
Cobh, Eire, 18
cocaine, 119
Cockerell, Miss, 235
Colebrook, Leonard, 169
Coleridge, Samuel Taylor, 66
Collins, Herbert, 258
Columbo, Sri Lanka, 158
combat fatigue, 274
Commissioners in Lunacy, 217, 219,
  312
Commissioner of Works, 81
Conservative Party, 37, 375, 377
Congo (river), 360
Conrad, Joseph, 360; *Heart of
  Darkness*, 15, 35, 216
Constable, John, 64–5, 81
Constable, Maria, 65
consumption – *see* tuberculosis
Cooper, Lady Diana, 53
Cork, Eire, 18, 127
Cottingley, Yorkshire, 207
Covent Garden, London, 353
Cow and Calf Rocks, Yorkshire,
  206
Coward, Sir Noël, 208, 247, 261,
  342, 348, 355
Cowes, Isle of Wight, *see
  frontispiece*, 48, 76, 249
Craiglockhart (war hospital),
  Edinburgh, 239, 254, 255
Cranbury Park, Winchester, 58, 80
Cranworth, Lady, 136
Crichton family, 83
Crimea War, 5, 121, 123, 151, 155,
  157, 199; folly of, 89, 120, 130–1;
  casualties of, 93, 95, 100, 137–8,
  236; *see also* Scutari Barracks
'Crippen', 32–3, 83

Cromwell, Oliver, Lord Protector,
  18, 83 *n*
Crooke-Lawless, Lady Emily, 190
Crooke-Lawless, Surgeon
  Lieutenant-General Sir Warren,
  190, 192, 244
Cruikshank, George, 207
The Crystal Palace, 8, 77, 303; *see
  also* Great Exhibition
Cumberland Infirmary, 321
Cyril (PH's uncle), 206, 310

Daily Sketch, 343
Daily Telegraph, 154
Dance-Holland, Sir Nathaniel, 60
'Dance of Death', 45
The Dancing Years, 213
Danel, Private, 144
Daniels, Simon, 244–5
Dante Alighieri, 21, 309
D'Arcy, Very Reverend Martin
  Cyril, 342
Dargai Heights, 156
Darling, 1ˢᵗ Baron, Charles John,
  389
Darwin, Charles, 8, 80, 166, 316,
  326
Davies, Dr Arthur Templer, 224–5
Davies, Colonel R., 330, 334
Davis, Private, 154
D Block (P Wing) (Victoria House),
  216–26, 238, 241, 244–5, 256, 257,
  258, 280, 286, 290–1, 303, 346,
  387, 392; Victorian and
  Edwardian history of, 216–223,
  219, 222, 334; & First World
  War, 223–6; between the wars,
  261, 307–9, 311–3, *310*; post-war,
  305, *314*, 314–28, 329–36;
  decayed, 330–3, *332*; renovated,
  333–4; contemporary, 345, 363;
  suicides at, 326, 329; *see also*
  Military Asylum
D-Day, 272, 273, 275
Dean, Terry, 330

Deeble, Mrs Jane, 145–7
Defence Act (1842), 378
Defence Act (1855), 98
Defence of the Realm Acts
  (DORA), 180
Defoe, Daniel, 67, 70, 208
De La Mennais Brothers (religious
  order), 31
Dennis, (PH's paternal grandfather),
  201–3, *202*, *203*
Deran, Ordinary Seaman Michael,
  92
de Sade, Marquis, 303
*Descriptive Catalogue
  of. . .Pathological
  Specimens. . .*(Netley), 6, 370
desertion, 186, 229, 389
Diamond Jubilee (1897), 155, 158–9
Dick, Lieutenant-Colonel William,
  163, 171
Dickens, Charles, 272; *Nicholas
  Nickleby*, 33; *The Pickwick
  Papers*, 207
Dietrich, Marlene, 362
HMS *Dilware*, 158
'Doecker' huts, 183
Dome of Discovery (1951), 277
Domesday Book, 15, 39
Dorchester, Dorset, 17
Doré, Gustav, 21
Dott, James, 70
Douglas, Lord Alfred, 342
Dover, 243
Doyle, Sir Arthur Conan, 119–20,
  207; *A Study in Scarlet*, 119; *The
  Lost World*, 120
Dracula, 202
Drake, Sir Francis, 35
drugs (medicinal), 246, 274–5, 324,
  329, 330
drugs (recreational) – *see* Opium,
  Morphine, Laudanum, Cocaine,
  Marijuana, LSD
Duchess of Malfi, 59
Dugdale, Thomas, 209, 262, *210*

Dummer, Thomas Lee, 37, 38, 58,
  60, 286
Dummer, Mrs Thomas, 60
HMS *Dunera*, 158
Dunkirk (retreat from), 271
Dunn, Dr, 234
Durban, South Africa, 126
Dutch elm disease, 362
dysentry, 133

The Eagle of the Ninth (Rosmary
  Sutcliff), 301
East India Company, 70
Eastleigh, Hampshire, *see
  frontispiece*, 357
E Block (PN Wing) (Albert House)
  (American Hospital), 214–5, 273,
  274, 314, 320, 330
Edward VI, 343
Edward VII, HM King (Prince of
  Wales), 84, 90
Edward VIII, HM King (Prince of
  Wales, Duke of Windsor), 208
Edwards, Fleetwood J., 15
Edwin Jones, 300
electro-convulsive therapy (ECT),
  313, 317, 318, 324
Eliot, T. S., 360; 'The Lovesong of
  Arthur Prufrock', 171; *Four
  Quartets*, 196, 352, 353
Elizabeth I, 35, 48
Elizabeth, HM Queen, The Queen
  Mother, 348, 359
Elliot, Maxine, 196
Elliot, Dr T. R., 225, 234
Ellis Island, New York Harbour,
  115
Embley Park, Hampshire, 103
Emerson, Ralph Waldo, 395
HMS *Empire Fowey*, 317
Empress Dock, Southampton, 158
SS *Empress of Britain*, 208
encephalitis lethargica ('sleepy
  sickness'), 264, 325
Enclosure Acts, 16, 50, 53 *n*

English Array, 287
Eno, Brian, 83
Enright, Miss, 26, 214
Erskine, General Sir George, 282
Esher, 355
Esler, Captain M. S., 184–6
Etretat, 250, 251, 253
eugenics, 240, 316
HMS *Euphrates*, 126

Fagley, Bradford, 205, 206
'Fairley Fieldhouses' 183, 273; *see also* Hutted Hospital
Fairy, (royal yacht), 90
Faraday, Michael, 383
Fareham, Hampshire, 55, 220
Fawcett, Colonel P. H., 370
Fawley Refinery, 277–9, 351, *278*
Ferry, Bryan, 83, 355
Festival of Britain (1951), 277
Findlater, Piper George, 156–7, 348
Fir Grove Road, 23
First World War, 19, 26, 156, 170, 175, 247, 311, 320, 323, 335–6, 338–9, 343, 360, 370, 388, 389, 390, 391, 394, 395–6; outbreak of, 176–7, 343; & Royal Victoria Military Hospital, 177–195, 223–262; & PH's family, 196–201, 204, 207
Fisherman's Spring, Westfield Common, 248, 390, 397; *248*
Fitzcarraldo, 360
Flannigan, Able Bodied Seaman Cornelius, 92
Fleming, Sir Alexander, 170, 264
Florence (PH's maternal grandmother), 198–200, *198, 199, 201*
Florence Nightingale (boat), 115
Folkestone, 255, 257
Fonthill Abbey, Wiltshire, 375
Foreign Office, 377
Fort Pitt, Chatham, 6, 93–4, 121, 217
Fountains Abbey, Yorkshire, 42, 58

Frazer, Sir James, 395–6
Frederick (PH's maternal grandfather), 196–200, *197, 198, 201*
Frederick, Prince of Wales, 69
freemasonry, 301, 320
French Revolution, 70, 73
Freud, Sigmund, 166, 235, 312, 316
Fyffe, Dr, 141–3

Gailly, 251
Gandhi, Mahatma, 395
Galbraith, Corporal, 141
Galloway, Sir James, 257
Ganges (river), 192
Gardener's Magazine, 114
Garrick, David, 70
Gas House Lane, Netley, 347
Gaukroger, 2nd Lieutenant, 252
Gawalior, Maharajah of, 190
Geneva Convention, 122
George II, HM King, 69
George V, HM King, 192
Georgiana, Duchess of Devonshire, 69, 89
German Secret Service, 240 *n*
The Ghosts of Versailles, 302–3
Glasgow, 310, 325
Glastonbury Festival, 362
Glenconner, 1st Baron, 343
Gloucester, Duke of, 69, 70
Goal, 341
Godwin Reading Room, Hutted Hospital, 194
Godwin, William, 63
Goering, Herman, 35
Gold Coast (Ghana), 151, 152
The Golden Bough, 395
The Golden Hind, 35
gonorrhoea, 322
Gormenghast, 85, 117
gothic, ancient origins of, 50–1; medieval origins of, 42–3, 45; 18th century conception of, 50–1, 52–67; 19th century conception of,

71–6, 78–82, 238, 375; 1920s conception of, 53, 264; 1940s conception of, 85, 287; 1960s conception of, 53–4, 286; 21st century conception of, 80–2, 389; as 'national style', 74; Gothic Revival, 78, 79, 98 *n*, 375, 377

Graham, Lieutenant-Colonel John, 158–161, 216

Grand Theatre, Southampton, 247

Gray, Thomas, 53–9, 68, 80, 305, 389; 'Elegy written in a Country Church-yard', 53 & *n*; at Netley, 54–8, 80

S.S. *Great Eastern*, 3–4

Great Exhibition (1851), 77, 80, 90, 277, 383

Great Famine (Ireland), 18, 202, 383

Great Plague (1665), 67

Great Stink, 105

Great War – *see* First World War

'The Green, Green Grass of Home', 32

Grey, Corporal, 154, 157

Grey of Fallodon, Lord (Sir Edward Grey), 343

Grey Lady, 245–6, 265, 267, 302, 303, 328, 389

Grimaldi, Carlo, 40, 362

Guide to Southampton (1781), 70

Guide to Southampton (1796), 65

Guernsey, 67

Guillaume, George, 82 *n*

Guinness, Edward (Viscount Iveagh), 183

Gumbley, Charles, 338

Gunard, Isle of Wight, 22

Gunston, Leslie, 253, 254

Hackett family, 123, 127, 128–30

Hackett, General Sir John, 130

Hackett, Major Robert, 123–30, 151

Hackett, Lieutenant-Colonel Thomas, 123, 128

Hall, Henry, 202

Hall, James, 50–1

Hall, Dr John, 138

Hall, Roger, 305–9, 311, 322

Hamble village, 381; river, 16, 36

Hamble Cliff House, 379–80

Hamburg, 318, N6

Hampshire, *see frontispiece*, 16, 17, 35, 52, 59, 71, 107, 148, 175, 184, 231, 249, 253, 277, 305, 309, 326, 335, 337, 357, 360, 395; origins of name, 40

Hampshire Chronicle, 157

Hampshire Constabulary, 334–6, 395; Police Museum, 335–6

Hampshire Independent, 89, 90, 92

Hampshire Record Office, 392

Hampshire Regiment (Royal Hampshires), 181, 196–7, 339

Hampton Court, 48

Hardy (gunboat), 92, 100

Hardy, Reverend C. J., 137

Harrow, 255

Hart, Dr Bernard, 234

Haslar Royal Naval Hospital, Gosport, 96

Hassall, Arthur Hill, 391

Hawkins, Benjamin Waterhouse, 8

Hawley, Brigadier-General P, 272

Haworth, 205

Hay, Lieutenant-General C., 140

Hazeley Down, Winchester, 254

'H' Blocks, 273

Head, Henry

Hearen, Private William, 131–2

Heine, Heinrich, 372

Henry III, 42

Henry VIII, 47, 48, 269

Henry, Roberta, 272, 274, 275

Heppleton, Corporal Charles, 132

Herbert of Lea, Sydney Herbert, Ist Baron, 101, 104, 105, 120, 385

herpes, 310

Herschel, Sir John, 383

Herstmonceux, Sussex, 96

Hess, Dame Myra, 342

Hess, Rudolph, 313–4
Highfield, Southampton, 258
High Royds Hospital, Menston, 201, 206
Hill, Southampton, 380
Hindenburg Line, 251
Hiroshima, 233
Hitler, Adolf, 314, 342
Hoare, Philip: birth & upbringing in Portswood, 24–5; upbringing in Sholing, 15, 18, 19–22, 25–29, 305; Irish background, 18; mother, 18, 24, 26, 28, 29, 196, 200, 204, 206, 207, 212–3, 264, 301; father, 18, 24, 27, 28, 30, 200–1, 202–214, 301, 358–9, *213*; brothers, 24, 29–32, 214, 301, 329; sisters, 27, 28, 30, 199, 359; aunts & uncles, 206, 214; great-uncles, 201; antecedents – *see* Frederick, Florence, Dennis, Josephine, Tom, Lucy; education, 26–8, 31–3, 299–300, 352, 355; & Catholicism, 27, 32; childhood holidays, 10–11, 204–7; leaves home, 355; leaves London, 355–7; as writer, 389; & memory of Netley, 211–12, 214–15, 331–3, 363; & death of brother, 29–31, 301; & Spring House, 339–44; & Stephen Tennant, 344
Hobbins, Private James, 219
Hogstead, Dr, 128–9
Holroyd, Michael, 169
holy wells, 81, 248
Home Guard, 214, 270
homosexual aversion therapy, 257, 320
homosexuality, 33, 54, 240, 254, 256, 257, 264, 319–20, 321
Hood, Lieutenant-General Sir Alexander, 272
Hopkins, Gerald Manley, 253
Hopkins, Miss, 61
Hitch, Private, 151

Hound, Hampshire, 43
Howitt, William, 49, 50, 78, 79, 80, 81
Hunt, George, 82 *n*
Huntingdon, 7th Earl of, 48
Hurst, Dr Arthur, 227, 230, 233–5, 237, 388, 391; ?229
Hurst Castle, 48
Hutted Hospital (Netley British Red Cross), 183–95, 247–9, 258–64, 273; *184, 255*
Huxley, Francis, 328
Huxley, Thomas, 80, 249
hyacinthoides non-scriptus (bluebell), 336–7
Hyacinthus, 336
Hyde Park, London, 242 *n*
hydrophobia (rabies), 67
hydrotherapy, 313
hypnosis, 226, 230, 234, 324
hysteria, 228, 232, 237
Hythe, Hampshire, 272

Ilkley Moor, Yorkshire, 206
'If You Go to San Francisco', 304
Illuminati, 65
Illustrated London News, 94 *n*
Imperial War Graves Commission, 339
Imperial War Museum, 356
Incledon, Charles, ('The Wandering Methodist') 62–3
Indian Medical Service, 158
Indian Mutiny (1857), 123
Industrial Revolution, 38, 65, 170
influenza, 264
Ingoldsby Legends, 75–6
Inkerman, battle of, 121
inoculation, 164, 167–70, 191, 383, 384
insulin coma therapy, 312–3, 315–6, 318, 324, 329, 330–1
Irish Hospital, 182, *184*; *see also* Hutted Hospital
Isandlwana, battle of, 124, 181

Isle of Wight, *see frontispiece*, 6, 22, 24, 32, 34, 42, 48, 56, 76, 93, 96, 99, 173, 250, 351, 391
Itchen (river), 16, 24, 25, 35, 36, 39, 269, 360
Itchen, Southampton, 375–6
Itchen Floating Bridge, 90
'It's a Long Way to Tipperary', 186, 200

Jacob family, 347
Jamaica, 362
Jannings, Emile, 316
Jarrow March, 209, 262; *210*
Jersey, 67
Jesus Chapel, Peartree, 375
Jackson, Private J., 143
Johansen, David, 353
Johnson, Nurse Francis, 143–4
Josephine (PH's paternal grandmother), 202–3, *202, 203*
Jourdain, Eleanor Frances, 302–3, 305
HMS *Jumna*, 126, 158
Jung, Carl, 310
Juvenile, Debbi (Debbie Wilson), 354

Kafka, Franz, 171
kala-azar, 168
Kambula Hill, battle of, 124–5
Karim, Abdul, 155
Kaufmann, Dr, 229 *n*, 313
Kelley, Navy Nurse Sara E. Marcum, 273
Kelly, Fr Henry Patrick, 26
Kensington Gardens, 39
Kensington Palace, 242 *n*
Kent, William, 38
Keogh, Sir Alfred, 133 *n*
Kierkegaard, Søren, 316
King John, 41, 56
Kingsley Hall, 327, 394–5
King's Road, Chelsea, 354
Kipling, John Lockwood, 158

Kipling, Rudyard, 158
Kitchener, Lord, 170
Kneebone, Colonel, 266–7
Kneebone, Nurse, 153, 267
Knighton, Henry, 45
Knowle Hospital, Hampshire, 220
Koch, Dr Robert, 131, 167
Korean War, 323
Kosovo, 233
Kraftwerk, 356

Laffan, Captain R. M., 95–8
Lahore School of Art, 158
Laing, R. D., 310–28, 329–31; background & character of, 310–11; at Netley, 311, 315–28; 'Personal Comment', 316–7, 326; *The Divided Self*, 327
Lance's Hill, 31, 299, 301
The Lancet, 98 *n*, 110 *n*, 225, 226, 233, 257, 380, 382, 387
Lansdowne, Marquis of, 374–5
Lawrence, T. E., 35, 251, 397
laudanum, 238
Leeds, Yorkshire, 206
Lee, Robert, 358
Leishman, William, 133 *n*, 168, 172
Lepe Beach, 279
leprosy, 44, 67, 337
leucotomy, 313, 330
Lewis, Matthew, 66; *The Monk*, 66; *Crazy Jane*, 66
Lewis, Percy Wyndham, 186; *see also* Vorticism
L'Hopital Lariboisiere, 105
Liberal Party, 375, 377; *see also* Whig Party
Lincoln, 9th Earl of, 54
Lister, Joseph, 105 *n*
Lester Sisters, 394
Little Chef, 355
Lloyd, David, 287
Lloyd George, David, 256, 258–9; *259*
Lloyd-Webber, Lord, 64

lobotomy – *see* leucotomy
Loch Ness, 10–11, 34, 303; Loch Ness Monster, 10–11, 303
Lodge, Sir Oliver, 166, 249, 303
Loos, battle of, 347
London, 24, 69, 77, 208, 254, 270, 277, 325, 327, 328; described, 352–6; PH leaves, 357; PH returns to, 358, 360
Longmore, Sir Thomas, 107, 163, 164, 165, 172, 175, 190; background, character & career, 121–3, 381; & case of Major Hackett, 126–130; gives evidence to Shaw Stewart enquiry, 140; *Gunshot Wounds*, 122; portrait, *122*
Longmore, Lady, 127, 381
Long Rooms, Southampton, 68, 70
Looby, Private, 141
LSD (lysergic acid), 328, 330
Lucifer (magazine), 237
Lucknow, 132
Lucy (PH's great aunt), 207
Lucy, Sir Berkeley, 49
Luftwaffe, 214, 287
SS *Luisitania*, 343
Luker, Esther Helen Audrey, 271–2, 286, 363
Lunacy Act (1845), 217, 218, 239
Luxmoore, Lieutenant-Colonel, 253

MacCormac, Private Patrick, 132–3
McDougall, William, 230
McGrigor, Sir James, 6
Machen, Arthur, 246
MacLean, Dr, 139
Mai, Aunt, 138
malaria therapy, 313
Mallarmé, Stefan, 80; 'A Phenomenon of the Future', 80
Mallik, Anne-Marie, 285–6; *286*
The Man Who Fell to Earth, 22
Map, Walter, 42
Mapleton, Dr, 96–7

Mapother, Dr, 234, 235
Marie-Antoinette, Queen, 302
marijuana, 316
Mark, 362
Marne, battle of, 230
Marvel Comics, 304–5
Mary, HM Queen, 192, 193; *193*
Mary, HRH Princess (Princess Royal), 192, 193; *192*
Mass Observation, 269
Mayfield Park, Weston, 36, 84, 193, 214
Mayflower, 175, 270
Mbenyesi, E., 339
Meades, Jonathan, 375
Meek, Private, 229–30, 237, 246; *229*
Meerut, India, 196, 383
meningitis, 207
Mennie, E. O., 2, 98, 107, 378
Mesmer, Friedrich Anton, 65, 237
Messel, Oliver, 53
Middlesex Hospital, 104
Mignonette (yacht), 375
Milford-on-Sea, Hampshire, 292
Military Lunatic Asylum, Netley, 134, 216–222; *219, 221*; *see also* D Block
Miller, Dr Jonathan, 285–6
Miller, Lee, 355
Miller, Private William, 133
Miller's Pond, Sholing, 22–3, 244; *23*
Mills, Sid, 245
Ministry of Pensions, 257
Ministry of Public Works, 81
Mintram, Alfred Maurice, 22–4
Mintram, Charles, 23
The Miracle, 53
Mitchell, R. J., 303 *n*, 397
Mitford, Mary Russell, 34
Moberly, Charlotte Anne Elizabeth, 302–3, 305
Moholy Nagy, László, 276
Monkey puzzle (*Araucaria aracana*), 24, 338

Montague, Mr, 74
Montesquieu, Robert, Comte de, 100
Montmarte, Paris, 316
Moore, Henry, 276
Morton, H. V., 175, 208; *In Search of England*, 175
Mouat, Deputy Inspector General, 136
Mowl, Timothy, 53
Mullan, Bob, 328
Munden, Joseph, 61
Mussolini, Benito, 342
Myers, Charles, 225, 228, 234, 235, 326
Myers, F.W.H., 249
Mythchett Place, Aldershot, 313

Napoleon, Prince Eugene Louis (Prince Imperial), 124
narcoanalysis, 275
Nash, Paul, 276
Nash, Surgeon-Major-General William, 155
National Hospital for Consumption, Ventnor, 391
National Service, 317, 318, 330
Natural History Museum, South Kensington, 9, 10, 377
Navy & Army Illustrated, 112, 117, 159–161, 370
Neal Street, Covent Garden, 353
Netley (village) *see frontispiece*, 1, 2, 4, 5, 6, 16, 26, 33, 34 *passim*, 115, 118, 122, 213, 397; origins of name, 39; climate of, 96–7, 108; development of, 77, 175; brothel in, 381; Roman presence in, 217, 336, 387
Netley Abbey, 38–85 *passim*, 138, 305; origins of, 39, 41; foundation of, 41–2; architecture of, 42–3; regime at, 44; financial state, 46; taxation of, 44; & lepers, 44, 337; & bubonic plague, 45–6;

dissolution of, 46, 48; conversion of, 48, 82; as house, 48–50; Elizabeth I visits, 48, 372; in ruins, 46, 49, 50; as gothic site, 50–67 *passim*; ghosts of, 47, 49–50, 57–8, 73, 239, 244, 389; in verse, 59–1, 75–6; on stage, 61–2; painted, 64–5; as *Northanger Abbey*, 71; & opening of hospital, 90; & origins of hospital, 95, 96, 107, 109, 118, 119, 181; contemporary, 79, 81, 82, 345; & time, 361; illustrated, *39, 55, 59, 61*
Netley Abbey – A Comic Opera, 61–4, 71
Netley Abbey, A Gothic Story, 64, 66
Netley British Red Cross – *see* Hutted Hospital, Red Cross
Netley British Red Cross Magazine, 247–9
Netley Castle, 56, 57, 82–3, 82 *n*
Netley station, 116, 122, 175–7, 244, 385
neurasthenia, 224, 225, 239; *see also* shell-shock
Neurological Section, Royal Victoria Military Hospital, 226, 387–8
New Forest, 17, 57, 211, 277, 278, 349, 351
New Malden, 177, 356
Newcastle United, 358
New York, 18, 47, 115, 325, 353
New York Dolls, 354
Nietzsche, Fredrich, 100, 111, 165, 166, 316
Nightingale, Florence, 89, 95, 118, 120, 121, 131, 143, 144, 146, 147, 148, 157, 158, 168, 188, 199, 217, 290; background & career, 100–1; portrait, *102*; & Netley, 100–105, 107, 109–110; & nursing at Netley, 134, 135–8, 145; death of,

Nightingale, Florence – *contd.*
178; myths of, 101, 109, 246;
*Notes affecting...the British
Army*, 101; *Notes on Hospitals*,
109; *Notes on Nursing*, 158
Nightingale Fund Council, 144–5
Nightingale Training Council, 145
Norman, Miss H. Campbell, 157
North-West Frontier, India, 156,
158
Norwich Hospital, 184
Novello, Ivor, 213
Novotel, Southampton, 361
HMS *Nubia*, 158

O'Brien, Colonel Terence, 106
O'Keefe, Tracy, 354
Old Bailey (Central Criminal
Court), 240 *n*
Ono, Yoko, 328
opium,134, 255
Ordnance Survey, 20, 96, 295
Orford, Earl of, 84
Organ, Ellen, 371
Orleans, Duke of, 70
Osborne House, IOW, 6, 24, 76, 89,
93, 99, 148, 149, 155, 173, 192, 377,
381, 382; described, 93; & Durbar
Hall, 158, 198; PH visits, 304
Osborne Road, Portswood, 24, 25,
214, 360
Owen, Richard, 8
Owen, Susan, 250, 253–5
Owen, Wilfred, 250–6, 360; at
Netley, 250, 253–5; 'Asleep', 254,
360; 'Dulce Et Decorum Est',
255; 'Mental Cases', 255;
'Disabled', 255; 'A New Heaven',
396; travels up Southampton
Water, 250; death of, 256, 339
Oxford, 286, 305; St Hugh's Hall,
302

'Pack Up Your Troubles', 200
The Paddock, Woolston, 381

Paderewski, Ignace Jan, 342
Page, William Bridgewater, 114,
345, 380
Palace of Westminster, 98 & *n*,
105
Palmerston, Lord, 103–4, 120, 377
Panmure, Lord, 90, 91, 94; &
Netley, 94–5, 98, 100, 101, 104,
107
Parker, Richard, 375
Paris, 316, 328
Parker, Ed, 330
Parkes, Dr Edmund Alexander, 383
Parratt, Private John, 220
Partridge (brig), 97
Pascal, Blaise, 316
Pasteur, Louis, 105 *n*
Pathé Brothers, 227, 236
*Paul Brothers' Guide to
Southampton* (1900), 5, 370
Paulet, Sir William (Ist Marquess of
Winchester), 47–8, 50, 71, 82,
112, 138
Paulet, Lord William, 138
Pavlov, Ivan Petrovich, 166
Paxton, Joseph, 77
Peabody Museum, Yale, 303
Peacock, Thomas Love, 66;
Nightmare Abbey, 66, 73
Peake, Mevyn, 85; *Gormenghast*, 85
Pearce, William, 63–4; *Netley
Abbey – A Comic Opera*, 61–3;
The Nunnery, 64; *Arrival at
Portsmouth*, 64; *Windsor Castle*,
64; *The Lock and Key*, 64; *see
also* Shield, Wm
Peartree, Southampton, 375, 378
penicillin, 170
Peninsula War, 73
Permain family, 341
Persuasion, 233, 323
Peter, 33, 47, 83–4, 331, 339
Petit Trianon, Versailles, 218,
302–3, 304
Pevsner, Nikolaus, 369; on Netley,

1; *The Buildings of England* – 20, 81, 287, 369
phthisis – *see* tuberculosis
'Piccadilly', Hutted Hospital, 185, 191, 261, 273
Pierrepoint, Albert, 208
Pietermaritzburg, South Africa, 126
Pirelli General Cable Works, Southampton, 210–11, 214
Playfair, Dr Lyon (1st Baron), 150, 165, 383
Plymouth, Devon, 95
Polygon Hotel, Southampton, 68
Ponsford, W., 127
Ponsford, Mrs W., 127
Ponsonby, Reverend Mr, 385
Pope, Alexander, 299
Pop, Iggy, 356
Porchester Castle, 96
Porton Down, 245
Portsmouth, *see frontispiece*, 16, 17, 19, 55, 64, 95
Portswood, Southampton, 24–25, 212
Power House Camp, Netley, 191
Preston, Private, 231, *231*
Pretoria, 169
Priestley, J.B., 203; on Southampton, 208–9
Prince Consort (public house), 83
Probable Nuclear Targets in the UK, 212
Public Record Office, 283, 392
Pugin, Augustus Welby, 77–8, 79–80, 98
Pugin & Pugin, Co., 85
punk, 85, 353–5
Putney, 352
psychoanalysis, 234, 235, 312; *see also* Laing, R.D.; shell-shock

Quanset hut, 312
Quarr, IOW, 42, 48
Queen Alexandra's Imperial Military Service, 271

Queen Alexandra's Royal Army Nursing Corps, 266

race, 169, 222–3, 239
Radiant Heat Department, 281
Radium Institute, Paris, 385
Ray, Surgeon Sidney Keyworth, 219
Radcliffe, Mrs Ann, 62, 63, 64, 66, 71
railways, 19, 77, 173, 175–7, 188–9, 210, 353–61, 385; *see also* Southampton, Netley, Sholing, Waterloo stations
Reading Gaol, 356
Red Cross, 122, 182, 184, 188, 194, 190, 191 *n*, 260, 263, 273, 385; *see also* Geneva Convention, Hutted Hospital
Read, Dr. C. Stanford, 257–8
Reed, Private, 227
're-education', 233, 234, 236
Reid, Private, 141
Richard I (The Lionheart), 175
Richmond, 352
Rivers, W. H., 225, 230, 234, 241, 257, 326
Riviera, French, 35
Robben Island, 18
Roberton, John, 103
Roberts, William, 187
Rock Scene, 353
Rogers, Lieutenant-Colonel, 234
Rolleston, Dr, 225
Røntgen, Wilhelm, 171, 238, 264
Rorke's Drift, battle of, 151, 156
Rose & Co., 270
'Roses of Picardy', 200, 260
'Rosina', 63
Ross, Dr T. A., 391
Rotten, Johnny (John Lydon), 85, 354
Roule, Private Fred, 132
Roxy Club, 353–4
Roxy Music, 83; *Roxy Music*, 83
Royal Academy, 255

411

Royal Army Medical Corps
(RAMC), 167–8, 173, 184, 191 *n*,
223, 240, 251, 257, 308, 316, 317,
322, 327, 348, 369, 388
Royal Commission to the Sanitary
Condition of the Army, 104–6
Royal Engineer Department, 2
Royal Garrison Artillery, 338
Royal Institute of British
Architects, 263, 276
Royal Military College, Sandhurst,
305–6
Royal Navy/Fleet Air Arm, 349
Royal Victoria Country Park
Royal Victoria Military Hospital, 1,
85, 89 *passim*; origins of, 89–111;
architecture of, 1–4, 9, 98–99,
102–111, 112–115, 118, 181;
museums, 5–9, 179, 349–51, *7*;
Officer's Mess, 6–8, 118, 303, *8,
9*; first patient admitted, 379;
described, 1–9, 112–121; daily
regime, 116–17, 160–2, 178–82,
380; nursing at, 113, 134–47, 382;
commodification of, 119; Royal
Chapel, 116–7, 180–1, 267, 282,
293, 349–50, 356, *117, 350*; pier,
115–6, 151, 172, *116, 173*;
illustrated, *3, 4, 7, 8, 9, 113, 178,
184, 228, 262, 274, 288, 289*;
shortcomings of, 2, 98 *n*, 99, 100,
103–7, 109, 110–1, 115, 118, 159,
178, 181, 182, 243, 263, 264, 266,
272–3, 279, 282–3, 287, 290, 293,
380; & South African War,
162–4, 168, 172, 183; & First
World War, 175–95, 212, 223–50,
253–5, 258; between the wars,
258–68; & Second World War,
212, 269–76; American
occupation of, 272–5, 280, *274*;
post-war, 280–351 *passim*;
demolition of, 286–95, *290, 292,
294, 295*; as country park,
345–51, 362–3, railway station,

173, 177–8, 189, 385; cemetary,
265, 308, 337–9, *314, 338*; filmed,
227, 231, 283–6, *228, 282, 285*;
German POWs at, 243, 244–5;
ghosts of, 245–6; experimentation
at, 167, 244–5, 283; *see also* D
Block, Military Asylum, Hutted
Hospital
Royal Warwick Regiment, 240, 241
Royal West Surreys, 311
Rufford & Finch, 2
The Ruins of Netley Abbey (verse),
59–60
Ruskin, John, 79–80, 277, 355; *The
Storm-Cloud of the Nineteenth
Century*, 79
Russell, Bertrand, 316

St Augustine, 361
St Bernard of Clairvaux, 42–3, 74
Abbey of Saint-Denis, 42
St John's Ambulance, 212
St John's Apocalypse, 45
St Mary's College, Southampton,
31–3, 47, 180, 299; *see also*
Bitterne Grove
St Mary's College, Strawberry Hill,
84, 352, 355
St Mary's Hospital, Paddington,
168, 169
St Mary's Island, Kent, 94 *n*
St Michael's Church, Southampton,
40
St Patrick's Church, Woolston, 26,
27, 35, 243, 269
St Patrick's School, Woolston, 26–7,
263, 299, 300
Saint-Quentin, France, 251
St Thomas's Hospital, Lambeth,
145, 168
St Veronica, 355
Sakel, Manfred, 312, 313
Salisbury, Wiltshire, 236, 269
Salisbury Plain, 89, 191
Saltaire, Bradford, 205

Salt, Sir Titus, 205
Sassoon, Siegfried, 250, 27, 264, 277, 344, 396; & Wilfred Owen, 255; & Stephen Tennant, 264, 344; at Craiglockhart, 238, 254–5; nightmares, 241, 261; travels down Southampton Water, 249
Satchell, Hampshire, 43
Savy Wood, 251
Schiele, Egon, 358
schizophrenia, 310, 321, 324
Schleswig-Holstein, Princess Victoria of, 173 & n
Scholz, Otto Paul Karl, 244–5, 283
Scott, Sir George Gilbert, 151, 377
Scott-Paine, Hubert, 397
Scutari Barracks, Crimea, 93, 96, 100, 109, 137–8, 148
Seale Hayne Military Hospital, Devon, 236, 391
Seaweed Hut, Weston Shore, 40–1, 305; 41
Sebastapol, Crimea, 100, 121
Second World War, 213–4, 268–76, 313, 318, 346; see also Royal Victoria Military Hospital, Hoare, Philip
Sedding, J. D., 82
'Seditionaries', 354
Seymour, Edward, Earl of Hertford, 48
Seymour family, 48
Shakespeare, William, 56, 340; King John, 56; Henry IV, Part I, 256
Shamrock Tea Rooms, 255
Shaw, George Bernard, 123, 168–9; The Doctor's Dilemma, 169
Shelley, Percy Bysshe, 205; character, 66; 'Ozymandias', 59; Zastrozzi, 66; 'Julian & Maddalo', 325
shell-shock, 223–42, 250, 254; early diagnosis of, 224–5; definitions & symptoms of, 225, 226, 227–33;

therapies for, 226–7, 228 & n, 230, 233–5, 236–9, 241, 311–2, 388; statistics of, 239 & n; post-war analysis of, 256–8, 262, 274
Shephard, Ben, 239 & n, 275, 395
Shepherd, Surgeon-Major Peter, 181
Shield, William, 61–4; Netley Abbey, A Comic Opera, 61–4, 71; for other works, see Pearce, William
Shipley, Yorkshire, 201
Shirley, Southampton, 271
Sholing, Southampton, see frontispiece, 25, 26, 31, 36, 39, 43, 96, 115, 122, 204, 209, 214, 217, 244, 305, 341, 360, 374; origins & description of, 15–24; see also Hoare, Philip
Sholing Common, 20, 96, 185, 270
Sholing station, 122, 175, 360, 361
Shoreditch, 328
Shorncliff Military Camp, Kent, 126–7
Shrapnel, Henry, 374
HMS Sicilia, 338
Simon's Town, South Africa, 126
Singh, Bhai Ram, 158
Sioux, Siouxsie, 355
Sitwell, Dame Edith, 342
Sitwell family, 53
Sitwell, Osbert, 335 n
Sixtus IV, 46
Skylon (1951), 277
smallpox, 384
Smith, Dr Andrew, 95, 109, 136, 137
Smith, Cecil Woodham, 102, 118
Smith, E., 2
Snowden, Arthur de Winton, 191 & n, 264
Smyth, Dame Ethel, 166–7
Soane, Sir John, 390
Society of St Vincent de Paul, 204
The Solent, see frontispiece, 6, 47, 89, 112, 174, 249, 362

Somme, battles of, 187, 230, 239, 247, 250, 251

Sotheby, William, 60; 'Ode, Netley Abbey; Midnight', 60

South African War, 120, 156, 162–4, 167–8, 172, 176, 183, 195, 198, 223; losses, 167–8; concentration camps, 167–8, 195; 165, 173; see also Royal Victoria Military Hospital

South Bank, London, 277

South Kensington museums, 377; see also Natural History Museum

South Wales Argus, 183

South Western Hotel, 208, 270

Southampton, 15–20, 24, 34, 38, 44, 55–6, 64–6, 82 n, 85, 136, 158, 175–7, 185–6, 196, 202, 206, 212, 243–4, 271, 341, 347, 352, 358; described, 176–7, 208–9, 210, 278, 361; origins, 40; attacked, 40, 268–70; vulnerability, 63; & bubonic plague, 45; as spa town, 62, 67–72, 76, 96; The Beach, 68, 70; High Street, 68, 176, 208, 236, 269, 362; the Avenue, 270; Western Esplanade, 361; in 19th century, 76–7, 374–5; snubs Victoria, 89–90; & First World War, 176–7, 189, 250; between the wars, 208–10, 258, 264; & Second World War, 268–70, 272, 349; post-war, 278; climate, 108; & sewage, 96; population (1851), 96; pier, 343; slums of, 208–9, 385; see also Bitterne, Highfield, Portswood, Shirley, Sholing, Woolston

Southampton Botanic Gardens (Old Spa Gardens), 76, 380

Southampton Corporation, 70, 92

Southampton Docks, 116, 158, 175, 177, 185–7, 209, 213, 250, 266, 338; 213

Southampton Guide, 67

Southampton station (Central), 243, 254, 360

Southampton Water, see frontispiece, 1, 3, 31, 44, 54, 55, 61, 64, 76, 81, 89, 96, 104, 106, 112, 127, 134, 167, 184, 185, 192, 217, 248, 268, 284, 338, 351; described, 34–5, 38, 55, 253, 277, 362–3; fortification of, 47, 270, 272; & First World War, 187, 189, 248, 250, 251; between the wars, 266; & Second World War, 268–9, 271, 276; post-war, 277–9, 304; as aerodrome, 397

Southern Command, 282

Speedwell, 175

Spencer, Stanley, 347

Spike Island (Bristol), 17

Spike Island (Ireland) (Inis Pich), 17–19, 370–1

Spike Island (Liverpool), 17, 28 n

Spike Island (Sholing), 36, 38, 39, 44, 107, 110, 185, 217, 243, 361; origins of, 16–19

Spion Kop, battle of, 163

Spiritualism, 120, 241–2, 249, 301

Sporting Life, 32

Spring House, 339–44, 396

Stafford-Clark, David, 315

Stalingrad, 342

Stalin, Josef, 342

Star Wars, 358

Station Hotel, Netley, 329

Sterling, Linder, 28 n

Steven, Captain, 191

Stevenson, Colonel, 171

Stevenson, Major, 247

Stewart, Jane Shaw, 137–147, 382

Stoker, Bram, 202

Stone Roses, 28 n

Strachey, Lytton, 103, 105 n

Strand Magazine, 126

Strange, Captain Benjamin, 130–1, 131

Strawberry Hill, Teddington, 52, 54, 78, 79, 84, 85, 352, 354
street shrines, 242 & 242 *n*
Strong, Mrs Rebecca, 147
suffrage, female, 166, 169
Suger, Abbot, 42, 43, 54, 78
Supermarine Aircraft Works, 360, 397
Sutton, Fred, 243
Suzuki, Dr Jiro, 190
Swanage, Dorset, 381
'Sweet Chariot', 355
Sydney House, Hamble, 390
Symns, Dr J, 227, 233, 388
syphilis, 131–3, 133 *n*, 221, 309, 13, 317, 321

'Take Me Back to Dear Old Blighty', 200
talking cure, 235, 312, 323
Taylor, A.J.P., 177, 303
Taylor, Major Pritchard, 234
Taylor, Walter (senior), 49
Taylor, Walter (junior), 38, 58, 293
Teddington, 352; *see also* Strawberry Hill
Tennant, Clare, 343, *344*
Tennant, David, 344
Tennant, Stephen, 35, 53, 208, 343–4, 348, 391; & Siegfried Sassoon, 264, 344; & PH, 344
Test (river), 35, 39
Thames (river), 15, 24, 35, 105, 305
Thatcher, Margaret, 395
Theatre Royal, Covent Garden, 61, 62
The Times, 68, 70, 119, 121, 168, 193, 194, 224, 278, 384
The Troubles, 330
Third Uhlans, 244
Third West General Hospital, Cardiff, 199, *199*
Thornycroft (shipbuilders), 243, 244
SS *Titanic*, 24, 35, 212, 390
Titchfield, Hampshire, 55

Tom (PH's great-uncle), 201, 202, 207, 224, *202*
Toplis, Percy (Monocled Mutineer), 335–6
Tory Party – *see* Conservative Party
Totton, Hampshire, 291
Tower of London, 35
Towne, Francis, 64
Toys 'Я' Us, 361
TransEurope Express, 356
transportation, 17, 18, 53 *n*
Trentham Hall, Staffs, 377
Truth, 312
tuberculosis, 131–3, 167–8, 191 & *n*, 205, 264–5, 316, 337, 391
Tufnell, Professor, 5
Twickenham, Middlesex, 353
2001: A Space Odyssey, 206, 362
Tyndall, John, 248
typhoid, 105 *n*, 133–4, 148, 167–70

überrumpellungsmethode, 229 *n*, 313
Ulex europeaus (gorse, furze), 16
Un Chien Andalou, 356
Union Castle Line, 341
US Army, 271, 272–6, 280, *274*
US Air Force, 349
US Medical Corps, 349
US Navy, 273–5, *274*
University of London, 119
Utrecht, South Africa, 124, 125

van der Rohe, Mies, 43
Vasari, Giogio, 52
venereal disease, 133 *n*, 223, 309; *A Manual of Venereal Disease*, 133 *n*; *see also* syphilis, herpes, gonorrhea
Venice, 325
Ventnor, IOW, 391
Verdun, battle of, 247
Versailles, Palace of, 1, 99, 218, 302–3
The Vibrators, 354

Vickery, Private Sam, 155–6, 348
Victoria, HRH Queen-Empress, 6,
    24, 83, 94 *n*, 111, 112, 117, 123,
    124, 136, 158, 192, 198, 347, 349,
    381; lays foundation stone of
    hospital, 89–93; at Osborne, 24,
    76, 89, 304; & origins of hospital,
    93–5, 100–1, 103, 110, 111; visits
    Netley, 89–93, 146, 147–157,
    170–3, 259, 292, 383; knits shawl,
    153, 246; Diamond Jubilee, 155;
    death of, 173–4; portrayed, *92,
    149, 156*
Victoria, Princess Royal, 90
Victoria and Albert (royal yacht),
    89, 93
Victoria Cross (honour), 91, 123,
    151, 155–7, 348
Victoria History of England
    (Hampshire), 40
Victoria station, 356
HMS *Victory*, 38
Vienna, 312
Vietnam, 323
Vincennes Military Hospital, 105
Vincent, Rifleman C.G., 339
Voluntary Aid Detachment (VAD),
    182, 188, 189, 199, 235, 249
Vorticism, 186, 276

Wagner, Richard, 2, 287; *Ring
    Cycle*, 2; *Götterdammerung*, 287
Waldegrave, 4th Earl, 84
Waldegrave, Lady Elizabeth, 84
Wallace, Edgar, 342
Walpole, Sir Edward, 84
Walpole, Horace, 4th Earl of
    Orford, 68; background & gothic
    taste, 52–4, 55–6, 66, 74, 78–9,
    80, 84–5; 'Committee of Taste',
    52, 53 & *n*, 54, 58, 74, 78–9;
    Castle of Otranto, 52, 66, 84, 372
Wardroper, Mrs, 145
Warhol, Andy, 53; *Electric Chair*,
    54

Warner, Reverend Richard, 64, 66
war neurosis – *see* shell-shock
War Neurosis (film), 227–233,
    235–7, 388; *228, 229, 231, 232,
    233*
War Office, 140, 169, 183;
    'Committee of Enquiry into
    Shell-Shock', 255–6
Washington, 349
Waterhouse, Alfred, 9
Waterloo Bridge, 353
Waterloo station, 177, 208, 213, 243,
    254, 352, 355
Watts, Isaac (senior), 49
Watts, Isaac (junior), 49
Waugh, Evelyn, 343; *Handful of
    Dust*, 371
Webster, John, 59
Wedden, Mrs, 146
Weekly News, 342
Welch, Denton, 85; *Voice Through
    a Cloud*, 85
Welch, Francis, 220
Welsh Hospital, 183, 250, 251, 253,
    254, *184*; *see also* Hutted Hospital
Welsh Ministry of Pensions, 183
Wellington, Duke of, 73
Wembley Empire Pool, 356
Westcott, Joan, 310
West Indies, 38, 133, 211, 277
Westminster Abbey, 42, 150
Weston, *see frontispiece*, 16, 35, 84,
    187, 193, 277, 287; described,
    35–8
Weston Grove, 36–8
Weston Shore, 35–6, 64, 108, 272,
    389
Westwood, 270
Weymouth, 69
Wharton, Dr, 54
Whistler, Rex, 53
Whitby, Yorkshire, 148, 202, 209
Whig Party, 62, 377; *see also* Liberal
    Party
White, Mr, 21,22

White, Arnold, 222–3, 224, 237, 239 & *n*, 258, 310, 328 *n*, 336; *The Views of Vanoc*, 328 *n*
White, Private Patrick, 334
The Whitehall Review, 77
White Star Line, 362
W.H. Smith, 176
Wilbraham, Major-General, 144
Wilde, Oscar, 240 *n*, 285, 355, 356; *Salome*, 53, 399
Wilde's Last Stand, 389
Williams, Private, 228
Willis, Walter Edwin, 338
Wiltshire, 264, 344
Winchester, *see frontispiece*, 17, 45, 55, 58, 80, 90, 204, 254, 357, 358, 359, 360, 372
Winchester, 14th Marquess of, 90
Winchester, Bishop of (des Roches), 41
Winchester, Bishop of (Wilberforce), 92, 95
Winchester Cathedral, 93
Winchester station, 357, 358, 359
Windsor Castle, 84, 170
Women in Love, 84

Woolston, Southampton, *see frontispiece*, 16, 18, 26, 115, 122, 129, 243, 263, 269, 360, 374, 381, 397; Woolston House, 37, 58; Woolston Library, 300
Wordsworth, William, 80; *The Borderers*, 216; *Lines written above Tintern Abbey*, 357
World's End, Chelsea, 354
Wright, Sir Almroth, 164–170, 172, 190, 224, 238, 264, 383, 384; background, 164–6; publications, 166, 170; anti-typhoid vaccine, 167–170, 384; & Bernard Shaw, 168–9; wives, 384; portrait, *166*
Wynne-Tyson, Esme, 247, 249, 271, 390

Yarmouth, IOW, 48
Yealland, Dr Lewis, 228 *n*
YMCA, 254, 347
Yorke, Hon. Eliot, 390
Yorkshire, 201, 205, 209

Zallinger, Rudolph, 303 & *n*, 347
Zululand (Kwazulu/Natal), 124, 181
Zulu Wars, 123–5, 151, 181

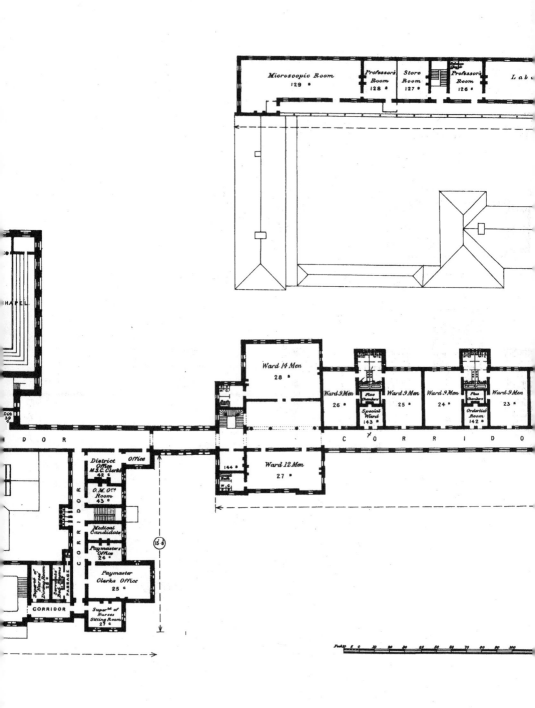

Microscopic Room
129 °

Professors
Room
128 °

Store
Room
127 °

Professors
Room
126 °

L a b

CHAPEL

Ward 14 Men
28 °

Ward 9 Men
26 °

Flue
Chamber

Special
Ward
143 °

Ward 9 Men
25 °

Ward 9 Men
24 °

Flue
Chamber

Orderlies
Room
142 °

Ward 9 Men
23 °

D   O   R

C   O   R   R   I   D   O

District
Office
M.S.C. Clerks
42 °

Office

O.M. Offs
Room
43 °

Medical
Candidates

Paymasters
Office
24 °

Paymaster
Clerks Office
25 °

Ward 12 Men
27 °

144 °

Supertt of
Nurses
Sitting Room
27 °

CORRIDOR

PASSAGE

CORRIDOR

15·6

Feet 10   5   0   10   20   30   40   50   60   70   80   90   100